THE FUTURE OF
DRUG SAFETY

PROMOTING AND PROTECTING THE HEALTH OF THE PUBLIC

Committee on the Assessment of the US Drug Safety System

Board on Population Health and Public Health Practice

Alina Baciu, Kathleen Stratton, Sheila P. Burke, *Editors*

INSTITUTE OF MEDICINE
OF THE NATIONAL ACADEMIES

THE NATIONAL ACADEMIES PRESS
Washington, D.C.
www.nap.edu

THE NATIONAL ACADEMIES PRESS   500 Fifth Street, N.W.   Washington, DC 20001

NOTICE: The project that is the subject of this report was approved by the Governing Board of the National Research Council, whose members are drawn from the councils of the National Academy of Sciences, the National Academy of Engineering, and the Institute of Medicine. The members of the committee responsible for the report were chosen for their special competences and with regard for appropriate balance.

This study was supported by Contract No. 223-01-2460, Task Order No. 23; HH-SP23320042509XI, Task Order No. 3; and HHSM-500-2005-00026C between the National Academy of Sciences and the Department of Health and Human Services (the Food and Drug Administration, the Agency for Healthcare Research and Quality, the Centers for Medicaid and Medicare Services, the National Institutes of Health), and the United States Department of Veterans Affairs. Any opinions, findings, conclusions, or recommendations expressed in this publication are those of the author(s) and do not necessarily reflect the view of the organizations or agencies that provided support for this project.

Library of Congress Cataloging-in-Publication Data

Institute of Medicine (U.S.). Committee on the Assessment of the US Drug Safety System.
  The future of drug safety : promoting and protecting the health of the public / Committee on the Assessment of the US Drug Safety System, Board on Population Health and Public Health Practice ; Alina Baciu, Kathleen Stratton, Sheila P. Burke, editors.
    p. ; cm.
  Includes bibliographical references.
  ISBN 978-0-309-10304-6 (pbk.)
  1. Pharmaceutical policy—United States. 2. United States. Food and Drug Administration. 3. Drugs—Safety measures—United States. I. Baciu, Alina. II. Stratton, Kathleen R. III. Burke, Sheila P. IV. Title.
  [DNLM: 1. United States. Food and Drug Administration. 2. Drug Approval—United States. 3. United States Government Agencies—United States. QV 771 I5852f 2007]
  RA401.A3.I568 2007
  362.17'82—dc22
                            2006039224

Additional copies of this report are available from the National Academies Press, 500 Fifth Street, N.W., Lockbox 285, Washington, DC 20055; (800) 624-6242 or (202) 334-3313 (in the Washington metropolitan area); Internet, http://www.nap.edu.

For more information about the Institute of Medicine, visit the IOM home page at: **www.iom.edu.**

The serpent has been a symbol of long life, healing, and knowledge among almost all cultures and religions since the beginning of recorded history. The serpent adopted as a logotype by the Institute of Medicine is a relief carving from ancient Greece, now held by the Staatliche Museen in Berlin.

"Knowing is not enough; we must apply.
Willing is not enough; we must do."
—Goethe

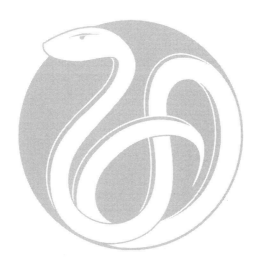

INSTITUTE OF MEDICINE
OF THE NATIONAL ACADEMIES

Advising the Nation. Improving Health.

THE NATIONAL ACADEMIES
Advisers to the Nation on Science, Engineering, and Medicine

The **National Academy of Sciences** is a private, nonprofit, self-perpetuating society of distinguished scholars engaged in scientific and engineering research, dedicated to the furtherance of science and technology and to their use for the general welfare. Upon the authority of the charter granted to it by the Congress in 1863, the Academy has a mandate that requires it to advise the federal government on scientific and technical matters. Dr. Ralph J. Cicerone is president of the National Academy of Sciences.

The **National Academy of Engineering** was established in 1964, under the charter of the National Academy of Sciences, as a parallel organization of outstanding engineers. It is autonomous in its administration and in the selection of its members, sharing with the National Academy of Sciences the responsibility for advising the federal government. The National Academy of Engineering also sponsors engineering programs aimed at meeting national needs, encourages education and research, and recognizes the superior achievements of engineers. Dr. Wm. A. Wulf is president of the National Academy of Engineering.

The **Institute of Medicine** was established in 1970 by the National Academy of Sciences to secure the services of eminent members of appropriate professions in the examination of policy matters pertaining to the health of the public. The Institute acts under the responsibility given to the National Academy of Sciences by its congressional charter to be an adviser to the federal government and, upon its own initiative, to identify issues of medical care, research, and education. Dr. Harvey V. Fineberg is president of the Institute of Medicine.

The **National Research Council** was organized by the National Academy of Sciences in 1916 to associate the broad community of science and technology with the Academy's purposes of furthering knowledge and advising the federal government. Functioning in accordance with general policies determined by the Academy, the Council has become the principal operating agency of both the National Academy of Sciences and the National Academy of Engineering in providing services to the government, the public, and the scientific and engineering communities. The Council is administered jointly by both Academies and the Institute of Medicine. Dr. Ralph J. Cicerone and Dr. Wm. A. Wulf are chair and vice chair, respectively, of the National Research Council.

www.national-academies.org

Reviewers

This report has been reviewed in draft form by individuals chosen for their diverse perspectives and technical expertise, in accordance with procedures approved by the NRC's Report Review Committee. The purpose of this independent review is to provide candid and critical comments that will assist the institution in making its published report as sound as possible and to ensure that the report meets institutional standards for objectivity, evidence, and responsiveness to the study charge. The review comments and draft manuscript remain confidential to protect the integrity of the deliberative process. We wish to thank the following individuals for their review of this report:

J. Lyle Bootman, College of Pharmacy–Pulido Center, The University of Arizona
John E. Calfee, American Enterprise Institute, Washington, DC
Dan Carpenter, Center for Government and International Studies, Harvard University
Ralph Edwards, The Uppsala Monitoring Centre, World Health Organization
David W. Feigal, NDA Partners, LLP and Arizona Biodesign Center
Garrett Fitzgerald, University of Pennsylvania School of Medicine
Henry G. Grabowski, Department of Economics, Program in Pharmaceuticals and Health Economics, Duke University
Sean Hennessy, University of Pennsylvania School of Medicine
Peter Barton Hutt, Covington & Burling

Anne Khademian, Center for Public Administration and Policy, Virginia Tech

Debra R. Lappin, B&D Sagamore, Washington, DC

Arthur Aaron Levin, Center for Medical Consumers, New York

Steven M. Paul, Lilly Research Laboratories, Eli Lilly and Company

Richard Platt, Department of Ambulatory Care and Prevention, Harvard Medical School

Wayne A. Ray, Department of Preventive Medicine, Vanderbilt University School of Medicine

Joshua M. Sharfstein, Health Department, City of Baltimore

Panos Tsintis, Unit for the Post-Authorisation Evaluation of Medicines for Human Use, European Medicines Agency, London

Eleanor M. Vogt, School of Pharmacy, University of California, San Francisco

Alastair J.J. Wood, Vanderbilt University Medical School

Although the reviewers listed above have provided many constructive comments and suggestions, they were not asked to endorse the conclusions or recommendations nor did they see the final draft of the report before its release. The review of this report was overseen by **Neal A. Vanselow**, Tulane University, Professor Emeritus and **Joseph P. Newhouse**, Harvard University. Appointed by the National Research Council and Institute of Medicine, they were responsible for making certain that an independent examination of this report was carried out in accordance with institutional procedures and that all review comments were carefully considered. Responsibility for the final content of this report rests entirely with the authoring committee and the institution.

Preface

The year 2006 marks the 100th anniversary of the signing of the Pure Food and Drug Act. During that century, drug regulation at the Food and Drug Administration (FDA) has evolved enormously, both in terms of statutory reforms (with major legislation in 1938, 1962, 1992, 1997, and 2002) and due to internal restructuring and growth in staff. Past changes have frequently been responses to problems in the functioning of the drug regulatory process. Although the agency has gained great respect and importance as one of the world's premier regulatory bodies, recent drug safety events have called into question FDA's regulatory decision-making and oversight processes, and caused the public to question its ability to accomplish a balanced evaluation of the safety and efficacy of the drugs it reviews and after their approval, of their performance under real-life conditions. In light of these developments, the Institute of Medicine (IOM) was asked by FDA to examine in detail the system of drug safety in this country. Our committee has, in the course of the last 15 months, undertaken this assessment.

The result of our review is a series of recommendations that we believe will improve the drug safety system by strengthening clinical and epidemiological research, and the scientific basis of regulatory action. Although mindful of recent actions by FDA to improve its postmarketing decision-making process, the committee believes a more comprehensive response is required that acknowledges the need for vigilance throughout the lifecycle of a drug. Underlying our 25 recommendations is the fundamental view that the interests of the public are best served when safety and efficacy are considered together. However, factors including, but not limited to, the current organizational culture of the Center for Drug Evaluation and

Research (CDER), combined with severe resource constraints and a problematic funding mechanism have impeded the development of a system that optimally integrates the safety and efficacy assessments along a drug's lifecycle, particularly with regard to safety issues arising postmarketing. Further complicating this problem is the lack of a clearly established and consistently applied systematic process of making risk-benefit assessments, and an adequate base of human and technological resources required to meet the center's critical responsibilities.

The committee believes that CDER staff are a dedicated and talented group of public servants who currently lack the organization and resources to address all of the challenges before them and perform the crucial role of advancing and protecting public health in an increasingly complex environment.

We believe that Congress needs to ensure that CDER is given the authority and assets (human, financial, technological) it requires. The center's leaders have to be prepared to address the underlying cultural problems that divide and impair the optimal functioning of center staff, and to effectively use existing and new authorities and resources to achieve the center's public health and regulatory mission. The committee's recommendations pertaining to these issues must be viewed as a coherent package of solutions or strategies rather than a menu of choices.

I would like to thank my colleagues on the committee for their extraordinary efforts. They have committed countless hours over the last 15 months in meetings, weekly conference calls, and a continuous stream of emails. They have passionately argued their positions, but also accommodated their colleagues and sought responsible consensus. I thank them for all they have done. I would also like to acknowledge the contributions of the IOM staff team—Kathleen Stratton, Alina Baciu, Amy Grossman, Ruth Kanthula, Andrea Pernack Anason, and consultant Renie Schapiro. Their dedication, guidance, and experience were of inestimable value to us in examining the highly complex process of drug evaluation and regulation. We could not have produced this report without them. The committee is grateful to everyone who spoke at our public meetings and who sent material for consideration. I also wish to thank the current and former staff at FDA and particularly CDER who spoke frankly with the committee and provided much needed insight into the workings of this agency.

Sheila P. Burke, *Chair*

Contents

SUMMARY   1

1   INTRODUCTION   15
    Changes in the Broad Context of Drug Regulation, 19
    Defining and Meeting the Charge, 21

2   NATURAL HISTORY OF A DRUG   31
    Economic Impact of Drugs, 32
    The Investigational New Drug, 33
        Investigational New Drug Submission and Review, 33
    New Drug Application, 39
    Postmarket Period, 51

3   A CULTURE OF SAFETY   65
    Organizational Challenges, 65
        The External Environment, 68
        Structural Factors, Policies, and Procedures, 75
        Proposed Solutions to CDER's Organizational Dysfunction, 90

4   THE SCIENCE OF SAFETY   105
    Generating the Science, 106
        Understanding Risk and Benefit for Approval Decisions, 106
        Reducing Uncertainty About Risk and Benefit After Approval, 107
        Risk Minimization Action Plans, 119
        Risk-Benefit Analyses Throughout the Lifecycle, 121

Credibility of the Science, 126
  Expertise in the Center for Drug Evaluaiton and Research, 127
  Advisory Committees, 131
  Transparency, 142

5   REGULATORY AUTHORITIES FOR DRUG SAFETY   151
    History of FDA Drug Regulation, 152
    An Aging and Inadequate Statutory Framework, 153
      FDA Authority Preapproval, 154
      FDA Authority After Approval, 155
      Rationale for Strengthening Drug Regulation, 164
    Strengthening FDA's Regulatory Authorities, 167

6   COMMUNICATING ABOUT SAFETY   177
      Roles and Needs of Providers and Patients, 178
      How Industry Communicates to the Public and Patients, 184
      FDA's Challenges in Communicating to the Public and
        Patients, 184

7   RESOURCES FOR THE DRUG SAFETY SYSTEM   193

APPENDIXES

A   Moving Target: Changes at FDA During the Course of the Study   205
B   Acronyms   217
C   PDUFA Performance Goals—All Years   221
D   Committee on the Assessment of the US Drug Safety System
    Meeting Agendas   255
E   Summary, *Preventing Medication Errors: Quality Chasm Series,*
    Institute of Medicine   267
F   Committee Biographies   309

INDEX   319

THE FUTURE OF
DRUG SAFETY

Summary

Every day the Food and Drug Administration (FDA) works to balance expeditious access to drugs with concerns for safety, consonant with its mission to protect and advance the public health. The task is all the more complex given the vast diversity of patients and how they respond to drugs, the conditions being treated, and the range of pharmaceutical products and supplements patients use. Reviewers in the Center for Drug Evaluation and Research (CDER) at the FDA must weigh the information available about a drug's risk and benefit, make decisions in the context of scientific uncertainty, and integrate emerging information bearing on a drug's risk-benefit profile throughout the lifecycle of a drug, from drug discovery to the end of its useful life. These processes may have life-or-death consequences for individual patients, and for drugs that are widely used, they may also affect entire segments of the population. The distinction between individual and population is important because it reflects complex determinations that FDA must make when a drug that is life-saving for a specific patient may pose substantial risk when viewed from a population health perspective. In a physician's office, the patient and the provider make decisions about the risk and benefits of a given drug for that patient, whereas FDA has to assess risks and benefits with a view toward their effects on the population. The agency has made great efforts to balance the need for expeditious approvals with great attention to safety, as reflected in its mission—to protect and advance the health of the public.

In the first years of the 21st century, the issue of prescription drug safety came to the attention of the public with renewed intensity. Drug withdrawals, apparent delays in warning the public about important drug risks, a perceived rush to approve drugs without sufficient attention to safety, and press coverage of internal problems in CDER may have contributed to a deterioration of public confidence in FDA. Academics, consumer organizations, professional societies, and legislators debated the possible causes and solutions of what was seen by many as a major problem (Consumers Union, 2005; Grassley, 2005; NCL, 2005; US PIRG, 2006). FDA and the Department of Health and Human Services (DHHS) announced a series of steps to address drug safety, including asking the Institute of Medicine (IOM) to convene a committee to assess the US drug safety system and to make recommendations to improve risk assessment, surveillance, and the safe use of drugs.

In its report, the committee considered the drug safety system as the sum of all activities conducted by FDA and other stakeholders to monitor, evaluate, improve, and ensure drug safety. (See the committee's Statement of Task in Box S-1.) Although much of the committee's work was focused on drug review, safety surveillance, and related activities of CDER, the committee also reviewed some key aspects of the roles and considered the potential contributions of the pharmaceutical industry, the academic research enterprise, Congress, the health care delivery system, patients, and the public.

Some observers believe that drug withdrawals (which are only one potential indicator of drug safety) represent de facto failures of the drug regulatory system, or that newly identified unusual and serious adverse events indicate that someone made a mistake in approving the drug. This is not so. FDA approval does not represent a lifetime guarantee of safety and efficacy, and what is newest is not always the best. For several related reasons, even the best drug safety system would not prevent adverse reactions to pharmaceuticals on the market. It is impossible to know everything about a drug at the point of approval because drugs' mechanisms of action are complex, and because the clinical testing that happens before approval is generally conducted in controlled settings in defined, carefully selected populations that may not fully represent the wide range of patients who will use the drug after approval, some chronically, and in combination with other drugs. Thus, the understanding of a drug's risk-benefit profile necessarily evolves over the drug's lifecycle. CDER staff who review regulatory submissions, such as new drug applications, must strike a delicate balance in judging the drug's risks and benefits, and whether the need for more study to increase certainty before approval warrants delaying the release of the drug into the marketplace and into the hands of health care providers and their patients.

Legitimate questions have arisen about CDER's handling of drug safety. Are safety signals recognized and addressed in a timely fashion? Is the public informed about safety problems in a clear and timely manner? Do the interactions of pre- and postmarketing center staff facilitate effective action

BOX S-1
The Statement of Task

In response to growing public concern with health risks posed by approved drugs, the FDA has requested that the Institute of Medicine (IOM) convene an ad hoc committee of experts to conduct an independent assessment of the current system for evaluating and ensuring drug safety postmarketing and make recommendations to improve risk assessment, surveillance, and the safe use of drugs. As part of its work, the IOM committee will:

- examine the FDA's current role and the role of other actors (e.g., health professionals, hospitals, patients, other public agencies) in ensuring drug safety as part of the US health care delivery system;
- examine the current efforts for the ongoing safety evaluation of marketed drug products at the FDA and by the pharmaceutical industry, the medical community, and public health authorities;
- evaluate the analytical and methodological tools employed by FDA to identify and manage drug safety problems and make recommendations for enhancement;
- evaluate FDA's internal organizational structure and operations around drug safety (including continuing postmarket assessment of risk vs. benefit);
- consider FDA's legal authorities for identifying and responding to drug safety issues and current resources (financial and human) dedicated to postmarketing safety activities;
- identify strengths, weaknesses, and limitations of the current system; and
- make recommendations in the areas of organization, legislation, regulation, and resources to improve risk assessment, surveillance, and the safe use of drugs.

on drug safety? Does the center have the mix of expertise, technology, scientific capacity, authority, and resources to achieve its share of FDA's mission, to protect and advance the health of the public? Do the political, social, and economic aspects of the external environment and the expectations of other stakeholders affect the agency's functioning? To answer some of these questions, the committee reviewed aspects of the drug safety system that it believes can be transformed to improve the monitoring and evaluation of drug safety signals and restore public confidence in the system, including:

- The organizational **culture** of CDER and its determinants, and how organizational culture may affect the center's performance in assessing and acting on the evolving understanding of risk and benefit over the drug lifecycle;
- Key factors of regulatory **science** and processes (methods, data resources, expert advice, independence) necessary to enhance drug safety;
- The **regulatory authorities** necessary to provide for drug safety;
- The **communication** structure needed to support an effective drug safety system; and
- The financial **resources** required to enable CDER to meet its responsibilities in supporting the FDA mission.

In its information gathering, the committee became aware of multiple proposals to strengthen the drug safety system that have been made in the past and have addressed many of the areas outlined. In its work, the committee has attempted to develop a coherent and integrative approach to transforming drug safety programs that encompasses the categories described above. The committee made several overarching findings. First, there is a perception of crisis that has compromised the credibility of FDA and of the pharmaceutical industry (Harris Interactive, 2005; Pricewaterhouse-Coopers' Health Research Institute, 2005). Second, the committee learned that most stakeholders—the agency, the industry, consumer organizations, Congress, professional societies, health care entities—appear to agree on the need for certain improvements in the system. Third, the committee found that the drug safety system is impaired by the following factors: serious resource constraints that weaken the quality and quantity of the science that is brought to bear on drug safety; an organizational culture in CDER that is not optimally functional; and unclear and insufficient regulatory authorities particularly with respect to enforcement. Fourth, the committee found that FDA, contrary to its public health mission, and the pharmaceutical industry, contrary to its responsibility to the users of its products (and its shareholders), do not consistently demonstrate accountability and transparency to the public by communicating safety concerns in a timely and effective fashion.

The committee's vision of a transformed drug safety system has at its core a lifecycle approach to drug risk and benefit—not a new concept, but one that has been implemented, at best, in a limited and fragmented manner. For FDA, attention to risk and benefit over a drug's lifecycle would require continuous availability of new data and ongoing, active reassessment of risk and benefit to drive regulatory action (responsive to the accumulating information about a given drug), and regulatory authority that is strong both before and after approval. For the industry, attention to risk and benefit over the lifecycle will require increased transparency toward FDA in the process of elucidating and communicating emerging information about a drug, and acceptance of changes intended to strengthen drug safety. Importantly, FDA's credibility is intertwined with that of the industry, and a more credible drug safety system is in everyone's best interest. For the health care delivery system, a lifecycle approach to risk and benefit implies the need to heed and follow FDA communication about drug safety matters and to exercise appropriate caution in drug-related decision making (from formularies to prescribing) in recognition of the limited information available at the time of drug approval. Also, the health care delivery system would benefit from consistently basing prescribing decisions on the science, and exercising caution in regard to the industry's influence on the practice of medicine. Health care organizations and professional societies could contribute to prescribers' understanding of the evolving science behind the assessment of drug risk and benefit. The academic research enterprise could enhance its contributions of data to the assessment of risk and benefit at all points in a drug's lifecycle, continue its crucial advisory relationship with FDA, and uphold the value of complete transparency in recognition of real and perceived conflicts associated with financial involvement with the industry. Other government agencies could contribute to the lifecycle approach to drug risk and benefit by collaborating with FDA and the private sector to ensure that data streams from publicly funded health care settings contribute to an improved drug safety system. The public and patients could do their part by communicating with their health care providers about the pharmaceutical products they are using, learning about and discussing with their providers drug risks and benefits in the context of their health needs and characteristics, informing their providers about side effects they experience, and calling for more useful and timelier information about drug benefits and risks associated with new drugs. The public and other stakeholders could also urge Congress to ensure and sustain adequate funding for FDA.

RECOMMENDATIONS

Organizational Culture

Instability in the Office of the Commissioner has been a serious problem for FDA and CDER in particular. A large, complex, science-based regulatory agency cannot perform optimally in the absence of stable, capable leadership, and clear, consistent direction.

3.1: The committee recommends that the FD&C Act be amended to require that the FDA Commissioner currently appointed by the President with the advice and consent of the Senate also be ap-

pointed for a 6-year term of office. The Commissioner should be an individual with appropriate expertise to head a science-based agency, demonstrated capacity to lead and inspire, and a proven commitment to public health, scientific integrity, transparency, and communication. The President may remove the Commissioner from office only for reasons of inefficiency, neglect of duty, or malfeasance in office.

A mechanism is needed to allow the agency and CDER leadership to benefit from the advice and support of individuals experienced in changing organizational culture and leading large and complex organizations.

3.2: The committee recommends that an external Management Advisory Board be appointed by the Secretary of HHS to advise the FDA commissioner in shepherding CDER (and the agency as a whole) to implement and sustain the changes necessary to transform the center's culture—by improving morale and retention of professional staff, strengthening transparency, restoring credibility, and creating a culture of safety based upon a lifecycle approach to risk-benefit.

3.3: The committee recommends the Secretary of HHS direct the FDA commissioner and Director of CDER, with the assistance of the Management Advisory Board, to develop a comprehensive strategy for sustained cultural change that positions the agency to fulfill its mission, including protecting the health of the public.

The Office of Drug Safety, now the Office of Surveillance and Epidemiology (OSE), has not had a formal role in drug regulation—neither formal opportunities to learn from and participate in relevant aspects of the review process nor the authority to take action regarding postmarketing safety.

3.4: The committee recommends that CDER appoint an OSE staff member to each New Drug Application review team and assign joint authority to OND and OSE for postapproval regulatory actions related to safety.

The Prescription Drug User Fee Act (PDUFA) mechanism that accounts for over half of CDER's funding and the reporting requirements associated with the user-fee program are excessively oriented toward supporting speed of approval and insufficiently attentive to safety.

3.5: To restore appropriate balance between the FDA's dual goals of speeding access to innovative drugs and ensuring drug safety over the product's lifecycle, the committee recommends that Congress should introduce specific safety-related performance goals in the Prescription Drug User Fee Act IV in 2007. (See Chapter 3 for suggested goals.)

Science and Expertise

FDA's Adverse Event Reporting System (AERS) is outdated and inefficient, and although CDER has begun a technological overhaul of the system, more work is needed to improve its usefulness in postmarketing surveillance.

4.1: The committee recommends that in order to improve the generation of new safety signals and hypotheses, CDER (a) conduct a systematic, scientific review of the AERS system, (b) identify and implement changes in key factors that could lead to a more efficient system, and (c) systematically implement statistical-surveillance methods on a regular and routine basis for the automated generation of new safety signals.

In addition, CDER's ability to test drug safety hypotheses is limited.

4.2: The committee recommends that in order to facilitate the formulation and testing of drug safety hypotheses, CDER (a) increase their intramural and extramural programs that access and study data from large automated healthcare databases and (b) include in these programs studies on drug utilization patterns and background incidence rates for adverse events of interest, and (c) develop and implement active surveillance of specific drugs and diseases as needed in a variety of settings.

The report makes several recommendations (4.3, 4.5, 4.8, and 5.4 below) intended to help CDER develop a more structured way to determine the level of postmarketing scrutiny and data requirements, in other words, to match the evaluation of drugs with the way that they will be used in the population. Short-term preapproval trials do not provide adequate information about the balance of risks and benefits of drugs that are used by many people for many years.

Various public- and private-sector organizations possess increasingly high-quality data resources and scientific capacity, and a concerted effort is needed to ensure that those resources are used efficiently and effectively in the service of drug safety.

> 4.3: The committee recommends that the Secretary of HHS, working with the Secretaries of Veterans Affairs and Defense, develop a public-private partnership with drug sponsors, public and private insurers, for-profit and not-for-profit health care provider organizations, consumer groups, and large pharmaceutical companies to prioritize, plan, and organize funding for confirmatory drug safety and efficacy studies of public health importance. Congress should capitalize the public share of this partnership.

> 4.4: The committee recommends that CDER assure the performance of timely and scientifically-valid evaluations (whether done internally or by industry sponsors) of Risk Minimization Action Plans (RiskMAPs).

The assessment of risks and benefits is an activity that does not end at approval, and risk and benefit cannot be considered in isolation of one another.

> 4.5: The committee recommends that CDER develop and continually improve a systematic approach to risk-benefit analysis for use throughout the FDA in the preapproval and postapproval settings.

The committee has made several recommendations to expand the data on drug risks and benefits to improve those decisions. However, in order to plan and use those data, appropriate expertise must be brought to bear. This expertise comes from the CDER staff as well as their advisory committees and other non-governmental experts. The committee believes there is a need to expand this expertise to take on the new responsibilities laid out in recommendations made in this report. CDER will need more expert staff, deeper expertise in the staff it already has, and different kinds of expertise.

With this expanded expertise and resources CDER can be a more effective steward of postmarketing safety and a more credible scientific partner with industry and academia by actively participating in defining important research questions and designing appropriate studies.

> 4.6: The committee recommends that CDER build internal epidemiologic and informatics capacity in order to improve the postmarket assessment of drugs.

Increasing the scientific sophistication of the CDER staff should not happen in isolation. Since the goal is to support good science-based regulatory decision making, a corollary goal is to support the research infrastructure of the agency. Expanded research opportunities should be linked explicitly to FDA's regulatory mission.

4.7: The committee recommends that the Commissioner of FDA demonstrate commitment to building the Agency's scientific research capacity by:

a. Appointing a Chief Scientist in the office of the Commissioner with responsibility for overseeing, coordinating, and ensuring the quality and regulatory focus of the agency's intramural research programs.
b. Designating the FDA's Science Board as the extramural advisory committee to the Chief Scientist.
c. Including research capacity in the Agency's mission statement.
d. Applying resources to support intramural research approved by the Chief Scientist.
e. Ensuring that adequate funding to support the intramural research program is requested in the Agency's annual budget request to Congress.

The fast pace of review does not allow CDER reviewers to solicit consistently needed input from the appropriate FDA advisory committee(s) on issues such as postmarketing safety and the need for additional studies.

4.8: The committee recommends that FDA have its advisory committees review all NMEs either prior to approval or soon after approval to advise in the process of ensuring drug safety and efficacy or managing drug risks.

4.9: The committee recommends that all FDA drug product advisory committees, and any other peer-review effort such as mentioned above for CDER-reviewed product safety, include a pharmacoepidemiologist or an individual with comparable public health expertise in studying the safety of medical products.

FDA's credibility is its most crucial asset and recent concerns about the independence of advisory committee members (who advise CDER in its regulatory decision making), along with broader concerns about scientific independence in the biomedical research establishment, have cast a shadow on the trustworthiness of the scientific advice received by the agency.

4.10: The committee recommends FDA establish a requirement that a substantial majority of the members of each advisory committee be free of significant financial involvement with companies whose interests may be affected by the committee's deliberations.

The committee believes strongly in the importance of increasing the availability of information about risks and benefits, whether specific study results or CDER staff analyses of concerns, to the public and to researchers. The National Library of Medicine hosts a Web site for registration of clinical trials, but with few exceptions, this is voluntary. In 2002, pharmaceutical companies that are members of the Pharmaceutical Research and Manufacturers of America (PhRMA) committed to voluntary disclosure of the results of hypothesis-testing clinical trials for marketed and investigational drugs and in 2004 PhRMA launched a Web site (ClinicalStudyResults.org) for this purpose. A review of the site shows great variability in the ease of accessibility and completeness of the information.

4.11: To ensure that trial registration is mandatory, systematic, standardized, and complete, and that the registration site is able to accommodate the reporting of trial results, **the committee recommends that Congress require industry sponsors to register in a timely manner at clinicaltrials.gov, at a minimum, all Phase 2 through 4 clinical trials, wherever they may have been conducted, if data from the trials are intended to be submitted to the FDA as part of an NDA, sNDA, or to fulfill a postmarket commitment. The committee further recommends that this requirement include the posting of a structured field summary of the efficacy and safety results of the studies.**

4.12: The committee recommends that FDA post all NDA review packages on the agency's Web site.

4:13: The committee recommends that the CDER review teams regularly and systematically analyze all postmarket study results and make public their assessment of the significance of the results with regard to the integration of risk and benefit information.

Regulation

FDA lacks the clear, unambiguous authority needed to enforce sponsor compliance with regulatory requirements and instead relies on the prospect of productive negotiations with industry. Although the agency historically has made effective use of its "bully pulpit" to compel sponsor compliance, this process leaves potentially critical regulatory action vulnerable to a subjective and highly variable process of exercising individual or agency influence, and to the vicissitudes of changing politics and attitudes toward regulation. That is why FDA's authorities must be clarified and strengthened to empower the agency to take rapid and decisive actions when necessary and appropriate.

> 5.1: The committee recommends that Congress ensure that the Food and Drug Administration has the ability to require such postmarketing risk assessment and risk management programs as are needed to monitor and ensure safe use of drug products. These conditions may be imposed both before and after approval of a new drug, new indication, or new dosage, as well as after identification of new contraindications or patterns of adverse events. The limitations imposed should match the specific safety concerns and benefits presented by the drug product. The risk assessment and risk management program may include:

> a. Distribution conditioned on compliance with agency-initiated changes in drug labels.
> b. Distribution conditioned on specific warnings to be incorporated into all promotional materials (including broadcast direct-to-consumer [DTC] advertising).
> c. Distribution conditioned on a moratorium on DTC advertising.
> d. Distribution restricted to certain facilities, pharmacists, or physicians with special training or experience.
> e. Distribution conditioned on the performance of specified medical procedures.
> f. Distribution conditioned on the performance of specified additional clinical trials or other studies.
> g. Distribution conditioned on the maintenance of an active adverse event surveillance system.

> 5.2: The committee recommends that Congress provide oversight and enact any needed legislation to ensure compliance by both the Food and Drug Administration and drug sponsors with the provisions listed above. FDA needs increased enforcement authority and better enforcement tools directed at drug sponsors, which should include fines, injunctions, and withdrawal of drug approval.

The agency's timely performance of the required postmarketing safety reviews could be listed as one of the goals associated with PDUFA and reported on in the goals letter to Congress (see Chapter 3).

5.3: The committee recommends that Congress amend the Food, Drug and Cosmetic Act to require that product labels carry a special symbol such as the black triangle used in the UK or an equivalent symbol for new drugs, new combinations of active substances, and new systems of delivery of existing drugs. The Food and Drug Administration should restrict direct-to-consumer advertising during the period of time the special symbol is in effect.

The symbol should remain on the drug label and related materials for 2 years unless FDA chooses to shorten or extend the period on a case-by-case basis.

5.4: The committee recommends that FDA evaluate all new data on new molecular entities no later than 5 years after approval. Sponsors will submit a report of accumulated data relevant to drug safety and efficacy, including any additional data published in a peer-reviewed journal, and will report on the status of any applicable conditions imposed on the distribution of the drug called for at or after the time of approval.

Communication

The public would benefit from more information about how drugs are studied before FDA approval, how drugs' risks and benefits are assessed, and what FDA review entails. Patients also need timely information about emerging safety concerns and about a drug's effectiveness. Such information would help patients make better decisions in collaboration with their health care providers. FDA does not have an adequate mechanism for seeking and receiving specific scientific and patient/consumer advice on communication matters.

6.1: The committee recommends that Congress enact legislation establishing a new FDA advisory committee on communication with patients and consumers. The committee would be composed of members who represent consumer and patient perspectives and organizations. The advisory committee would advise CDER and other centers on communication issues related to efficacy, safety, and use during the lifecycle of drugs and other medical products, and it would support the centers in their mission to "help the public get the accurate, science-based information they need to use medicines and foods to improve their health."

6.2: The committee recommends that the new Office of Drug Safety Policy and Communication should develop a cohesive risk communication plan that includes, at a minimum, a review of all center risk communication activities, evaluation and revision of communication tools for clarity and consistency, and priority-setting to ensure efficient use of resources.

Resources

The suite of recommendations put forward in this report—to improve the culture in CDER, attract and retain highly qualified staff, improve technological capacity, obtain and benefit from access to data and innovative scientific partnerships, and so on—are all dependent on adequate resources. An agency whose crucial mission is to protect and advance the public's health should not have to go begging for resources to do its job. Also, the effect on CDER's work of CDER's overdependence on PDUFA funding with the strings that are attached hurts FDA's credibility and may affect the agency's effectiveness.

7.1: To support improvements in drug safety and efficacy activities over a product's lifecycle, the committee recommends that the Administration should request and Congress should approve substantially increased resources in both funds and personnel for the Food and Drug Administration.

The committee favors appropriations from general revenues, rather than user fees, to support the full spectrum of new drug safety responsibilities proposed in this report. This preference is based on the expectation that CDER will continue to review and approve drugs in a timely manner and that increasing attention to drug safety will not occur at the expense of efficacy reviews but rather it will complement efficacy review for a life-cycle approach to drugs. Congressional appropriations from general tax revenues are a mechanism by which the public can directly, fairly, and effectively invest in the FDA's postmarket drug safety activities. However, if appropriations are not sufficient to fund these activities and user fees are required, Congress should greatly reduce current restrictions on how CDER uses PDUFA funds.

The year 2006 marks a major milestone in FDA's history, public interest in drug safety matters has reached a high point, negotiations in advance of the September 2007 sunset of PDUFA have begun, Medicare part D has enrolled millions of senior citizens in a system that has the potential to yield useful data about experience with drugs, and congressional attention to drug safety issues has become intense. Now is the time to renew and transform

CDER's culture, its authorities, its scientific capacity, and its ability to communicate with health care providers and the public. The committee believes that the recommendations contained in this report, implemented together and with adequate resources, will enable the center (and the agency) to function more effectively in the present and to position itself for an even more challenging future in advancing and protecting the health of patients and the public.

REFERENCES

Consumers Union. 2005. *NEWS—IOM Panel Urged to Immediately Recommend that Congress Toughen Drug Safety Laws to Save Lives: Consumers Union Testifies Today That Obvious Safety Problems Need Action Now.* [Online]. Available: http://www.pharmalive. com/news/print.cfm?articleid=247043 [accessed June 9, 2005].

Grassley C. 2005. S.930: A bill to amend the Federal Food, Drug, and Cosmetic Act with respect to drug safety, and for other purposes. 109th Congress.

Harris Interactive. 2005. *The Public Has Doubts About the Pharmaceutical Industry's Willingness to Publish Safety Information About Their Drugs in a Timely Manner.* [Online]. Available: http://www.harrisinteractive.com/news/printerfriend/index.asp?NewsID=882 [accessed March 10, 2006].

NCL (National Consumers League). 2005. *Comments of the National Consumers League to DKT. No. 2005N-0394, Communication of Drug Safety Information.* [Online]. Available: http://www.nclnet.org/advocacy/health/letter_drugsafety_01062006.htm [accessed September 16, 2006].

PricewaterhouseCoopers' Health Research Institute. 2005. *Recapturing the Vision: Integrity Driven Performance in the Pharmaceutical Industry.* [Online]. Available: http://www. pwc.com/extweb/pwcpublications.nsf/docid/EE74BACB6DE454768525702A00630CFF [accessed February 20, 2006].

US PIRG (United States Public Interest Research Group). 2006. *Drug Safety.* [Online]. Available: http://uspirg.org/uspirg.asp?id2=17568&id3=US& [accessed September 16, 2006].

1

Introduction

". . . [A]lmost every morning's newspaper and each evening's television news-casts include a new and more disturbing episode of pharmacological crisis and medical mayhem in the United States" (Markel, 2005).

". . . FDA has become synonymous with drug safety. In a sense, 'FDA ap-proved' is the brand that the entire $216 billion US drug market is founded upon. Dilute the confidence of the public in the agency, and many billions of dollars in current and potential sales vanish overnight. That's exactly what's happening right now in the wake of the biggest drug withdrawal ever" (Herper, 2005).

The recent highly publicized controversies surrounding the safety of some drugs have contributed to a public perception that the drug safety system is in crisis. It seems fair to say that this perception has created an opportunity for a thorough evaluation of the US drug safety system. News media coverage and congressional examination of the Center for Drug Evaluation and Research's (CDER's) handling of safety concerns have raised questions about the review and approval process and whether it has become so accelerated that adequate attention may not be given to safety, and about the completeness and timeliness of risk communication to the public. Questions also surfaced about the independence of the scientific expertise relied on by the Food and Drug Administration (FDA) (conflict of interest in its advisory committees) and about the possibility of undue industry influence related to CDER's increasing dependence on Prescription Drug User Fee Act (PDUFA) funding. It would be easy to conclude that FDA's most recent troubles are just a reflection of the swinging of the pendulum from tighter to looser regulation and back again (Applebaum, 2005; Geraghty, 2006). The committee believes that the reality is more complicated than that. The committee did not attempt to document whether or not a drug safety crisis exists, and this report should not be interpreted as commenting on that claim one way or the other. The committee also did not set out to—nor was it asked to—conduct in-depth reviews of the industry and the agency's handling of safety information and data for drugs with potential safety problems. Instead, the committee examined the existing drug safety system with a view to identify areas of vulnerability and facets of the system that could be strengthened in order to improve its overall functioning in meeting the needs of the American public.

Complaints about delayed patient access to drugs already approved in other countries and the AIDS advocacy movement of the 1980s are considered among the major factors that motivated legislative action to speed up FDA's drug approval process. However, criticism of the pace of drug approval may be traced to the early 1970s. At that time, pharmaceutical companies, scientists, and consumer organizations argued that the 1962 Drug Amendments to the Food, Drug, and Cosmetic Act, intended to strengthen the drug approval process by requiring that sponsors demonstrate efficacy, also stifled drug development and delayed drug approval (DHEW, 1977). In the 1990s, FDA attributed the delays to shortages of staff and computers (FDA, 2005b). Concern about the slow pace of drug review finally led to PDUFA.

The enactment of PDUFA in 1992 resulted from a potent combination of interests. Patient advocacy groups called for faster access to promising therapies, the industry desired a more efficient regulatory process to enable faster marketing of new drugs and a longer patent life, FDA needed more resources to expand its review staff to meet demand for greater regulatory expediency, and some members of Congress were concerned that new drug approvals in the United States lagged behind those of comparable European nations. With congressional oversight and input, PDUFA was enacted with the goal of meeting the needs of FDA, industry, and patients. Although the 1992 PDUFA succeeded greatly in decreasing review times (FDA, 2005b), its first two iterations (PDUFA I in 1992 and PDUFA II in 1997, see below) specifically prohibited the use of fees for any postmarketing drug safety activities. Also, the speeding up of the review process highlighted potential weaknesses and limited capability in the area of postmarketing safety. By the latter part of the 1990s, various observers, including consumer groups and researchers, became concerned that the increased pace of drug approvals had unintentionally led to a neglect of—or at least insufficient attention to—safety considerations, resulting in what was seen as a greater rate of drug withdrawals (Lurie and Wolfe, 1988; Hart, 1999; Tone, 1999). Numerous journal editorials and articles by scientists, consumer advocates, and agency leadership continued the dialogue (Kleinke and Gottlieb, 1998; Wood et al., 1998; Friedman et al., 1999; Landow, 1999; Lurie and Sasich, 1999). In response to mounting unease, FDA Commissioner Jane Henney convened "a Task Force to evaluate the system for managing the risks of FDA-approved medical products" (DHHS/FDA, May 1999). Although the task force found that rates of withdrawals were low (the limitations of treating withdrawals as a safety metric are discussed below), the group identified process, resource, and statutory constraints on FDA's ability to identify adverse events and made a series of substantive recommendations to strengthen risk management. Some of the recommendations of the task force have been implemented, including the convening of public meetings to solicit input on drug safety and risk management from various constituencies.

Drug safety concerns have continued to emerge, as have the proposals to address them. Alosetron was withdrawn and then returned to market with restrictions and a label warning. Troglitazone, propulsid, cerivastatin, rofecoxib, and valdecoxib have been withdrawn. Celecoxib and other non-selective non-steroidal anti-inflammatory drugs had boxed warnings added to their labels. Warnings have been added to all antidepressant labels. FDA's performance in approving drugs or monitoring their safety after approval has been questioned and criticized. Several major factors converged to create at the least the appearance of a crisis in drug safety, among them, CDER's limited resources, organizational and management challenges, seemingly long reaction times, poor external communication, questions about external influences on CDER's decision making, an ever more diverse information environment (news media, the Internet and the blogosphere, and advertising) coupled with increasing consumer awareness and engagement, and growing congressional concern.

The Committee on the Assessment of the US Drug Safety System believes that as more drugs are being approved faster with less time to intensively investigate premarketing safety data, FDA does not have adequate resources or procedures for translating preapproval safety signals into effective postmarketing studies, for monitoring and ascertaining the safety of new marketed drugs, for responding promptly to the safety problems that are discovered after marketing approval, and for quickly and effectively communicating appropriate risk information to the public. The committee is aware of promising components of the current drug safety efforts at CDER and of agency improvement initiatives (see Appendix A), but it believes that neither the agency's newly enhanced postmarketing safety initiatives nor the necessary contributions of other actors in the US drug safety system are equal to the task. Major obstacles remain. They include inadequate resources, the complexity of the science and technology involved in drug development and regulation (e.g., assessing risk and benefit), a dysfunctional organizational culture, problems with credibility and public trust, and the lack of adequate communication about and limited public awareness of drug risks and benefits.

The credibility of FDA, the industry, the academic research enterprise, and health care providers has become seriously diminished in recent years (Kaiser Family Foundation, 2005; Wall Street Journal and Harris Interactive, 2005). FDA's reputation has been hurt by a perceived lack of transparency and accountability to the public, a legacy of organizational changes that have not been completed or sustained, and an apparent slowness in addressing lack of sponsor compliance (US House of Representatives Committee on Government Reform Minority Staff, 2006). The industry's once sterling reputation has been blemished by reported compliance problems, delays in responding to safety concerns and complying with postmarketing commitments, highly publicized concerns about the effects of direct-to-consumer advertising, and the preponderance of "me-too" products, rather than truly pioneering therapies (PricewaterhouseCoopers Health Research Institute, 2005; Wall Street Journal and Harris Interactive, 2005). The integrity of the academic research enterprise has also been questioned, as universities and scientists are increasingly dependent on industry funding for their work. The behavior of prescribers, the gatekeepers for patient access to prescription drugs, are also under public and congressional scrutiny, as health care providers receive intense and targeted promotional ("detailing") efforts of pharmaceutical companies.

Of particular concern are the common but inaccurate perceptions that FDA approval represents a guarantee of safety, that approval is based on a high degree of clarity and certainty about a drug's risks and benefits, and that such safety actions as boxed warnings on drug labels and withdrawals reflect sponsor or agency failures.

Addressing weaknesses and missed opportunities in the drug safety system requires some fundamental changes in the organizational culture of CDER to support effective action on drug safety (Chapter 3), in the scientific approaches to drug safety (Chapter 4), in the regulations pertinent to drug safety (Chapter 5), in communication about drug safety (Chapter 6), and in the agency's funding structure (which currently leaves critical regulatory and public health functions inadequately resourced) (Chapter 7).

Some of the recommendations offered in this report echo proposals made over the last two decades by various groups convened by the agency or by the Department of Health and Human Services (DHHS) (DHEW Review Panel on New Drug Regulation, 1977; Joint Commission on Prescription Drug Use, 1980; DHHS/FDA, 1999). It is puzzling and troubling that despite this series of reviews and recommendations, some have not been fully implemented and some issues have resurfaced repeatedly. A primary obstacle, the committee suspects, may be the chronic underfunding of core FDA activities owing to inadequate attention to resource needs by Congress and by the Office of Management and Budget. The committee asserts that the piecemeal organizational modifications and short-lived programmatic initiatives of the past and the current, seemingly fragmented and reactive initiatives to improve CDER are not sufficient to meet the need to improve postmarket drug safety activities and protect the public health better. The present report endeavors to provide an integrative approach to transforming drug safety in FDA and in the agency's interactions with other stakeholders in five major areas: organizational culture and leadership, science, regulatory authority, communication, and the funding without which improvements in these areas would not be possible. No one in FDA, industry, or academic research enterprise would disagree with the importance of implementing a lifecycle approach to the assessment of drug risks and benefits. Nevertheless, a great deal of separation persists between premarket and postmarket activities and functions. The separation, both structural and cultural, is reinforced by user-fee funding that is predominantly devoted to premarket activities and funding from appropriations that has not kept up with need in vital areas of the agency's work, by regulatory authority that is stronger and clearer preapproval, and by data requirements that are more structured and intensive for approval than for the postmarketing period (see Chapter 3) (DHEW Review Panel on New Drug Regulation, 1977; FDA, 2005b).

The year 2006 is a good time for thoughtful attention to transforming the drug safety system to address existing areas of vulnerability, and to prepare for the challenges and opportunities of the future. In this year of FDA's centennial,[1] public attention to drug safety matters has reached a high point, negotiations in advance of the September 2007 sunset of PDUFA have begun, Medicare Part D has enrolled tens of millions of senior citizens in a system that is expected to yield a wealth of population data about experience with drugs, new research promises further progress against illness (including more targeted therapies), and congressional interest in drug safety is intense. Those are but some of the factors that make this a moment of opportunity to renew and transform CDER, to enable it to function more effectively and to position itself for a far more complex future.

Changes in the Broad Context of Drug Regulation

Prescription drug development, regulation, and use have changed greatly since the 1962 drug amendments and continue to evolve. The scientific and demographic changes of the future will present challenges and opportunities for drug development and regulation. The promise of personalized medicine shimmers on the horizon, but considerable work remains to identify candidate measures, validate them, and show that their use in a clinical setting improves health outcomes, reduces costs, or both. The population of the United States is aging and requires more therapeutics for prevention and treatment for the chronic diseases associated with older people. Increasing ethnic and cultural diversity will require better under-

---

[1]The year 2006 is technically the centennial of the 1906 Pure Food and Drug Act, but the FDA asserts that "the modern era of the FDA dates to 1906 with the passage of the Federal Food and Drugs Act" (CDER, 1998).

standing of disparities in health status and the development of appropriate means of communicating useful therapeutic and health care information to heterogeneous populations.

The science and technology that underpin drug discovery are in a process of dramatic transformation. Advances in the basic sciences have increased the number of targeted drugs, and technological advances promise to transform and expand the array of drugs available for the prevention and treatment of human disease (Gwynne and Heebner, 2001; Cockburn, 2004). Technologic and scientific developments also promise to enhance the prediction of safety problems and opportunities earlier in the development process, but much more work is needed to actualize these promises (FDA, 2004).

The practice of drug discovery and drug development research has also changed substantially in response to scientific and technological advances. Drug discovery research is funded by both industry and government, and takes place in academe, government—especially the National Institutes of Health (NIH)—and industry. Almost all drug development occurs in industry, but an increasing proportion of industry-funded studies is being conducted outside academic health centers by contract research organizations, and more clinical trials are being conducted abroad (Cockburn, 2004). Biomedical research accounts for 5.6 percent of health expenditures in the US, with 57 percent of the research is funded by industry, and 28 percent by NIH (Moses et al., 2005). Despite advances, the development of new pharmaceutical problems is facing challenges—in its Critical Path report (FDA, 2004), FDA asserted that the translation from the basic sciences of drug discovery to the applied sciences of drug development has become sluggish because "the development path is becoming increasingly challenging, inefficient, and costly."

The practice of medicine and the provider-patient interaction—the point where the pharmaceutical product traditionally "meets" the patient—also have undergone great transformation in the last two or three decades. First, use of prescription drugs has been increasing steadily (Ganslaw, 2005). Physicians and other health care providers have more therapeutic options at their disposal, and both polypharmacy[2] and the chronic use of drugs have become extremely common, especially in the rapidly growing segment of the population in late middle age and older. Use of drugs to treat chronic disease risk factors such as high blood pressure and high cholesterol has expanded immensely. Second, the role of the patient has changed as part of the larger shift toward consumer empowerment in the private sector. The health care system (like other sectors) places increased emphasis on consumer choice.

---

[2]The administration of multiple drugs concurrently, with the concomitant increased risk of drug interactions.

Quality of care also has become a major issue for consumers. Pharmaceutical and health plan offerings are promoted to consumers now empowered to be decision-makers. Patients have unprecedented access to information about drugs, their benefits, and side effects. This is due in part to changes in the information environment. Promotion of drugs to patients has increased, including broadcast direct-to-consumer advertising. Access to the Internet has become widespread; this powerful tool provides access to information that varies greatly in accuracy, quality, and completeness (Tatsioni et al., 2003). The relationship between patients and their physicians has changed as patients have become more engaged and knowledgeable. Third, a category of "lifestyle" drugs has arrived in the marketplace. Two decades ago, patients used drugs chronically for treatment for and control of serious diseases. Today, many fundamentally healthy people take drugs long-term for purposes ranging from cosmetic improvement (such as botox) to symptomatic management (such as antihistamines) to performance enhancement (such as erectile dysfunction). For people who need to take drugs for control or treatment of serious diseases, the potential of adverse drug effects may be of less concern than it is for people who take drugs for very minor issues (see Box 1-1 for some FDA milestones).

Defining and Meeting the Charge

The Charge

Given the changes outlined above and in response to growing public concern with health risks posed by prescription drugs, FDA requested that the Institute of Medicine (IOM) convene an ad hoc committee of experts to conduct an independent assessment of the current system for evaluating and ensuring drug safety and to make recommendations to improve risk assessment, surveillance, and the safe use of drugs (see Box 1-2). In recognition of their roles in the drug safety system, the Centers for Medicare and Medicaid Services (CMS), the Agency for Healthcare Research and Quality (AHRQ), NIH, and the Department of Veterans Affairs are also sponsors of the report.

In responding to the charge, the committee focused much of its attention on FDA's CDER. Although the report is addressed to the FDA as a whole, a considerable proportion of the committee's discussion and recommendations pertain to CDER's structure, organization, and scientific and regulatory activities. Given the study timeframe, the committee found it difficult to accord the same level of attention (in terms of a detailed assessment and recommendations) to all other important stakeholders in the drug safety system. The roles of industry, the health care delivery system, and health care

BOX 1-1
Some Key Milestones in FDA History

The Pure Food and Drug Act of 1906 gave FDA's predecessor, the Bureau of Chemistry in the Department of Agriculture, its first regulatory powers. At inception, the agency's pharmaceutical regulatory work focused largely on misbranding and adulteration of drugs. In 1937, elixir sulfanilamide caused more than 100 deaths and led to the passing of the 1938 Federal Food, Drug, and Cosmetic (FD&C) Act. The act prohibited false therapeutic claims for drugs and for the first time required premarket notification of FDA by the sponsor for all new drugs. This meant that a company submitted its New Drug Application (NDA) and, if FDA did not explicitly prohibit marketing, the company was free to market the product without any type of approval after 60 days (unless FDA extended that period to 180 days), when the NDA became "effective." Although the FD&C Act required a manufacturer to prove a drug's safety by conducting preclinical toxicity testing and gathering and submitting drug safety data, it did not require proof of efficacy (Swann, 1998; Stergachis and Hazlet, 2002). Some two decades later, thousands of children with birth defects were born to European mothers who had taken the popular sedative thalidomide for morning sickness. Marketing of thalidomide in the United States had been held up in the approval process and this so-called near miss led to the Drug Amendments of 1962. The drug amendments required companies to provide proof of efficacy of a drug for it to be considered for marketing approval, and the randomized controlled trial became established as the gold standard for demonstrating efficacy (Stergachis and Hazlet, 2002).

In the 1980s, the public health crisis of HIV/AIDS motivated a powerful advocacy movement whose aims included faster approval of drugs for patients with incurable disorders. Other consumer and patient advocacy groups began to call for changing the drug approval process to speed up the availability of potentially life-saving or life-sustaining drugs to patients in need of them. Consumer groups, regulators, the regulated industry, and others contributed to and Congress passed the PDUFA legislation that aimed to ensure that FDA had adequate resources to expand its drug review staff and capabilities, and so to increase the pace of drug reviews. Agreements among FDA, industry, and Congress are crystallized in a series of performance goals for FDA. These are not part of the PDUFA statute, so they lack the force of law (Tauzin, 2002) but they reflect activities the agency considers its obligations—"The letter outlines goals that the agency must meet, which help frame the basis to judge the user fee programs success" (Tauzin, 2002). These goals are contained in the "PDUFA Reauthorization Performance Goals and Procedures," or the PDUFA "goals letter" (a letter with enclosures), which is transmitted by the Secretary of HHS to Congress annually.

PDUFA required that FDA and specifically CDER review staff meet certain performance goals and report annually to Congress on their progress in meeting those goals. PDUFA also required that companies pay three types of fees to FDA, including a one-time fee submitted with each NDA, an establishment fee, and a product fee (FDA, 2005a,b).* Congress reauthorized PDUFA in 1997 (as part of the FDA Modernization Act) and in 2002 as part of the Bioterrorism and Preparedness and Response Act. In PDUFA I and II, funds were limited to use to the review of sponsor applications for new drugs and indications. No PDUFA funds were allocated to postmarketing drug safety activities until 2002, when limited funds were allocated for limited safety activities. The 1992 PDUFA Amendments to the FD&C Act stipulated that PDUFA user fees must not be used in lieu of but to supplement appropriations. FDA was authorized to assess user fees only if appropriations for drug review were equal to or greater than appropriations for salaries and other FDA expenses in 1992 (Zelenay, 2005). PDUFA II set the trigger at 1997 levels: "Fees under subsection (a) of this section shall be refunded for a fiscal year beginning after fiscal year 1997 unless appropriations for salaries and expenses of the Food and Drug Administration for such fiscal year (excluding the amount of fees appropriated for such fiscal year) are equal to or greater than the amount of appropriations for the salaries and expenses of the Food and Drug Administration for the fiscal year 1997 (excluding the amount of fees appropriated for such fiscal year) multiplied by the adjustment factor applicable to the fiscal year involved" (21 US Code 379h(f)). The adjustment factor is based on the Consumer Price Index (Zelenay, 2005), and that may help explain why, although the agency has always met the trigger that allowed the collection of user funds, appropriations have grown at a much lower rate than user fees (FDA, 2005b). Appropriations have not only not kept pace, but they have declined since 2003, as FDA's payroll costs have increased (FDA, 2005b).

---

*For FY 2006, the application fee is $767,400, the establishment fee is $264,000, and the product fee is $42,130 (FDA, 2005a).

BOX 1-2
The Statement of Task

In response to growing public concern with health risks posed by approved drugs, the FDA has requested that the IOM convene an ad hoc committee of experts to conduct an independent assessment of the current system for evaluating and ensuring drug safety postmarketing and make recommendations to improve risk assessment, surveillance, and the safe use of drugs. As part of its work, the IOM committee will:

- examine the FDA's current role and the role of other actors (e.g., health professionals, hospitals, patients, other public agencies) in ensuring drug safety as part of the US health care delivery system;
- examine the current efforts for the ongoing safety evaluation of marketed drug products at the FDA and by the pharmaceutical industry, the medical community, and public health authorities;
- evaluate the analytical and methodological tools employed by FDA to identify and manage drug safety problems and make recommendations for enhancement;
- evaluate FDA's internal organizational structure and operations around drug safety (including continuing postmarket assessment of risk vs. benefit);
- consider FDA's legal authorities for identifying and responding to drug safety issues and current resources (financial and human) dedicated to postmarketing safety activities;
- identify strengths, weaknesses, and limitations of the current system; and
- make recommendations in the areas of organization, legislation, regulation, and resources to improve risk assessment, surveillance, and the safe use of drugs.

---

providers, patients, the public, Congress, the academic research enterprise, and other government agencies are discussed in much less detail. However, the committee's recommendations have implications for those stakeholders, and are discussed in the report where appropriate.

What This Study Is Not

This report does not address the related area of medication errors. That was the purview of the IOM Committee on Identifying and Preventing Medication Errors, whose report was released July 2006 (see Appendix E for that report summary). The present report does not treat several very important issues that were not in the charge given to the committee, including the regulation or safety of medical devices or biological products other than those regulated by CDER; pharmaceutical product abuse, overuse, or misuse; over-the-counter (OTC) drugs or the switch from prescription to OTC status; generic drugs; drug pricing; or the causes and consequences of the current challenges in pharmaceutical innovation. Finally, although the postapproval stage of a drug's life cannot be discussed in isolation from the preapproval stages, this report does not consider in any detail the complex ethical, practical, economic, and scientific issues related to the Investigational New Drug process or the clinical trial conduct in the testing of drugs.

Study Process

The committee gathered information to address its charge through a variety of means. It held three information-gathering meetings and one workshop that were open to the public. The first meeting focused on obtaining background on the committee charge from a number of perspectives, including FDA's. This and all other meeting agendas can be found in Appendix D. The second meeting focused on hearing from the public on day 1, and learning about the role of FDA, AHRQ, and CMS in US drug safety activities on day 2. The committee also held a workshop on Advancing the Methods and Application of Risk-Benefit Assessment of Medicines and held a final information-gathering meeting to hear opinions on proposals to improve drug safety in the United States. The committee met in executive sessions for deliberative discussions throughout the study process.

All the open meetings were Webcast in real time so that members of the public could listen to the proceedings and send questions to the committee by e-mail. The committee also received public submissions of material for its consideration at the meetings and by mail, e-mail, and fax throughout the course of the study. A Web site (http://www.iom.edu/drugsafety) and a listserv were created to provide information to the public about the committee's work and to facilitate communication with the committee. Many of the speakers' presentation slides from the three information-gathering meetings and workshop are available in electronic format on the project's Web site.

A few committee members and staff visited FDA to gain a better understanding of the background and daily operations of CDER. The committee and staff also conducted over 30 discussions with present and past FDA staff, managers, and leadership. Those discussions were confidential, but a summary of the main themes and points of discussion is provided in the public access file for this project (see IOM Staff Notes, 2005–2006).

The committee also commissioned two papers to inform it about industry's views of drug safety in the United States (written by Hugh Tilson) and those of academe (written by Brian Strom); these papers were based in part on small meetings convened by the authors and can be found in the public access file.[3]

Moving Target—The Shifting Landscape of Drug Safety in the United States

The committee has worked in the context of continuing change and proposals for change: modifications in the organizational structure of CDER and in the evaluation and monitoring of drug safety undertaken by FDA and to a lesser extent other stakeholders; multiple legislative proposals for changing the structure, resources, and authorities of CDER in FDA; and consumer and patient organizations' calls for changes in CDER. Those efforts have, in some cases, informed the work of the committee during its deliberations. Some of these changes have closed gaps, others have raised new questions and concerns, and still others have helped to increase the knowledge base of the committee. The efforts are described in greater detail in Appendix A.

Toward a New Vision of Drug Safety

The increasingly complex interface between innovation and regulation has been characterized by binary opposites: speed vs. safety, tight preapproval regulation vs. loose postapproval regulation, active collection of data before approval vs. passive surveillance after approval, and an abundance of clinical efficacy data before approval compared to much fewer safety data after approval. The polarity of approach and emphasis is inconsistent with the widely accepted notions that risk must be considered in the context of benefits, that understanding of the risks and benefits associated with a drug changes over a drug's lifecycle (FDA, 2004), and that the attention paid to safety and efficacy before approval must therefore be sustained as a drug enters and diffuses through the market and is used by a growing number and diversity of patients. Timely approval and attention to safety can become complementary rather than antithetical goals as postapproval surveillance becomes more effective, and regulatory authority and its exercise is commensurate with how a drug performs in real-life conditions over its lifecycle.

---

[3]A list of materials reviewed by the committee (in the form in which they were reviewed), including all submissions of information from the public and many items not cited in this report, can be found in the study's public access file, obtained from the National Academies Public Access Records Office at (202) 334-3543 or http://www8.nationalacademies.org/cp/ManageRequest.aspx?key=162.

The approval decision does not represent a singular moment of clarity about the risks and benefits associated with a drug—preapproval clinical trials do not obviate continuing formal evaluations after approval. However, the approval decision is a critical juncture in a product's lifecycle because it releases a drug to the market, where the public will gain broad exposure to it. In a strengthened drug safety system, that juncture should mark the beginning of another important stage in the lifecycle, when regulators, sponsors, health insurers, health care providers, and independent researchers actively pursue and manage emerging knowledge about risk-benefit relationships and uncertainty and they communicate that knowledge to patients, and health care organizations in a timely manner. Regulatory, health insurance coverage, and treatment decisions over a drug's lifecycle depend on the quality and timeliness of data collected, evaluated, and transmitted by trustworthy stakeholders in the health care system. In short, a drug safety system oriented around the new paradigm requires:

- A **culture** of safety in CDER supported by strong leadership, effective management, science-based decision making that is, insofar as possible, insulated from outside influences, and a healthy organization that encourages debate, teamwork, and independent scientific inquiry.
- **Science** that is rigorous and that through the individual and joint efforts of sponsors, academic researchers, and health care organizations describes a drug's risk-benefit profile, patterns of drug use, comparative effectiveness of drugs, behaviors of prescribers and users, and behaviors of institutions that affect prescribers and users.
- A **regulatory process** that is flexible, dynamic (e.g., proactive, responsive), and attentive to safety throughout the lifecycle of a drug, and a regulatory agency that is sufficiently empowered to take actions necessary to protect the public health.
- **Communication** about safety that is timely and effective and that facilitates transparency and enhances credibility.

The committee's vision of a transformed drug safety system has at its core a lifecycle approach to drug risk and benefit—not a new concept, but one that has been implemented, at best, in a narrow and fragmented manner. For FDA, attention to risk and benefit over the life of a drug requires continuous availability of new data and ongoing, active reassessment of risk and benefit to drive regulatory action (in response to the accumulating information on a given drug), and regulatory authority that is strong both before and after approval. For the industry, attention to risk and benefit over the lifecycle will require more careful assessments of emerging information about possible new risks and timely communication of this information to

FDA, and acceptance of changes intended to strengthen drug safety. FDA's credibility is intertwined with that of the industry, and a more credible drug safety system is in everyone's best interest. For the health care delivery system, a lifecycle approach to risk and benefit implies the need to heed and follow FDA communication about drug safety matters and to exercise appropriate caution in drug-related decision making (from formularies to prescribing) in recognition of the limited information available at the time of drug approval. The health care delivery system will benefit by consistently basing prescribing decisions on the science, and by exercising caution in regard to the industry's influence on the practice of medicine. Health care organizations and professional societies can contribute to prescribers' understanding of the evolving science behind the assessment of drug risk and benefit. The academic research enterprise can enhance its contributions of data to the assessment of risk and benefit at all points in a drug's lifecycle, continue its crucial advisory relationship with FDA, and uphold the value of complete transparency in recognition of real and perceived conflicts associated with financial involvement with the industry. Other government agencies can contribute to the lifecycle approach to drug risk and benefit by collaborating with FDA and the private sector to ensure that data streams from publicly funded health care settings contribute to an improved drug safety system. The public and patients can do their part by communicating with their health care providers about the pharmaceutical products they are using, learning about and discussing with their providers a drug's risks and benefits in the context of their health needs and characteristics, informing their providers about side effects they experience, and calling for more useful and timelier information about drug benefits and risks associated with new drugs.

REFERENCES

Applebaum A (The Washington Post). 2005. *The Drug Approval Pendulum.* [Online]. Available: http://www.washingtonpost.com/wp-dyn/articles/A48135-2005Apr12.html [accessed April 21, 2005].

CDER (Center for Drug Evaluation and Research). 1998. *Guideline for the Format and Content of the Clinical and Statistical Sections of an Application.* Rockville, MD: CDER.

Cockburn IM. 2004. The changing structure of the pharmaceutical industry. *Health Aff (Millwood)* 23(1):10-22.

DHEW (Department of Health Review Panel on New Drug Regulation), Dorsen N, Weiner N, Astin AV, Cohen MN, Cornelius CE, Hamilton RW, Rall DP. 1977. *Final Report.* Washington, DC: DHEW.

DHHS (Department of Health and Human Services), FDA, Task Force on Risk Management. 1999. *Managing the Risks from Medical Product Use: Creating a Risk Management Framework.* [Online]. Available: http://www.fda.gov/oc/tfrm/riskmanagement.pdf [accessed October 10, 2005].

FDA (Food and Drug Administration). 2004. *Innovation Stagnation: Challenge and Opportunity on the Critical Path to New Medical Products.* [Online]. Available: http://www.fda. gov/oc/initiatives/criticalpath/whitepaper.html [accessed October 10, 2005].

FDA. 2005a. Establishment of Prescription Drug User Fee rates for fiscal year 2006. *Fed Reg* 70(146):44106-44109.

FDA. 2005b. *White Paper, Prescription Drug User Fee Act (PDUFA): Adding Resources and Improving Performance in FDA Review of New Drug Applications.* [Online]. Available: http://www.fda.gov/oc/pdufa/PDUFAWhitePaper.pdf [accessed December 5, 2005].

Friedman MA, Woodcock J, Lumpkin MM, Shuren JE, Hass AE, Thompson LJ. 1999. The safety of newly approved medicines: do recent market removals mean there is a problem? *JAMA* 281(18):1728-1734.

Ganslaw LS. Drug safety: new legal/regulatory approaches. *FDLI* July/August (4):7-10.

Geraghty LN (The New York Times). 2006. *Doctors Fear Acne Drug Rules Go Too Far.* [Online]. Available: http://www.nytimes.com/2006/01/12/fashion/thursdaystyles/12skin. html [accessed January 13, 2006].

Gwynne P, Heebner G. 2001. Technologies in drug discovery/drug development: the next generation. *Science* Aug:1-17.

Hart C. 1999. Drug approvals: safe at any speed? *Mod Drug Disc* 2(5):25-26, 28.

Herper M. 2005. *Five Ways to Fix the FDA.* [Online]. Available: http://www.forbes.com/ healthcare/2005/01/12/cx_mh_0112fdaintro.html [accessed July 1, 2005].

Joint Commission on Prescription Drug Use. 1980. *Report of the Joint Commission on Prescription Drug Use.* KF3869.R4. Rockville, MD.

Kaiser Family Foundation. 2005. *Kaiser HealthPoll Report Views on Prescription Drugs and the Pharmaceutical Industry.* [Online]. Available: http://www.kff.org/healthpollreport/ feb_2005/upload/full_report.pdf [accessed September 22, 2005].

Kleinke JD, Gottlieb S. 1998. Is the FDA approving drugs too fast? Probably not—but drug recalls have sparked debate. [see comment]. *BMJ* 317(7163):899.

Landow L. 1999. FDA approves drugs even when experts on its advisory panels raise safety questions. *BMJ* 318(7188):944.

Lurie P, Wolfe SM. 1998. *FDA Medical Officers Report Lowers Standards Permit Dangerous Drug Approvals.* [Online]. Available: http://www.citizen.org/publications/release. cfm?ID=7104 [accessed October 15, 2005].

Lurie P, Sasich LD. 1999. Safety of FDA-approved drugs. *JAMA* 282(24):2297-2298.

Markel H. 2005. Why America needs a strong FDA. *JAMA* 294(19):2489-2491.

Moses H, Dorsey ER, Matheson DHM, Their SO. 2005. Financial anatomy of biomedical research. *JAMA* 294(11):1333-1342.

PricewaterhouseCoopers' Health Research Institute. 2005. *Recapturing the Vision:Integrity Driven Performance in the Pharmaceutical Industry.* [Online]. Available: http://www. pwc.com/extweb/pwcpublications.nsf/docid/EE74BACB6DE454768525702A00630CFF [accessed March 10, 2006].

Stergachis A, Hazlet T. 2002. Pharmacoepidemiology. In: DiPiro JT, Talbert RL, Yee GC, Matzke GR, Wells BG, Posey LM. *Pharmacotherapy: A Pathophysiologic Approach.* New York: McGraw-Hill Medical. Pp. 91-97.

Swann JP. 1998. *History of the FDA.* [Online]. Available: http://www.fda.gov/oc/history/ historyoffda/fulltext.html [accessed January 14, 2006].

Tatsioni A, Gerasi E, Charitidou E, Simou N, Mavreas V, Ioannidis JP. 2003. Important drug safety information on the internet: assessing its accuracy and reliability. *Drug Saf* 26(7):519-527.

Tauzin B. 2002. *Reauthorization of the Prescription Drug User Fee Act. Statement at the March 6, 2002 Hearing of the Committee on Energy and Commerce.* [Online]. Available: http:// energycommerce.house.gov/107/action/107-93.pdf [accessed September 14, 2006].

Tone B. 1999. *Rushing Through? Questioning the Safety of Drug Approvals.* [Online]. Available: http://www.nurseweek.com/features/99-11/fda.html [accessed July 1, 2005].

US House of Representatives Committee on Government Reform Minority Staff. 2006. *Prescription for Harm: The Decline in FDA Enforcement Activity.* [Online]. Available: http://www.democrats.reform.house.gov/Documents/20060627101434-98349.pdf [accessed August 26, 2006].

Wall Street Journal, Harris Interactive. 2005. *The Public Has Doubts About the Pharmaceutical Industry's Willingness to Publish Safety Information About Their Drugs in a Timely Manner.* [Online]. Available: http://www.harrisinteractive.com/news/printerfriend/index.asp?NewsID=882 [accessed March 10, 2006].

Wood AJ, Stein CM, Woosley R. 1998. Making medicines safer—the need for an independent drug safety board. *N Engl J Med* 339(25):1851-1854.

Zelenay JL. 2005. The Prescription Drug User Fee Act: is a faster Food and Drug Administration always a better Food and Drug Administration? *Food and Drug Law J* 60(2):261-338.

2

Natural History of a Drug

This chapter describes some key steps in reviewing potential new therapies and monitoring drugs once they are in the marketplace, with an emphasis on how safety considerations are handled throughout the process. The elements of the drug regulatory system have been well described elsewhere (Lipsky and Sharp, 2001; Randall, 2001; Meadows, 2002; FDA, 2006c). The committee also reviewed some of the factors that shape how the understanding of a drug's safety and efficacy profile evolves during the lifecycle and what regulatory action is taken. Those factors include scientific uncertainty; resources at the Food and Drug Administration (FDA); statutory requirements, including both limitations in authority and deadlines that shape the timing and scope of regulatory activities; and workload and staffing.

This discussion is intended to provide a reference point for subsequent chapters that provide the committee's findings about the strengths and weaknesses of the drug safety system and recommendations for strengthening it. A number of the points addressed in this chapter are related directly to the committee's recommendations. The material in this chapter is drawn largely from Center for Drug Evaluation and Research (CDER) documents—both guidance documents for sponsors and internal manual of policies and procedures that describe a wide variety of official policies—and from conversations with current and former FDA staff.

CDER reviews various types of drug applications and supplements. This chapter focuses on New Drug Applications (NDAs), although some of the processes also apply to supplemental NDAs, which are most often submitted for new indications of approved drugs. The chapter traces the work of the NDA review process in CDER's Office of New Drugs (OND) and its offices of drug evaluation which conduct premarket reviews, and in CDER's Office of Drug Safety (ODS) (which is now called the Office of Surveillance and Epidemiology, OSE, because of a restructuring of CDER in May 2005[1]) and its Division of Drug Risk Evaluation (DDRE), which monitors postmarket risks and undertakes risk assessments. (Other divisions and offices of ODS/OSE address safety issues, such as medication errors and drug names.[2]) The chapter does not address Abbreviated NDAs for generic drugs that go through CDER's Office of Generic Drugs. Nor are drugs that are on special tracks, such as accelerated approval or orphan-drug status, specifically addressed in this general description of how a new drug moves through the system.

Economic Impact of Drugs

Prescription drugs play a major role in American health and economy. For example, prescription drugs for controlling blood pressure and blood cholesterol levels were partly responsible for one of the ten great public health achievements of the 20th century: the 5 percent decline in death rates for coronary heart disease since 1972 (CDC, 1999). Prescription drugs are among the innovations that have replaced some highly invasive measures (such as surgery) with less invasive preventive and health maintenance therapies (DHHS, 2002). Prescription drugs also can help reduce health care costs by decreasing hospitalization. National survey data show that 44 percent of Americans take at least one prescription drug in any given month (NCHS, 2004). In economic terms, the investment and return on investment of drug discovery and development are vast. Although methodologies used for estimating the cost of bringing a drug to market are a matter of some controversy, some estimates are provided here as an illustration (Epstein, 2004). The cost of drug development has been estimated at approximately $800 million and at between $500 and $2,000 million (DiMasi et al., 2003; Adams and Brantner, 2006). The Bain report provided the estimated cost of development at $1.7 billion (Gilber et al., 2003). In 2005, the biopharmaceutical industry spent approximately $51.3 billion in drug discovery and development (PhRMA, 2006). A great deal is spent on prescription drugs. Due to cost-containment strategies, the rate of increase of spending on prescription drugs has slowed down, but still totaled $179.2 billion in 2003, and comprised 11 percent of national health spending (Kaiser Family Foundation, 2005; Smith et al., 2005).

---

[1]For the remainder of this chapter, we will refer to this office as ODS/OSE.
[2]Division of Surveillance, Research and Communication Support and Division of Medication Errors & Technical Support.

THE INVESTIGATIONAL NEW DRUG

As discussed in Chapter 1 and throughout the report, FDA has initiated or is initiating many changes related to drug safety in its internal procedures and organization. Some of the changes may supersede the descriptions in this chapter. Also on the horizon is FDA's Critical Path Initiative, announced in 2004, which is intended to stimulate the development and use of new scientific tools to better assess the safety and effectiveness of drugs under study (FDA, 2004a; DHHS/FDA, 2006).

Investigational New Drug Submission and Review

The vast majority of chemical molecules and candidate drugs screened for therapeutic potential and toxicity never show sufficient promise to enter human trials (PhRMA, 2006). But when preclinical data indicate that a compound is reasonably safe for initial testing in humans, shows promising pharmacologic activity, and has commercial prospects, the sponsor submits an Investigational New Drug (IND) Application to FDA, and the agency's oversight begins (FDA, 2006c).

IND sponsors can be companies, research institutions, or individual investigators. Often the sponsor has been in frequent contact with FDA throughout the development process prior to submission of the IND, and has participated in FDA's pre-IND consultation program (FDA, 2006c). FDA produces numerous guidance documents to steer sponsors through the regulatory process. Those documents are prepared and updated continually. Some are very specific, for example, describing appropriate methods for a specific type of study; others provide more general guidance about preparing submissions to the agency (FDA and CDER, 2006b). Some reflect international harmonization efforts among European, Japanese, and US regulators.

The average new commercial IND submission totals about 28 volumes of about 500 pages each—about 14,000 pages (Henderson, 2006). It contains manufacturing and chemical information about the drug and the results of animal tests, toxicology studies, and other preclinical tests. The IND also contains protocols for small phase 1 human studies intended to document the drug's metabolism and excretion, determine a safe dose, and identify acute side effects (FDA and CDER, 2006b). Local institutional review boards (IRBs) must review the protocols to ensure protection of human subjects. If a sponsor has already begun human trials outside the United States, it also includes their results.

By law, FDA has 30 days from the date an IND is received to place a hold on the proposed human trials (FD&C Act, SEC. 505(i)(2)) if it deems it to be necessary. CDER can take up to about 2 weeks of that period to process the IND, assign it to a review division within OND on the basis of the drug's likely indication, and assemble a review team. The team includes a project manager and several scientific reviewers from OND and other CDER offices as required (CDER et al., 1998). The reviewers then have the remainder of the 30-day period to determine whether safety concerns justify placing a hold on the human trials. In the absence of FDA action to delay or prevent a trial, the sponsor can begin testing the compound in humans on day 31 (FDA and CDER, 2006b).

FDA typically allows human trials to proceed if no serious safety concerns have surfaced (FDA and CDER, 2001a). As occurs throughout the review process, safety assessments and regulatory actions are influenced by evidence of the potential benefit of the product. For example, reviewers are likely to tolerate a higher threshold of toxicity for a drug that will be used to treat life-threatening cancer than for a new antihistamine similar to those on the market.

Early Clinical Trials and Related Studies

The sponsor typically begins phase 1 trials by testing several increasing dosages in healthy volunteers (see Box 2-1 for definitions of all phases of clinical trials). About 20–80 subjects are usually involved in one or more of these trials (FDA, 2006c). Animal and other toxicology studies and phase 1 studies may be concurrent. If the initial phase 1 results do not show unacceptable toxicity, the sponsor moves to larger, phase 2, trials which involve from a few dozen to hundreds of patients who have the condition for which the drug is being studied (CDER et al., 1998; FDA, 2006c). Efficacy and safety are evaluated by continuing to test various dosages of the compound in patients (FDA, 2006c).

Clinical trials are conducted under the sponsor's auspices by commercial, academic, or other entities in the United States or, increasingly, overseas. In trials, an active product is compared with a placebo or occasionally with an existing drug for the condition (FDA, 2006c). Sponsors increasingly include genetic studies in the premarket period as part of a personalized-medicine approach to identifying target populations for a drug. The developing science of pharmacogenomics is generating strong interest and attention in and outside FDA as a way to improve drug safety through predictive techniques, but any widespread use of these techniques in clinical practice is well into the future.

Sponsors develop study protocols and undertake, fund, and oversee studies. The OND review team and sponsor consult as the trials and studies are under way, new protocols are developed, and new data emerge. The review team can play a critical role in how the studies proceed. The extent of consultation varies among drugs and sponsors. The sponsor is required to notify FDA and all investigators in written safety reports of "any adverse

BOX 2-1
Phases of Clinical Trials and Medicine Development

Phase 1
Clinical pharmacology studies in healthy volunteers (sometimes subjects) to determine the safety and tolerability of the drug/product, other dynamic effects, and the pharmacokinetic profile (absorption, distribution, metabolism, and excretion).

Phase 2
Clinical investigation studies in subjects with the target disease, to determine efficacy, safety, and tolerability in carefully controlled dose-ranging studies. Phase 2 studies are typically well controlled and closely monitored.

Phase 3
Formal clinical trials. Large-scale placebo controlled and uncontrolled studies in subjects to gather further information on efficacy and on the safety and tolerability of the drug or product.

Phase 4
Postmarketing surveillance to expand safety and efficacy data in a large population, including further formal therapeutic trials and comparisons with other active comparators.

SOURCE: Adapted from 21 CFR 312.21 (2005).

experience associated with the use of the drug that is both serious and unexpected" or "any finding from tests in laboratory animals that suggests a significant risk for human subjects including reports of mutagenicity, teratogenicity, or carcinogenicity" (21 CFR 312.33). The sponsor also submits annual progress reports on the IND to FDA.

The regulators may direct the sponsor to undertake specific studies or laboratory evaluations in studies to look for possible markers of safety problems (such as liver toxicity or cardiovascular changes) on the basis of previous experience or questions about the class of drugs or the mechanism of action.

End of Phase 2 Meeting and Phase 3 Trials

If the results of the early trials are promising, the sponsor and the review team typically meet for an "end of phase 2 meeting" to discuss the upcoming phase 3 trials. The phase 3 trials can involve fewer than 100 patients in some cases or many thousands in others, depending on the target population and the endpoints being evaluated (on the average, they involve about 600–3,000 patients). The drug is tested against a placebo or sometimes against another drug (FDA, 2006c). The trials are designed and powered to evaluate selected efficacy outcomes, not safety end points, although they can generate safety signals to pursue. The "end of phase 2 meeting" can be an important early point in the lifecycle of the drug to identify and track potential safety issues and to ensure that the sponsor's protocols address key questions.

Roles of the Office of New Drugs and the Office of Drug Safety/Office of Surveillance and Epidemiology Premarket Period

OND is responsible for premarket reviews, makes approval decisions, and retains authority for regulatory decisions after a drug is marketed. OND clinical reviewers typically are physicians, some with epidemiology training, who are skilled in review of clinical trials. DDRE staff are mostly pharmacists and epidemiologists whose expertise tends to be in observational studies and whose primary focus has been on monitoring and evaluating postmarket data. Traditionally, the OND review team has drawn on ODS/OSE, and particularly DDRE, as safety consultants when they determined a need for a specific safety review.

DDRE staff routinely participate in a limited number of premarket activities; they have historically functioned in a consultation capacity to OND, called on to perform specific safety reviews. In a recent report on postmarketing drug safety, the Government Accountability Office characterized ODS/OSE as a consultant to OND in the postmarket period and described a problematic working relationship between the two offices (GAO, 2006). In its official response to that report, FDA asserted that the "consultant" term understates the importance of ODS/OSE and referred to the agency's efforts to "foster a partnership" between ODS/OSE and OND that makes them equals in the postmarket identification and timely resolution of drug safety issues (GAO, 2006). FDA's recent efforts to integrate the work of the two offices better may also extend to the premarket period. Chapter 3 discusses the challenges in the OND and ODS/OSE relationship and recent efforts to address them.

One of the 17 drug-evaluation divisions (see organization chart), the Division of Neurology Products (DNP),[3] has a safety team in the unit. The

---

[3]DNP and the Division of Psychiatry Products were combined in the past and were separated in the 2005 reorganization of OND. They both continue to use the safety team, which now officially reports to DNP.

safety team's role is to quantify and set priorities among potential risks posed by the drug they are reviewing. They do not make recommendations on a drug's approvability (Racoosin, 2006). The committee was told that discussions have occurred in FDA about including a full-time safety officer in the other ODS/ODE divisions. Two possible explanations for why that has not occurred were offered: shortage of safety officers and the fact that some divisions do not review enough applications to support a full-time safety officer.

Completion of Clinical Trials and Their Limitations

Clinical trials typically take 2–10 years to complete (PhRMA, 2006), depending on such factors as the rate of the event of primary interest, the length of patient followup, the staging of trials, and the difficulty of accruing patients. When data from phase 2 trials seem extremely promising, particularly in the context of serious or life-threatening diseases or conditions, an NDA may be filed without proceeding to or completing phase 3 trials.[4] For example, azidothymidine (AZT) was approved for treatment of HIV infection on the basis of phase 2 trials (Grassley et al., 2004).

Only about 20 percent of drugs that enter phase 1 trials go on to be approved and marketed (lower estimates have been provided by others so the true percent is unknown) (DiMasi et al., 2003; PhRMA, 2006). A sponsor may decide to halt trials for various scientific or commercial reasons. A recent study found that the number of clinical trials being conducted in the United States leveled off in 2000 and then started to decline in 2002. The author attributes the decline to cancellation of late-stage trials (Kaitin, 2005).

Even when a sponsor completes its trials and submits the resulting data in support of an NDA, important safety information about the drug is not yet available. That point is essential for an understanding of the drug regulatory system and the incomplete safety profiles of the drugs that enter the marketplace.

The gaps in critical information, such as safety data, are due to a number of factors, including the limited number of subjects studied and the ways in which the subjects and the research setting differ from the conditions of use when the drug is marketed (CDER et al., 1998). Preapproval trials typically are too small to detect even significant safety problems if they are rare. An adverse event (even a serious one) that occurs in less than one in 1,000 patients cannot be reliably detected except in the largest premarket trials but can pose a serious public health problem when hundreds of thousands

---

[4]FDA may grant accelerated approval on the basis of surrogate endpoints, but approval is conditional on sponsors' undertaking or completing validation trials.

or millions of people use the drug (GAO, 1990; Okie, 2005; Racoosin, 2006). For example, bromfenac, a non-steroidal anti-inflammatory drug (NSAID) marketed for 11 months in 1997–1998, was found to have serious and sometimes fatal liver toxicity in about one in 20,000 people who used the drug (Friedman et al., 1999); the NDA clinical trial base would have had to include 60,000 patients to detect such an effect before marketing (Friedman et al., 1999).

Preapproval clinical trials also have little information on the effects of long-term exposure to the drug due to their often short duration. Furthermore, clinical trials usually do not represent the full array of patients who will use the product once it is approved. Trials often exclude patients with comorbidities or those taking other medications, although both may be common among future users of the marketed drugs. Elderly patients, ethnic and racial minorities, and the very sick are underrepresented, and pregnant women are generally excluded from trials. Drugs generally have not been tested in children as part of the NDA, although patent-extension incentives are aimed specifically at encouraging pediatric testing in children (Meadows, 2003).

Those limitations are inherent in the system and cannot be changed without adding considerably to the time and expense of drug approvals, which would delay patient access to potentially beneficial drugs. It is generally understood that it is not routinely realistic to require premarket trials on tens or hundreds of thousands of subjects. Thus, inherent in the fundamental design of the drug approval system is the delayed availability of important safety data until a drug is used in larger and more diverse populations after marketing. That approach means that the initial postmarket period is a critical time for developing a fuller understanding of a drug's safety profile.

Premarket clinical trials are designed primarily with efficacy. Safety issues sometimes surface, but the challenge is the possibility of unusual, unexpected, undocumented risk. If sponsors and CDER reviewers are not vigilant about identifying and pursuing safety signals in the trials, the opportunity to evaluate safety in the premarket trial period may be lost.

In the premarket period there usually is a shortage of information on how a new drug compares with other treatments for the same indication. Sponsors are not routinely required to submit such comparative trials to obtain approval. Once a drug is on the market, it can be difficult to compel sponsors or others to undertake appropriate comparative trials. Sponsors usually do not initiate such trials unless they believe that their product has a readily identified or demonstrable advantage. A postmarket comparative trial of newer hypertension agents—angiotensin-converting enzyme (ACE) inhibitors—against older diuretic drugs, for example, found the older drugs to be more effective in reducing blood pressure (Appel, 2002). In addition, comparative trials are expensive, and cost-benefit considerations are not part of FDA's statutory purview. (Chapter 4 addresses this topic in greater detail.) Thus, premarket studies typically do not answer questions of great concern to health care providers, patients, and payers: Which drug in a class works work best for most patients? Which is the best first line of treatment? Which is most cost-effective?

By definition, premarket trials do not address the implications of expansive off-label use, that is, use for conditions in which the given compound was not studied (or not approved) in tests submitted to FDA (Beck and Azari, 1998). A recent study found that 21 percent of the 725 million prescriptions written in 2001 were for off-label uses (Boodman, 2006).

Pre-New Drug Application Submission Meeting

As trials are completed and analyzed, the sponsor meets with the review team to go over the impending NDA submission; it is in the sponsor's and FDA's interest to anticipate issues so that the NDA is complete when submitted. For example, a 2006 report indicated that when sponsors met with CDER staff before submitting an NDA, there was a greater likelihood that the drug was approved on the first cycle (FDA News, 2006b).

According to FDA documents, the discussions include development of strategies to manage known risks (CDER, 2005b). ODS/OSE staff sometimes participate in the meetings; it may be the first time that ODS/OSE staff become involved in the IND. (When OND is reviewing a supplemental NDA for new labeling or manufacturing, ODS/OSE may be active in reviewing available postmarket data on the approved indication.)

NEW DRUG APPLICATION

In the last couple of years, FDA has received 110–120 NDAs per year (FDA and CDER, 2005). The average size is 235 MB with 250 files, the equivalent of almost 400 volumes of 500 pages each, or about 200,000 pages (Henderson, 2006). Often, an NDA does not arrive all at once—FDA allows gradual submission for fast track[5] studies (rolling review). Sponsors are also required to provide additional data that become available during the review process.

Data management is a critical task with a project of this size. Scientific reviewers need sophisticated knowledge of and access to programs for managing and analyzing the data. In addition, because sponsors have some

---

[5]"Fast track is a process designed to facilitate the development, and expedite the review of drugs to treat serious diseases and fill an unmet medical need. The purpose is to get important new drugs to the patient earlier. Fast Track addresses a broad range of serious diseases" (FDA, 2006c).

leeway in how they present their summary safety and efficacy data and where in this massive file they are found, reviewers must sometimes devote considerable time to finding the critical safety data needed for the review. ODS/OSE involvement is typically limited to meeting attendance and providing consults at this point in the process. The arrival of data on a rolling basis can further complicate the process. Sponsors can submit materials to the NDA fewer than two dozen times, as was the case with cinacalcet hydrochloride[6] (Meyer, 2004), or as many as 70 (or even more) times, as occurred with sibutramine[7] (Bilstad, 1997).

Prescription Drug User Fee Act Timetables and Performance Goals Triggered

When FDA receives the final piece of an NDA the Prescription Drug User Fee Act (PDUFA) clock begins ticking (FDA, 2005f). PDUFA was enacted in 1992 and reauthorized in 1997 (PDUFA II) and 2002 (PDUFA III). It is up for reauthorization in 2007. The law provides for the pharmaceutical industry to pay user fees to FDA to be used primarily to staff and resource new drug (and biologic) review divisions, in exchange for which FDA agrees to expedite drug reviews according to specific timetables. PDUFA has also established deadlines to expedite the premarket review process, to schedule meetings requested by industry, resolve disputes, to respond to questions about study protocols, and develop guidances (see Box 2-2 and Appendix C for the goals, and see Chapter 3 for additional discussion of PDUFA).

The PDUFA II and III goals call on FDA to review and act on 90 percent of standard original NDAs within 10 months and 90 percent of priority NDAs in 6 months. A priority NDA review is intended for drugs that "represent significant improvements compared with marketed products" (FDA and CDER, 2005). PDUFA has resulted in a dramatic decline in new drug review time. For standard NDA reviews, the median FDA review time was 11.9 months in 2004, down from 20.8 months in 1993 (FDA, 2005d; CDER, 2006). For priority NDA reviews, the median review time was 6.0 months in 2004, down from 16.3 months in 1993 (Weiss Smith, 2006).

Initial Filing Review

CDER does an initial review of an NDA to determine whether it is acceptable for review. Within 60 days, CDER informs the sponsor if there are

---

[6]Sponsor submitted data to FDA 19 times from September 8, 2003, through March 5, 2004.

[7]Sponsor submitted data to FDA 85 times from August 7, 1995, through November 22, 1997.

substantive deficiencies in the file that cause FDA to "refuse to file" the application (CDER et al., 1998). That occurs when the NDA has such critical deficiencies that it clearly is not approvable as submitted. When submitted, the NDA is also designated as a standard (10-month timetable) or priority (6-month timetable) review by the division office or office director. A minority of NDAs have been designated as priority reviews. In 2004, for example, 29 of the 119 NDAs submitted were priority reviews, and the remaining 90 were standard reviews. Most priority reviews involve new molecular entities (NMEs). An NME is defined as "a medication containing an active substance that has never before been approved for marketing in any form in the United States" (FDA and CDER, 2001b). Of the 119 NDAs submitted in 2004, 36 were for NMEs, and 21 of these were assigned priority status. (See Table 2-1 for past NME priority and standard approval numbers.)

Assembly of Review Team and Beginning of Review

Within about 2 weeks of receiving an NDA, CDER names a review project manager and primary scientific reviewers. Although reviewers who were involved with the IND are strong candidates for the review, the team does not necessarily include all those involved earlier. Some members of the original team may be too busy with other work, may have moved on to other positions, or may have left FDA.

Reviewers' workloads typically include premarket reviews and supplemental NDA reviews and issues arising with marketed drugs that they previously reviewed. They may also be involved in writing guidance documents or may be participating in other CDER or FDA initiatives; in the wake of highly publicized concerns about safety, CDER has launched a number of initiatives in the last year to evaluate, articulate, and improve procedures. Obstacles in hiring new staff due to a change in Department of Health and Human Services human resources policies have placed added strain on the workforce.

The review team includes OND staff with expertise in various medical and scientific specialties—including clinical medicine,[8] pharmacology, and toxicology—and CDER reviewers from outside OND with expertise in such fields as chemistry, manufacturing and controls, microbiology, and statistics. In some cases, outside experts (special government employees) may participate in reviews (CDER et al., 1998; FDA, 2006c).

In consultation with the clinical team leader and perhaps other team members, the primary clinical reviewer will ultimately be responsible for

---

[8]There are inconsistencies in CDER documents in the use of medical review or clinical review. They appear to be interchangeable terms. It has been suggested that use of clinical review indicates that a primary reviewer need not necessarily be a physician, although most of them are. In this report, we will use the more inclusive term clinical review or clinical reviewer.

BOX 2-2
Select PDUFA Goals

Clinical Development
Under PDUFA, FDA's goal is to reply to a sponsor's complete response to a clinical hold within 30 days of the agency's receipt of the submission of such sponsor response, and do this for at least 90% of such submissions. Rapid resolution of safety issues that lead to clinical hold helps ensure patient safety while enabling access to the experimental treatment.

FDA Oversight and Review of Clinical Trial Protocols During Development
Under PDUFA, FDA will evaluate specific questions about the sponsor's special study protocol designs for carcinogenicity, stability and phase 3 for clinical trials that will form the primary basis of an efficacy claim.

- FDA will review scientific and regulatory requirements for which the sponsor seeks agreement.
- FDA's goal is to provide a succinct written response, within 45 days of receipt of the protocol and specific questions, and do this for at least 90% of such submissions.

Sponsor-Requested Meetings with FDA During Clinical Development
Under PDUFA FDA's goal is to review all filed original NDA/biologics license application (BLA) submissions within the following time frames:

TABLE 2-1 Numbers of Priority and Standard NME and New BLA Approvals, 1995–2004

Year	Priority	Standard	Total
1995	10	19	29
1996	18	35	53
1997	9	30	39
1998	16	14	30
1999	19	16	35
2000	9	18	27
2001	7	17	24
2002	7	10	17
2003	9	12	21
2004*	21	15	36
2005*	15	5	20

*Includes BLAs for therapeutic biologics.

SOURCE: Adapted from the 2004 and 2005 CDER Report to the Nation.

- Review and act on 90% of priority applications within 6 months.
- Review and act on 90% of standard applications within 10 months.

For all NDA/BLA resubmissions:

- Review and act on 90% of Class 1 resubmissions within 2 months.
- Review and act on 90% of Class 2 resubmissions within 6 months.

FDA Filing and Review of Submitted Marketing Applications (NDA/BLA)

Under PDUFA FDA's goal is to review all filed original NDA/BLA submissions within the following time frames:

- Review and act on 90% of priority applications within 6 months.
- Review and act on 90% of standard applications within 10 months.

For all NDA/BLA resubmissions:

- Review and act on 90% of Class 1 resubmissions within 2 months.
- Review and act on 90% of Class 2 resubmissions within 6 months.

Under PDUFA FDA's goal is to review all filed original Efficacy Supplements within the following timeframes:

- Review and act on 90% of priority efficacy supplements within 6 months.
- Review and act on 90% of standard efficacy supplements within 10 months.

preparing and signing the written review of the NDA. The primary review summarizes and analyzes the clinical data in the NDA and provides the reviewer's assessment and conclusions regarding the effectiveness and safety data. It also sets out the reviewer's assessment of the proposed directions for use and includes a recommendation for regulatory action. The other scientific reviewers will each write and sign "discipline reviews" that evaluate the NDA from the point of view of their expertise, and the primary review includes a summary of those reviews. The team leader will sign off on the primary review, sometimes adding a memo that summarizes broader issues or professional disagreements raised by the NDA (CDER, 2004).

If the NDA is for an NME—that is, an active substance that has not been approved before—the OND office director or deputy director must sign off on the approval. When it is not for an NME, the director or deputy director of the review division in OND can sign off on the approval decision.

The NDA contains data from animal and human studies; it is illegal to exclude any pertinent data. It also has information on product manufacturing and characteristics, packaging and labeling for both physician and consumer, IND data, and the results of any additional toxicologic studies that were not included in the IND (21 CFR 314.50) (CDER et al., 1998). Data on the use of the drug outside the United States may be included in the NDA. In the early 1980s, only about 2 or 3 percent of new drugs were first marketed in the United States, so useful safety data on use abroad could sometimes be included (Friedman et al., 1999). By 1998, that proportion grew to 50 percent and the proportion of drugs launched in the United States first has increased with each reauthorization of PDUFA: I, 25.23 percent; II, 47.19 percent; and III, 50 percent (FDA, 2005d; Okie, 2005).

Unlike their European counterparts who generally rely on the sponsor's summaries, FDA reviewers compile and reanalyze the data submitted by the sponsor and use the analyses, as well as the one done by the sponsor, to inform their decision about the drug.

Throughout the review process, the sponsor may be submitting amendments in response to FDA requests or to complete work identified in the pre-NDA meeting. If major amendments arrive in the last 3 months of the review, the PDUFA clock may be extended (FDA, 2002). As issues arise, the sponsor or FDA may request formal meetings during the process to resolve disputes or discuss pending concerns. The number of such meetings varies, but it is not uncommon for several meetings to be held while the application is under review.

PDUFA establishes specific timelines for FDA to respond to an industry request for a meeting, schedule the meeting, and distribute minutes from it (FDA, 2005g). The PDUFA goals were associated with about a 33 percent increase in sponsor-requested meetings from fiscal year (FY) 1999 to FY 2004 (FDA, 2005d). That has required FDA staff to devote many hours to planning, conducting, and following up on the meetings. Although time-consuming and resource-intensive, the meetings can clarify issues and improve the review process by reducing the risk of misunderstandings late in the review process.

Advisory Committees

During the review process, a decision may be made, usually by the division director, to convene an advisory committee meeting (see Box 2-3 for deadlines to convene an advisory committee meeting). Advisory committees are used as a source of independent advice from experts outside FDA (FDA, 2006b). Chapter 4 discusses advisory committees in more detail.

BOX 2-3
Timeline for Planning an Advisory Committee Meeting

Planning of an advisory committee meeting takes roughly 4 months and involves the following:

- Advisory committee members must fill out a "Conflict of Interest Disclosure Report for SGEs" (form 3410) for each topic to be discussed.
- FDA staff (advisory committee oversight and management) must determine whether existing advisory committee members have a conflict of interest (COI) regarding the current topic and what other expertise they need (if not already on the committee, or to replace a committee member with a COI in that topic).
- Five weeks before the meeting: proposed waivers need to be submitted for approval. Waivers are reviewed by
    - committee members
    - the executive secretary
    - the committee management specialist
    - the program officer
    - the chief of scientific advisers and consultants staff
    - the ethics specialist
    - the director of advisory committee oversight
    - the senior associate commissioner.
- The dockets office needs a few days to a week to prepare the posting for the *Federal Register.*
- Fifteen days before the meeting: FDA must post notice of the advisory committee meeting, including the topic to be discussed and any waivers obtained for the meeting on its Web site (Hinchey Amendment). FDA also posts this information in the *Federal Register.*
- No later than the day of the meeting: if the Secretary of Health and Human Services or FDA discovers a COI less than 15 days before the advisory committee meeting, the agency must make a disclosure as soon as possible but in any event no later than the date of the meeting (Hinchey Amendment).

CDER has 17 topic-specific advisory committees,[9] each composed mainly of clinical experts in a specific field, such as gastrointestinal or onco-

---

[9]Number of advisory committees in other units of FDA: Center for Biologics Evaluation and Research = 5, Center for Devices and Radiological = 21, Center for Food Safety and Applied Nutrition = 1, Center for Veterinary Medicine = 1, National Center for Toxicological Research = 2, Office of the Commissioner = 2.

logic drugs (FDA, 2006a). Advisory committees roughly match the medical specialties of the review divisions in OND. In addition, the Drug Safety and Risk Management Advisory Committee provides guidance on issues related to safety and research methods (CDER, 2005a).

Typically, advisory committees are convened when applications involve new or complex technologies or to address controversies (FDA, 2006b). Sometimes, they are used to address general concerns not related to the approval of a specific product, such as the acceptability of a particular study design or the use of a particular endpoint as a surrogate (FDA, 2006b). Committees convened to assess an NDA may be asked to comment on whether the data support product approval; on some unique aspect of safety, effectiveness, or clinical development of the product; on whether additional studies are needed; or on whether changes should be made in a drug's label or other action should be taken in response to new risk information after a drug is approved.

After presentations by the sponsor and agency representatives and a public comment period, the committee members usually vote on the questions posed to them by FDA staff. The votes are not binding (FDA, 2006b), but FDA decisions usually are consistent with the majority vote. The meetings can lead FDA to request additional information from the sponsors.

Safety Tracking

As described in Chapter 1, FDA has been under pressure to speed drug reviews and get promising therapies to patients sooner (Lurie et al., 1999) for at least two decades. PDUFA established goals for speed that, as noted, have resulted in substantial decreases in review time. However, no comparable safety goals drive the review process. Case studies of specific drugs point out both the strengths and the weaknesses of FDA's investigation of safety signals in specific instances, but there seems to be no overall metric in place comparable with measures of speed to track how safety is being monitored and assessed.

Individual drug evaluation offices in OND seem to differ in how and the extent to which they track safety issues regarding drugs that they are reviewing. The committee has been told that for the last 2–3 years OND's senior leadership has listed and tracked safety issues by office at its weekly meetings (IOM Staff Notes, 2005–2006). Difficult or controversial safety issues are sometimes discussed at "regulatory briefings," which are attended by staff from various parts of CDER and allow wider input on important questions faced by individual divisions, promote consistency in approach and decision-making, and raise awareness of emerging issues throughout CDER.

In response to congressional and public concerns, CDER has expanded its safety-oversight infrastructure over the last 2 years. In 2006, a new position of associate center director for safety policy and communications was created in CDER with responsibility for overseeing safety issues (FDA, 2006c). In early 2005, the Drug Safety Oversight Board was created to increase both oversight and transparency in matters of safety (CDER, 2005c). It is too early to know whether those highly publicized initiatives will strengthen oversight of and communication about safety.

Dispute Resolution

Differences of opinion among reviewers may surface at various points during the review process or in the postmarket period. Sometimes, they reflect different professional perspectives on how to assess and weigh the types of data available and draw a conclusion. The evaluation of drugs is a team process, incorporating experts in a wide array of disciplines who must work together effectively. Furthermore, reviewers rarely have all the information they would like to have to make the required scientific determinations; in this environment of scientific uncertainty, legitimate differences of opinion on the appropriate course of action are inevitable. But a regulatory decision must be reached and must incorporate the most persuasive and compelling scientific assessments, while leaving all participants feeling that they have been heard.

Disparate views may be discussed at global assessment meetings when the whole review team tracks the review in progress or in other informal or official meetings. Where disagreement persists, upper-level supervisors have traditionally had responsibility for evaluating the options and making a decision to resolve the disagreement.

In a few high-profile cases, internal disagreements about CDER's handling of safety issues on particular drugs or in general have been aired in the mass media or in congressional hearings (Graham, 2004; Hensley et al., 2005; Neergaard, 2005). Surveys of CDER staff reveal some concern about decision-making regarding postmarketing safety (DHHS/OIG, 2003). (See Chapter 3 for more information on this topic.)

In November 2004, CDER created a pilot program in the CDER ombudsman's office to provide a forum to discuss and resolve differences (MAPP 4151.2[10]). It provides for dispute resolution at the center direc-

---

[10]This MAPP provides a new pilot procedure for CDER staff to express their differing professional opinions (DPOs) concerning regulatory actions or policy decisions with substantial public health implications in instances when the normal procedures for resolving internal disputes are not sufficient. The DPO procedure provides short timeframes for hearing a differing professional opinion so that it can be resolved expeditiously, review of the DPO by qualified staff not directly involved in the decisions, and evaluation of the pilot after 1 year to determine whether it adds value to the regulatory decision-making process.

tor level. No CDER employees have used the program as of early 2006, however.

The inclination of senior management at CDER to intervene at earlier stages when disputes occur in CDER may be a function of management style and the existence of processes that make them aware of developing issues, as well as competing demands on their time. Senior managers are responsible to constituencies both in CDER and outside CDER, such as the Office of the Commissioner and Congress.

Key Review Meetings

Reviewers, consultants, and supervisors interact throughout the review process, but the midcycle review at the end of the 5th month for standard or the 2nd month for priority drugs is a prescribed time to make a more formal assessment of findings and to raise questions about the application.

Later, the results of the various review activities are integrated during an internal "wrap-up" meeting that begins the "action phase" of the NDA. The meeting is intended to occur by the end of month 8 for standard or month 5 for priority drugs, by which time the team should have a comprehensive understanding of the safety, efficacy, and quality of the drug under review (CDER et al., 1998, 2005). An FDA guidance document states that a preliminary decision is made on the regulatory action at the meeting (CDER et al., 2005). Critical elements—such as risk management, major labeling issues, and postmarket commitments—are considered. If PDUFA deadlines are to be met, actions must be developed expeditiously and, as noted below, plans can sometimes be developed hurriedly.

The preapproval safety conference, held near the time of approval, is a key meeting in the safety review process. It is a time for the team to review the NDA safety base comprehensively and explore safety issues that could warrant careful monitoring after approval. Discussions may lead the regulators to ask the sponsor to conduct additional safety studies either before or after approval. ODS/OSE staff are typically involved in this meeting.

Risk Minimization Plans

Some approval plans for NDAs include risk minimization action plans (RiskMAPs), strategic plans developed by the sponsor to minimize known risks posed by a product while preserving its benefits (DHHS et al., 2005). They go beyond the requirements for all sponsors to minimize risks through such efforts as accurate labeling and adverse event reporting. RiskMAPs apply primarily to products that "may pose a clinically important and unusual type or level of risk" (DHHS et al., 2005). PDUFA (III) requires ODS/OSE to be involved in reviewing RiskMAPs.

As part of PDUFA (III), OND and ODS/OSE (and FDA's Center for Biologics) developed guidance documents for industry on how to develop RiskMAPS to assess, manage, and monitor known risks posed by a product (both before and after approval). In its guidance (FDA, 2005b), FDA notes that risk management (defined as risk assessment and minimization) is an iterative process and sets out four steps: (1) assessing a product's benefit/risk balance, (2) developing and implementing tools to minimize the risks associated with it while preserving its benefits, (3) evaluating the effectiveness of the tools and reassessing the benefit-risk balance, and (4) making appropriate adjustments to the risk minimization tools to improve the benefit-risk balance further. FDA calls for those four steps to be ongoing throughout a product's lifecycle, with the results of risk assessment informing the sponsor's decisions regarding risk minimization (FDA, 2005b).

RiskMAPS are relatively new and still a work in progress. CDER staff have challenging scientific, policy, and resource issues to work out, both in general and for specific drugs or classes of drugs.

Postapproval Requirements and Labeling

The final days of NDA review typically involve negotiations between the sponsor and the regulators about the drug label and postmarket requirements. It is the sponsor's responsibility to develop a study protocol when it is agreed that a postmarket study will be undertaken and to draft label language; it is CDER's job to provide input and review and to comment on the sponsor's plans or suggested product labels.

CDER usually seeks commitments from sponsors to undertake postmarket (phase 4) trials or other studies to define risks further in some populations or under some conditions of use. Despite their importance, discussion of such studies is often delayed until late in the review process, when little time is available to consider the specifics of the protocol. With FDA facing a PDUFA deadline and with approval at stake for the sponsor, agreement is sometimes reached on studies that later prove to be infeasible or unjustified for a variety of reasons. It may be because ethical concerns preclude obtaining IRB approval or because of inability to recruit study subjects. Study designs may also be superseded by new treatments or findings that would undermine the value of a trial.

FDA may ask sponsors to take other actions, such as establishing a registry of patients who are taking the drug. An example is pregnancy registries, which are surveillance studies in which women who take a particular medication or have a particular condition during pregnancy answer questions before and after childbirth. There are eight registries for specific medical conditions (while taking a certain class of drugs to treat that condition), such as asthma and epilepsy (as of July 2004) and 14 for specific medicines (as of July 2003) (Kennedy et al., 2004; FDA and Office of Women's Health, 2006).

Negotiations about the wording of a drug label also come late in the process, when all the information about the drug has been pulled together. The label specifies conditions of safe use of the drug (CDER et al., 1998). It is the official description of a drug product and includes the drug's indication; who should take it; adverse effects; special instructions for use of the drug in pregnant women, children, and other populations; and safety information for the patient. Although FDA can refuse to approve a drug if the sponsor fails to agree to what the regulators want in the label, the final label is typically a result of negotiations between regulators and sponsor.

In the case of serious safety concerns, FDA may direct the sponsor to highlight a safety warning in the label by putting a black box around it. These may be added to marketed drugs when new data become available. A recent example are antidepressant medications, which now require a black box warning describing the risk and emphasizing the need for close monitoring of suicidality of patients (FDA News, 2004).

Although the product labeling is intended to guide prescribers in use of a drug, studies show that prescribers often fail to follow the label (Public Health Newswire, 2006). For example, cisapride was contraindicated in patients at increased risk for cardiac arrhythmias, but 20 percent of its use was in such patients (Ray and Stein, 2006). The label for troglitazone specified that liver-function tests were required, but often they were not performed (Ray and Stein, 2006).

Some approved drugs (such as cisapride) have a narrow therapeutic index; that is, the toxic dose is close to the effective dose so that there is a small margin of error for triggering safety problems. Such drugs make it incumbent on the sponsor and FDA to develop careful risk management strategies and incumbent on practitioners to be cognizant of proper use. The Institute of Medicine report *Preventing Medication Errors* discusses matters related to patient comprehension of and adherence to medication labeling (IOM, 2007). In an effort to improve awareness of labeling directions, FDA in January 2006 announced a revision of the label format (FDA News, 2006a) (see Appendix A for more detail).

FDA requires sponsors to provide patient medication guides (known as MedGuides) for drugs with "special risk management information" (FDA and CDER, 2006a). There are 42 medications marketed by brand name and 38 by active ingredient that have MedGuides that must accompany them when they are dispensed (Wolfe and Public Citizen's Health Research Group, 2005; CDER, 2006) (see Chapter 6 for additional discussion).

FDA has imposed restrictions on the distribution of some new drugs (such as drugs containing isotretinoin) which are discussed in Chapter 4. But there appears to be a lack of clarity about the scope of FDA's authority under the Food, Drug, and Cosmetic (FD&C) Act to restrict distribution. General counsels to FDA have apparently differed in their interpretation of the FD&C Act in that regard over the last decade. The statute governing medical-device regulation, which was enacted more recently than the FD&C Act, is more explicit about FDA's authority to restrict product distribution to protect the public health.

Site Inspections

Before an NDA can be approved, FDA usually inspects the facilities and manufacturing processes that will be involved in producing the product (FDA, 2006c). That process usually occurs toward the end of the NDA process and it is likely that the records of at least some of the clinical trial investigators will be inspected (Huddleston, 1999). Often sponsors continue to refine their manufacturing processes after the product is approved; those changes must approved by FDA. In FY 2004, 1,610 chemical and manufacturing control supplements were submitted.

Letter Sent to Sponsor

FDA may send the sponsor a "not approvable" letter that explains why an application cannot be approved on the basis of current information, an "approvable" letter stating that the product could be approved if specified additional actions were taken, or an "approval" letter indicating that the product has been approved with specified labeling and postmarket requirements (21 CFR 314.100a [2001]). The review team participates in the drafting of the letter, and it is signed by the division director or office director, depending on the product. (See Box 2-4 for a list of NDA review elements.)

POSTMARKET PERIOD

Historically, drugs undergoing premarket review have received more attention in and outside FDA than drugs that are in the marketplace. There is now growing awareness that a robust drug safety system requires a life-cycle approach (Crawford, 2005) and that drug approval triggers a critical period for monitoring safety. The budget for postmarketing surveillance and assessment is not commensurate with FDA's growing scope.

DDRE in ODS/OSE monitors marketed drugs and prepares safety reviews and risk assessments. Although ODS/OSE staff may contribute to the development of risk management plans, it is OND that has responsibility for deciding what regulatory action to take in response to new safety information. ODS/OSE has undergone enormous change in the last decade, with

BOX 2-4
Current Review Elements for New Drug Approval

- Periodic team progress check-ins
- Midcycle review meeting
- Team or subgroup interaction on particular issues
- Primary review completion
- Secondary (team leader or branch chief) review
- Review division director, or higher level, review
- Consult review input
- Advisory committee meetings
- Internal briefings for signatory authority
- Wrap-up (integration of review, consult, and inspection input)
- Preapproval safety conference (CDER)
- Preapproval facility inspections (BLAs)
- Labeling negotiation
- Issuance of action letter by PDUFA goal date

numerous leaders and acting leaders, name changes, and reorganizations (GAO, 2006). In recent years, it has also assumed expanded responsibilities, and its pharmacists and safety officers are monitoring more products and conducting more assessments, relying on the array of data sources and technologies described below (FDA and CDER, 2005) (see Chapters 3 and 4 for additional discussion of ODS/OSE and OND functions and relationship).

Drug Promotion and Information

The Division of Drug Marketing and Communication (DDMAC) in ODS/OSE is charged with reviewing sponsor promotional materials. The DDMAC staff of 35 reviews more than 53,000 promotional pieces every year, including print and broadcast direct-to-consumer (DTC) advertising (see Chapter 5 for detailed discussion) and materials prepared for professional conferences and for health care providers. FDA does not have the authority to review or sanction promotional material before launch or release (or to review instructions given by sponsors to their sales force) unless they are voluntarily submitted by the sponsor; it often reviews material after it has been released or broadcast, and it can then require corrective action in letters sent to the sponsor. However, many sponsors submit their promotional material in advance to ensure that they will not encounter regulatory problems later.

Since 1997, when FDA eased rules for DTC advertising, companies have greatly expanded their use of it to promote drugs via the mass media (Gahart et al., 2003; Gilhooley, 2005). According to a 2004 study (Brownfield et al., 2004), the average television viewer spends 100 minutes watching DTC advertising for every minute in a doctor's office. Typically, less is known about the safety of a new drug than of an older drug on the market, but the public is not likely to be aware of this and may simply assume that a new drug is a better drug.

Spontaneous Adverse Event Reporting System

The FDA's primary source for managing and monitoring new adverse effects of marketed drugs is the Adverse Event Reporting System (AERS), an automated system for storing and analyzing safety reports. ODS/OSE has primary responsibility for AERS (FDA, 2004c).

Adverse event reports have several sources. When an adverse event is both serious[11] and unexpected (not listed in the drug product's current labeling), drug sponsors are required to report it to FDA within 15 calendar days ("15-day reports"). Sponsors must also submit periodic reports that summarize all adverse events quarterly for the first 3 years after the NDA was approved and annually over multiple years (FDA, 2005a).

Another source of spontaneous reports is FDA's voluntary reporting system, MedWatch, which covers drugs and other FDA-regulated products. MedWatch enables health care professionals and consumers to file adverse event reports directly to FDA via telephone, completion of FDA Form 3500 online, or via fax or mail (FDA, 2003).

FDA receives more than 400,000 spontaneous reports each year as part of the surveillance system. In FY 2004, for example, ODS/OSE received 422,889 adverse event reports (see Box 2-5 for a breakdown) (FDA and CDER, 2005). Although exact figures are not available, that is assumed to represent a small fraction of all adverse effects of drugs. The system contains 3–4 million reports accumulated from multiple years (FDA and CDER, 2005).

Most adverse event reports arrive on paper via fax. ODS/OSE has placed a high priority on increasing the number of reports filed electronically to both expedite and reduce the cost of receiving and processing the report. In FY 2004, 16 percent of all reports were submitted electronically, up from 10 percent in FY 2003 (FDA and CDER, 2005). In the European

---

[11]A serious adverse event is any untoward medical occurrence that at any dose: results in death, is life threatening, requires inpatient hospitalization or prolongs existing hospitalization, results in persistent or significant disability/incapacity, is a congenital anomaly/birth defect (CFR 312.32).

BOX 2-5
Adverse Event Reporting in 2004

In 2004, FDA received 422,889 reports of suspected drug-related adverse events:

- 21,493 MedWatch reports directly from individuals (patients or providers).
- 162,107 manufacturer 15-day (expedited) reports.
- 89,960 serious manufacturer periodic reports.
- 149,329 nonserious manufacturer periodic reports.

SOURCE: FDA and CDER (2005).

Union, where electronic reporting to the European Medicines Agency has been mandatory since November 2005, over 90 percent of adverse reactions involving European-authorized medicines have been electronically reported by manufacturers.

ODS/OSE safety officers are expected to review the "15-day reports" when they arrive. They continually review incoming reports from Med-Watch, redirecting those related to other regulated products, and contractors enter all the MedWatch reports into AERS. Some adverse events (AEs) from companies, such as those in periodic reports for drugs that have been approved for more than 3 years or those considered non-serious, are not are routinely entered into AERS.

The structure of the AERS database complies with a guidance issued by the International Conference on Harmonisation (ICH E2B). FDA codes AEs with a standardized international terminology, the Medical Dictionary for Regulatory Activities (MedDRA). AERS allows for the on-screen review of reports, the use of searching tools, and various output reports. FDA is making limited use of data mining software to identify early drug safety signals in the AERS database via automated searching.

AERS is an important component of the postmarket surveillance system, particularly for identifying unexpected and rare adverse events (Rodriguez et al., 2001). For example, aplastic anemia and the rare skin disorder Stevens-Johnson syndrome have been linked to drugs through AE reporting (FDA, 1994). However, AERS is not efficient in distinguishing between signal and noise from adverse events, such as heart disease, which has a high background rate in the population (see Chapter 4 for a more comprehensive discussion). Some of the limitations of AERS data are the lack of denominator data on number of users to delineate the frequency of an event, lack of control groups, recall bias of patients and reporters, poor case documentation in the reports (critical details that could contribute to an understanding of an event are missing), and substantial underreporting of AEs (Ahmad et al., 2005).

Other Postmarket Data

Although AERS data may provide the initial signal of a safety problem, other studies and databases are typically needed to investigate associations. Those data include results of clinical trials and epidemiologic studies that are conducted, or whose results are available, after a drug is approved.

The sponsors' phase 4 trials are intended to expand the understanding of the safety and efficacy profile, of selected drugs. However, many of these studies are not completed (or even begun), for various reasons described above. FDA lacks the regulatory tools to adequately compel sponsors to complete appropriate studies (see Chapter 5 for more information). According to a March 2006 report, out of 1,231 agreed-on (by the sponsor) open postmarket commitments of drugs and biologics, 797 (65 percent) have yet to be started[12] (FDA, 2006d).

Another source of postmarket safety data is studies of marketed drugs designed to investigate new or expanded indications. Sponsors may include these studies in an efficacy supplement submitted to FDA seeking expanded label indications. Sometimes these studies may yield important data. For example, the APPROVe (Adenomatous Polyp Prevention on Vioxx) trial was designed to identify a new application for rofecoxib and showed an increased risk of serious cardiovascular events with rofecoxib compared with placebo—this cardiovascular impact was a secondary consideration (FDA, 2004b). Post-marketing safety information may also be generated by sponsors through the establishment of active surveillance systems, such as pregnancy-exposure registries (Ackermann Shiff et al., 2006).

The National Institutes of Health (NIH) or other agencies may also sponsor trials to gain new information about marketed drugs. Examples are the NIH-funded randomized controlled primary prevention trial, the Women's Health Initiative, which reported on adverse health effects of and benefits from use of combined estrogen and progestin (Rossouw et al., 2002). An earlier NIH-funded study, the cardiac arrhythmia suppression trial, found that drug treatment for asymptomatic ventricular arrhythmia in patients who had a heart attack did not prevent—and in fact substantially increased the risk of—sudden cardiac death. FDA had used a drug's effect on

---

[12]231 (19%) are ongoing; 28 (2%) are delayed; 3 (1%) have been terminated; 172 (14%) have been submitted.

arrhythmia as a surrogate marker of efficacy, but although the drug reduced arrhythmia, it also increased cardiac death (NHLBI, 2005).

Additional information on the safety of marketed drugs may come from large, automated databases. FDA purchases access to some of those databases as a resource for pharmacoepidemiologic studies designed to test hypotheses, particularly those arising from AERS. (Chapter 4 contains a more detailed discussion of relevant programs and agreements with academic research institutions.) FDA also obtains information from IMS Health, a provider of market research services to the pharmaceutical and health care industries. Among the services obtained from IMS Health are the National Disease and Therapeutic Index, which provides data on diagnoses, patients, and treatment patterns; Integrated Promotional Services, which measures professional and consumer promotional activity in the pharmaceutical industry; and the National Prescription Audit, which tracks pharmaceutical products dispensed in retail, mail-order, and long-term care channels.

Trained staff and (often expensive) supportive technology are typically needed to use some of those databases fully. CDER's limited resources for such activities have precluded taking full advantage of their potential contribution to understanding the safety of approved drugs (see further discussion in Chapter 4).

Resources also severely constrain their external research program. DDRE has about 18 epidemiologists. They work with the safety officers (who are also referred to as safety evaluators and generally are pharmacists) on assessments, determining for example the background risk of a condition to determine whether reported rates may be above expected levels. They also oversee agency-sponsored epidemiologic research.

Identifying and Evaluating Spontaneous Safety Signals

As CDER receives new information related to a drug's safety profile, it makes risk assessments and determines how risks can best be managed. For monitoring purposes, every marketed drug is assigned to a safety evaluator, usually a pharmacist in DDRE. Generally, one safety evaluator oversees all drugs in a class, such as statins, so he or she tends to work consistently with a specific OND division that handles those drugs. AE reports on a drug are automatically forwarded by e-mail to the appropriate safety evaluator and to the OND reviewer with responsibility for that drug.

ODS/OSE employs about 25 safety evaluators, and each receives about 500–800 reports a month to monitor, including some that are designated as "serious" on the basis of criteria established by FDA. The committee was told that safety evaluators now have less time than before to keep up with their inboxes as they are spending more time on OND consultations, in developing complex postmarket risk assessments, and in such activities as

RiskMAP development and assessments required by the Best Pharmaceuticals for Children Act (FDA and CDER, 2005).

Safety officers begin the process of building on initial reports either when requested by an OND reviewer to pursue a signal or on the basis of their own review of reports. Initial safety signal information is generally incomplete or uncertain; for example, a case report has few details, a patient is taking several drugs at once and a reaction could be related to the combination or to one of the drugs alone, could be related to the disease rather than to any of the drugs, or the effect may be so common in the population that it is difficult to determine whether it is associated with drug use. Only through additional investigations—including data mining searching with MedDRA codes, review of premarket studies, and analysis of available data from sources described above—might a picture begin to emerge. Increasingly, ODS/OSE is undertaking assessments not just regarding the drug that may have generated reports but regarding the class of drugs that it belongs to.

Rare is the story that builds as clearly and completely as one would like for making scientific evaluations and regulatory decisions. Adequate information to quantify risk or to compare the safety of a drug with the safety of alternative therapies in its class may not be readily available. Not uncommonly, uncertainties and professional disagreements about the significance of signals persist.

OND and ODS/OSE are expected to work together to assess risk and determine how to manage it, but OND has authority to make regulatory decisions related to the findings. A recent Government Accountability Office report noted problems in the relationship between ODS/OSE and OND staff, including lack of clarity about roles and responsibilities and communication barriers (GAO, 2006). As noted earlier, FDA's official response to those findings cited its commitment to making ODS/OSE and OND "co-equal partners in the post-market identification and timely resolution of drug safety issues" (GAO, 2006) (see discussion in Chapter 3).

Another challenge facing FDA is to decide when to alert the public and providers of AE reports that are under investigation. On one hand, reporting at the earliest stages could confuse and perhaps unduly alarm patients and providers and lead patients to inappropriately avoid or stop using a drug that they need. On the other hand, waiting too long to alert providers and users about potentially serious problems with a marketed drug can put patients at risk. FDA has been criticized for waiting too long and has proposed a Drug Watch Web site that would give the public and providers information about potential problems with marketed drugs earlier than in the past. The proposed Drug Watch program has been subject to criticism from the pharmaceutical industry. One reason given by industry against the program is that it is not useful to look at one study in isolation, as would be the case in Med Watch; they would prefer that similar studies be published together giving physicians and patients the opportunity to see the data in context (Agres, 2006). This has prompted FDA to rethink the program, so launch of that program has been delayed (FDA, 2005c,e).

To help to resolve uncertainties, discuss issues publicly, or consider regulatory strategies to address a risk, an advisory committee meeting may be held. Members of the Drug Safety and Risk Management Advisory Committee and the committee with expertise in the specific class of drugs are typically involved.

Regulatory Actions

FDA's regulatory authority is grounded in the FD&C Act and its amendments (21 USC 301). The historical origins of the act lie in the many 19th- and 20th-century incidents of widespread injury caused by ingestion of items that were either tainted versions of otherwise safe substances or unsafe substances marketed as something else entirely.

Fundamentally FDA's authority is limited to prohibiting the marketing of a drug that is adulterated or misbranded. With the middle-20th-century amendments came an expansion of the notion of misbranding, in which any failure to prove efficacy and safety before marketing would result in a finding of misbranding, because the marketing of the product would be a form of deception. Similarly, failure to adhere to agreed-on labeling or advertising requirements was viewed as a form of misbranding. The result is that FDA's remedies for the marketing of dangerous or mislabeled drugs is limited largely to withdrawing them from the market. The threat of such an action (although for critical or popular therapies such a threat may not be credible) and the agency's ability to use the mass media to call attention to the controversy give the agency some teeth in getting sponsors to comply with regulatory actions. Actions may include mandatory postmarketing surveillance, limitations on distribution, special education programs, or labeling changes, including use of a black box warning to call attention to serious risks. FDA also uses "Dear Health Practitioner" letters to inform providers of new information related to the safe and effective use of a marketed drug.

Such actions have been taken numerous times although enforcement activities have varied over the years. Decisions about use of enforcement tools, especially such aggressive ones as seizing products deemed to be misbranded, are not CDER's alone. The general counsel and the commissioner, both political appointees, are key to those decisions. FDA has come under criticism from some external stakeholders for not acting quickly enough or appropriately in the face of serious safety questions in specific cases (Wolfe, 2004; Curran, 2005). Some surveys also indicate concerns among CDER staff respondents about how safety issues are handled (DHHS/OIG, 2003) although senior management has strongly defended controversial actions (IOM Staff Notes, 2005–2006). FDA does not routinely conduct "postmortems" of drug withdrawals as a basis for examining and possibly improving its procedures. Drugs withdrawn from the market have been reinstated by FDA for use with restrictions at the request of the sponsor (see Box 2-6 for summary of this case).

One important issue for FDA and all other stakeholders in drug safety is the limited effectiveness of these regulatory warning tools in promoting drug safety. Although changes in the information provided in a label is a key tool for responding to and communicating new safety information, studies show that many patients are at risk because providers and the patients do not consistently heed labels, including the most serious black box warnings (Lasser et al., 2006).

It is worth underscoring that the fundamental design of the drug approval system described above—separate from the quality of the data that sponsors generate in compliance with it—inevitably puts drugs on the market when safety information is incomplete. The obvious corollary is that the postmarket monitoring system, as well as the premarket review processes, must be as effective and efficient as possible.

BOX 2-6
The Story of Alosetron (Lotronex)

November 1999—FDA advisory committee recommends approval
February 2000—FDA approves Alosetron for treatment of "diarrhea-predominant irritable bowel syndrome" in women
June 2000—FDA advisory committee meeting discusses evidence of serious adverse events and votes to retain the drug on the market
November 2000—FDA and the sponsor meet, sponsor withdraws Alosetron
December 2001—sponsor proposes returning Alosetron to market with restrictions
April 2002—FDA advisory committee recommends return to market with restrictions
June 2002—FDA approves Alosetron's return to market, with less rigorous restrictions than those recommended by the advisory committee

SOURCE: Moynihan (2002).

REFERENCES

Ackermann Shiff S, Mundkur C, Shamp J. 2006. *iPLEDGE: Isotretinoin Pregnancy Risk Management Program. Presented to DSaRM.* [Online]. Available: http://www.fda.gov/ohrms/dockets/ac/06/slides/2006-4202S2_05-Sponsor.ppt# [accessed February 10, 2006].

Adams CP, Brantner VV. 2006. Estimating the cost of new drug development: is it really $802 million? *Health Aff* 25(2):420-428.

Agres T. 2006. *Drug Safety Reshaping FDA Monolith.* [Online]. Available: http://www.ddd-mag.com/ShowPR.aspx?PUBCODE=016&ACCT=1600000100&ISSUE=0504&RELTYPE=PR&ORIGRELTYPE=PNP&PRODCODE=00000000&PRODLETT=AF [accessed September 15, 2006].

Ahmad SR, Goetsch RA, Marks NS. 2005. Chapter 9: spontaneous reporting in the United States. In: Strom BS, Ed. *Pharmacoepidemiology.* Fourth ed. West Sussex, England: John Wiley & Sons. Pp. 135-159.

Appel JL. 2002. The verdict from ALLHAT-thiazide diuretics are the preferred initial therapy for hypertension. *JAMA* 288(23):3030-3042.

Beck JM, Azari ED. 1998. FDA, off-label use, and informed consent: debunking myths and misconceptions. *Food Drug Law J* 53(1):71-104.

Bilstad J (HHS, FDA, CDER, Office of Drug Evaluation II). 1997. Letter to Knoll Pharmaceutical Company. Rockville, MD.

Boodman SG. 2006. *Many Drug Uses Don't Rest on Strong Science.* [Online]. Available: http://www.washingtonpost.com/wp-dyn/content/article/2006/05/22/AR2006052201428.html?referrer=emailarticle [accessed July 3, 2006].

Brownfield ED, Bernhardt JM, Pham JL, Williams MV, Parker RM. 2004. Direct-to-consumer drug advertisements on network television: an exploration of quantity, frequency, and placement. *J Health Commun* 9(6):561-562.

CDC (Centers for Disease Control and Prevention). 1999. Ten great public health achievements—United States 1900–1999. *MMWR* 48(12):241-243.

CDER (Center for Drug Evaluation and Research). 2004. *Clinical Review Template, MAPP 6010.3.* [Online]. Available: http://www.fda.gov/cder/mapp/6010.3.pdf [accessed May 19, 2006].

CDER. 2005a. *Drug Safety and Risk Management Advisory Committee (DSaRM).* [Online]. Available: http://www.fda.gov/OHRMS/DOCKETS/AC/05/agenda/2005-4143A1_Final.htm [accessed May 19, 2005].

CDER. 2005b. *Review Management: Risk Management Plan Activities in OND and ODS, MAPP 6700.1.* [Online]. Available: http://www.fda.gov/cder/mapp/6700.1.pdf [accessed November 14, 2005].

CDER. 2005c. *Drug Safety Oversight Board (DSB), MAPP 4151-3.* [Online]. Available: http://www.fda.gov/cder/mapp/4151-3.pdf [accessed June 20, 2005].

CDER. 2006. *Medication Guides.* [Online]. Available: www.fda.gov/cder/offices/ods/medication_guides.htm [accessed July 6, 2006].

CDER, FDA, DHHS. 1998. *The CDER Handbook.* [Online]. Available: http://www.fda.gov/cder/handbook/handbook.pdf [accessed November 14, 2005].

CDER, FDA, DHHS. 2005. *Reviewer Guidance: Conducting a Clinical Safety Review of a New Product Application and Preparing a Report on the Review.* [Online]. Available: http://www.fda.gov/cder/guidance/3580fnl.pdf [accessed December 30, 2005].

Crawford LM, Acting Commissioner of the FDA. 2005. *Speech Before FDA All-Hands Briefing with New HHS Secretary Mike Leavitt.* [Online]. Available: http://www.fda.gov/oc/speeches/2005/safedrugs0215.html [accessed February 23, 2005].

Curran J. 2005. *Merck Fought Vioxx Warning.* [Online]. Available: http://www.philly.com/mld/philly/business/12707648.htm [accessed October 10, 2005].

DHHS (Department of Health and Human Services). 2002. *Securing the Benefits of Medical Innovation for Seniors: The Role of Prescription Drugs and Drug Coverage.* [Online]. Available: http://aspe.hhs.gov/health/reports/medicalinnovation/innovation.pdf [accessed October 10, 2005].

DHHS, FDA (Food and Drug Administration). 2006. *Critical Path Opportunities Report.* [Online]. Available: http://www.fda.gov/oc/initiatives/criticalpath/reports/opp_report.pdf [accessed June 2, 2006].

DHHS, FDA, CDER, CBER (Center for Biologics Research). 2005. *Development and Use of Risk Minimization Action Plans.* [Online]. Available: http://www.fda.gov/cder/guidance/6358fnl.htm [accessed April 14, 2006].

DHHS, OIG (Office of Inspector General). 2003. *FDA's Review Process for New Drug Applications: A Management Review. OEI-01-01-00590.* Washington, DC: OIG.

DiMasi JA, Hansen RW, Grabowski HG. 2003. The price of innovation: new estimates of drug development costs. *J Health Econ* 22(2):151-185.

Epstein RA. 2004. *Issue Brief: Does America Have a Prescription Drug Problem? The Perils of Ignoring the Economics of Pharmaceuticals.* [Online]. Available: http://www.ipi.org/ipi/IPIPublications.nsf/PublicationLookupFullTextPDF/E6214F2C0ADBC86C86256F260069D1E2/$File/EpsteinDrugProblem.pdf [accessed July 27, 2006].

FDA (Food and Drug Administration). 1994. *Clinical Therapeutics and the Recognition of Drug-Induced Disease.* [Online]. Available: http://www.fda.gov/medwaTCH/articles/dig/recognit.htm [accessed July 12, 2006].

FDA. 2002. *Enclosure: PDUFA Reauthorization Performance Goals and Procedures.* [Online]. Available: http://www.fda.gov/oc/pdufaIIIGoals.html [accessed June 21, 2006].

FDA. 2003. *MedWatch Reporting by Consumers.* [Online]. Available: http://www.fda.gov/medwatch/report/consumer/consumer.htm [accessed May 24, 2005].

FDA. 2004a. *Innovation Stagnation: Challenge and Opportunity on the Critical Path to New Medical Products.* [Online]. Available: http://www.fda.gov/oc/initiatives/criticalpath/whitepaper.pdf [accessed October 10, 2005].

FDA. 2004b. *FDA Statement on Vioxx and Recent Allegations and the Agency's Continued Commitment to Sound Science and Peer Review.* [Online]. Available: http://www.fda.gov/bbs/topics/news/2004/NEW01136.html [accessed May 12, 2005].

FDA. 2004c. *Adverse Event Reporting System (AERS).* [Online]. Available: http://www.fda.gov/cder/aers/default.htm [accessed May 24, 2005].

FDA. 2005a. *Chapter 53—Postmarketing Surveillance and Epidemiology: Human Drugs.* [Online]. Available: http://www.fda.gov/cder/aers/chapter53.htm [accessed July 12, 2006].

FDA. 2005b. *Guidance for Industry: Development and Use of Risk Minimization Action Plans.* March 2005. Rockville, MD: FDA.

FDA. 2005c. *Questions and Answers (Qs & As) Proposed Drug Watch Program.* [Online]. Available: http://www.fda.gov/cder/guidance/6657qs&asext5-2.pdf [accessed May 6, 2005].

FDA. 2005d. *White Paper, Prescription Drug User Fee Act (PDUFA): Adding Resources and Improving Performance in FDA Review of New Drug Applications.* [Online]. Available: http://www.fda.gov/oc/pdufa/PDUFAWhitePaper.pdf [accessed December 5, 2005].

FDA. 2005e. *FDA Fact Sheet: FDA Improvement in Drug Safety Monitoring.* [Online]. Available: http://www.fda.gov/oc/factsheets/drugsafety.html [accessed February 23, 2005].

FDA. 2005f. *Guidance for Review Staff and Industry Good Review Management Principles and Practices for PDUFA Products.* April 2005. Rockville, MD: FDA.

FDA. 2005g. *Enclosure: PDUFA Reauthorization Performance Goals and Procedures.* [Online]. Available: http://www.fda.gov/cder/news/pdufagoals.htm [accessed July 3, 2006].

FDA. 2006a. *FDA Advisory Committees.* [Online]. Available: http://www.fda.gov/oc/advisory/default.htm [accessed July 3, 2006].

FDA. 2006b. *From Test Tube to Patient: Advisory Committees: Critical to the FDA's Product Review Process, 4th Edition.* [Online]. Available: http://www.fda.gov/fdac/special/testtubetopatient/advisory.html [accessed June 29, 2006].

FDA. 2006c. *From Test Tube to Patient: The FDA's Drug Review Process: Ensuring Drugs Are Safe and Effective, 4th Edition.* [Online]. Available: http://www.fda.gov/fdac/special/testtubetopatient/drugreview.html [accessed June 29, 2006].

FDA. 2006d. Report on the performance of drug and biologics firms in conducting postmarketing commitment studies. *Federal Register* 71(42):10978-10979.

FDA, CDER. 2001a. *Frequently Asked Questions on Drug Development and Investigational New Drug Applications.* [Online]. Available: http://www.fda.gov/cder/about/smallbiz/faq.htm#IND [accessed June 29, 2006].

FDA, CDER. 2001b. *FDA's Drug Review and Approval Time.* [Online]. Available: http://www.fda.gov/cder/reports/reviewtimes/default.htm [accessed June 16, 2006].

FDA, CDER. 2005. *Office of Drug Safety Annual Report FY 2004.* [Online]. Available: http://www.fda.gov/cder/offices/ods/annrep2004/ [accessed June 23, 2005].

FDA, CDER. 2006a. *Drugs@FDA Instructions.* [Online]. Available: http://www.fda.gov/cder/drugsatfda/instructionsPrint.htm [accessed July 3, 2006].

FDA, CDER. 2006b. *Investigational New Drug (IND) Application Process.* [Online]. Available: http://www.fda.gov/cder/regulatory/applications/ind_page_1.htm#preIND [accessed June 29, 2006].

FDA, Office of Women's Health. 2006. *Information About Pregnancy Registries.* [Online]. Available: http://www.fda.gov/womens/registries/general.html [accessed July 3, 2006].

FDA News. 2004 (October 15). *FDA Launches a Multi-Pronged Strategy to Strengthen Safeguards for Children Treated with Antidepressant Medications.* [Online]. Available: http://www.fda.gov/bbs/topics/news/2004/NEW01124.html [accessed September 15, 2006].

FDA News. 2006a (Janaury 18). *FDA Announces New Prescription Drug Information Format to Improve Patient Safety.* [Online]. Available: http://www.fda.gov/bbs/topics/news/2005/NEW01272.html [accessed March 9, 2006].

FDA News. 2006b (February 9). *Report Demonstrates Benefits of Earlier Meetings with FDA to Make Drug Review Process More Efficient.* [Online]. Available: http://www.fda.gov/bbs/topics/news/2006/NEW01312.html [accessed June 15, 2006].

FDA News. 2006c (April 18). *FDA Names First Associate Center Director for Safety Policy and Communication in the Center for Drug Evaluation and Research FDA Centralizes Drug Safety Policy and Communication.* [Online]. Available: http://www.fda.gov/bbs/topics/NEWS/2006/NEW01359.html [accessed May 25, 2006].

Friedman MA, Woodcock J, Lumpkin MM, Shuren JE, Hass AE, Thompson LJ. 1999. The safety of newly approved medicines: do recent market removals mean there is a problem? *JAMA* 281(18):1728-1734.

Gahart MT, Duhamel LM, Dievler A, Price R. 2003. Examining the FDA's oversight of direct-to-consumer advertising. *Health Aff (Millwood)* Suppl Web Exclusives:W3-120-123.

GAO (Government Accountability Office). 1990. *FDA Drug Review: Postapproval Risks 1976–85.* GAO/PEMD-90-15. Washington, DC: GAO.

GAO. 2006. *Drug Safety: Improvement Needed in FDA's Postmarket Decision-Making and Oversight Process.* GAO-06-402. Washington, DC: GAO.

Gilber J, Henske P, Singh A. 2003. Rebuilding big pharma's business model. *Bus Med Rep* 21(10):1-10.

Gilhooley M. 2005. Heal the damage: prescription drug consumer advertisements and relative choice. *J Health Law* 38(1):Winter.

Graham DJ. 2004. *Testimony of David J. Graham, M.D., M.P.H., November 18, 2004 Before the Committee on Finance.* [Online]. Available: http://www.senate.gov/~finance/hearings/testimony/2004test/111804dgtest.pdf [accessed October 10, 2005].

Grassley C, Baucus M, Graham D, Singh G, Psaty B, Kweder S, Gilmartin R. 2004. *FDA, Merck and Vioxx: Putting Patient Safety First?* Statements at the November 18, 2004 hearing before the United States Senate Committee on Finance, United States Senate.

Henderson D. 2006 (February). *Doc Room Stats for IOM.* Personal Communication: E-mail to Stratton K (IOM Staff).

Hensley S, Davies P, Martinez B. 2005. *Vioxx Verdict Stokes Backlash That Hit FDA, Manufacturers.* [Online]. Available: http://online.wsj.com/article/0,,SB112467370587619279-email,00.html [accessed October 10, 2005].

Huddleston, RD. 1999. *FDA Clinical Investigator Site Inspections: The Sponsor's Role.* [Online]. Available: http://www.findarticles.com/p/articles/mi_qa3899/is_199907/ai_n8868995/print [accessed August 1, 2006].

IOM (Institute of Medince). 2007. *Preventing Medication Errors.* Washington, DC: The National Academies Press.

Kaiser Family Foundation. 2005. *Prescription Drug Trends.* [Online]. Available: http://www.kff.org/insurance/upload/3057-04.pdf [accessed March 10, 2006].

Kaitin KI. 2005. Numbers of active investigators in FDA-regulated clinical trials drop. *Tufts Center for the Study of Drug Development Impact Report* 7(3).

Kennedy DL, Uhl K, Kweder SL. 2004. Pregnancy exposure registries. *Drug Saf* 27(4): 215-228.

Lasser KE, Seger DL, Yu DT, Karson AS, Fiskio JM, Seger AC, Shah NR, Gandhi TK, Rothschild JM, Bates, DW. 2006. Adherence to black box warnings for prescription medications in outpatients. *Arch Int Med* Feb(166):338-344.

Lipsky MS, Sharp LK. 2001. From idea to market: the drug approval process. *J Am Board Fam Pract* 14(5):362-367.

Lurie P, Woodcock J, Kaitin KI. 1999. FDA drug review: the debate over safety, efficacy, and speed. *Medical Crossfire* 1(3):52-60.

Meadows M. 2002. The FDA's drug review process: ensuring drugs are safe and effective. *FDA Consum* 36(4):19-24.

Meadows M. 2003. *Drug Research and Children.* [Online]. Available: http://www.fda.gov/fdac/features/2003/103_drugs.html [accessed July 12, 2006].

Meyer R. 2004. *Letter to Amgen Inc and Danagher P, March 8, 2004.* [Online]. Available: http://www.fda.gov/cder/foi/appletter/2004/21688ltr.pdf [accessed August 28, 2006].

Moynihan R. 2002. FDA fails to reduce accessibility of paracetamol despite 450 deaths a year. *BMJ* 325(7366):678.

NCHS (National Center for Health Statistics). 2004. *Health, United States, 2004: With Chartbook on Trends in the Health of Americans with Special Feature on Drugs.* Hyattsville, MD: NCHS.

Neergaard L. 2005. *FDA Looking into Blindness-Viagra Link.* [Online]. Available: http://abcnews.go.com/Health/wireStory?id=796471 [accessed May 27, 2005].

NHLBI (National Heart, Lung and Blood Institute). 2005. *Cardiac Arrhythmia Suppression Trial (CAST).* [Online]. Available: http://www.clinicaltrials.gov/ct/show/NCT00000526 [accessed July 12, 2006].

Okie S. 2005. Safety in numbers—monitoring risk in approved drugs. *N Engl J Med* 352(12): 1173-1176.

PhRMA (Pharmaceutical Research and Manufacturers of America). 2006. *Pharmaceutical Industry Profile.* Washington, DC.

Public Health Newswire. 2006. *Drugs' Black Box Warning Violations in Outpatient Settings Putting Patients at Risk.* [Online.] Available: http://www.medicalnewstoday.com/medicalnews.php?newsid=37735 [accessed July 13, 2006].

Racoosin JA. 2006 (January 17). *Pre-Marketing Assessment of Drug Safety.* PowerPoint presentation, presented at the Institute of Medicine Workshop on Advancing the Methods and Application of Risk-Benefit Assessment of Medicines, Washington, DC. Insitute of Medicine Committee on the Assessment of the US Drug Safety System.

Randall, B. 2001. *The US Drug Approval Process: A Primer.* [Online]. Available: http://www. thememoryhole.org/crs/more-reports/RL30989.pdf [accessed June 27, 2005].

Ray WA, Stein CM. 2006. Reform of drug regulation—beyond an independent drug-safety board. *N Engl J Med* 354(2):194-201.

Rodriguez EM, Staffa JA, Graham DJ. 2001. The role of databases in drug postmarketing surveillance. *Pharmacoepidemiol Drug Saf* 10(5):407-410.

Rossouw JE, Anderson GL, Prentice RL, LaCroix AZ, Kooperberg C, Stefanick ML, Jackson RD, Beresford SA, Howard BV, Johnson KC, Kotchen JM, Ockene J; Writing Group for the Women's Health Initiative Investigators. 2002. Risks and benefits of estrogen plus progestin in healthy postmenopausal women: principal results from the Women's Health Initiative randomized controlled trial. *JAMA* 288:321-333.

Smith C, Cowan C, Sensenig A, Catlin A, the Health Accounts Team. 2005. Health spending growth slows in 2003. *Health Aff* 24(1):185-194.

Weiss Smith S. 2006. *Summary of Issues: January 17, 2006 IOM Workshop.* Paper Commissioned by the IOM Committee on the Assessment of the US Drug Safety System. Washington, DC.

Wolfe S. 2004. *Take Drugs Off the Market.* [Online]. Available: http://www.usatoday.com/ news/opinion/editorials/2004-12-26-oppose_x.htm [accessed March 8, 2005].

Wolfe S, Public Citizen's Health Research Group. 2005. *Statement by Sidney M. Wolfe, M.D., Director, Public Citizen's Health Research Group*, at the Public Hearing on CDER's Current Risk Communication Strategies for Human Drugs, December 7, 2005. Washington, DC.

3

A Culture of Safety

The Committee on the Assessment of the US Drug Safety System has examined three determinants of organizational culture in the Food and Drug Administration (FDA) Center for Drug Evaluation and Research (CDER): the external environment, structural factors, and management. The committee believes that cultural changes are urgently needed to support a stronger, more systematic and more credible approach to drug safety in CDER, and it recommends solutions to problems created or exacerbated by elements of CDER's management, structure, and environment. However, implementing some of these recommendations may require additional resources, as discussed in greater detail in Chapter 7.

ORGANIZATIONAL CHALLENGES

A number of highly publicized events, including the Vioxx withdrawal and concern about other cox-2 inhibitors, and ongoing drug safety problems including those related to salmeterol, Ketek, and others have brought FDA's, and specifically CDER's, performance under the scrutiny of the American public (via the mass media) and Congress (Harris, 2006b; Hendrick, 2006; Washington Drug Letter, 2006). Critics have charged that there were failures or delays in informing patients about important drug risks, inadequate postmarketing assessment of drug safety, and failures to follow up and enforce sponsors' postmarketing study commitments agreed on at the time of approval. Others have expressed concern that the recent focus on safety could reverse considerable gains in the pace of drug review and the speed of approving new therapies.

Mass media coverage of perceived organizational problems in CDER has been frequent and detailed, for example, describing an apparent lack of mutual respect and tension between preapproval review staff and postmarketing safety staff, and a work environment thought to be marginalizing dissenting voices on drug safety (Mathews, November 10, 2004; Harris, February 20, 2005; Henderson, December 6, 2005). As questions about culpability mounted, a series of organizational and programmatic problems in the center highlighted in the mass media were also examined in government reports, including the reports of the DHHS Inspector General that surveyed CDER staff (DHHS/OIG, 2003) and reviewed the state of postmarketing commitments (DHHS/OIG, 2006), respectively, and the reports of the Government Accountability Office that assessed the impact of the Prescription Drug User Fee Act (PDUFA) on CDER staff's morale and workload (GAO, 2002) and examined the structure and effectiveness of CDER postmarketing decision-making processes (GAO, 2006). Many observe signs of an organizational culture in crisis. It has also become apparent that drug safety events, whether indicative of or associated with organizational and cultural problems, have led to diminished agency credibility among the public. Drug safety experts, members of Congress (including Senators Michael Enzi, Edward Kennedy, and Charles Grassley, and Representatives Rosa DeLauro and Maurice Hinchey), consumer organizations (such as Consumers Union, Public Interest Research Group, the National Consumers League, Public Citizen), and others have called for organizational, statutory, and resource changes in the agency. Proposals have included restructuring the agency to segregate the drug review and postmarketing safety functions by creating an independent drug safety center (Fontanarosa et al., 2004; Consumers Union, 2005; Grassley, 2005; Ray and Stein, 2006; Wolfe S, 2006). FDA itself has undertaken a series of initiatives and changes, described in detail in Appendix A, including the commissioning of this Institute of Medicine report (see discussion in Chapter 1) (Crawford, 2004; Wall Street Journal and Harris Interactive, 2006).

In its discussions with current and recent FDA staff and managers (see Box 3-1), and on the basis of its review of relevant government reports, the committee found that the organizational culture in CDER confirms some of the adverse perceptions conveyed in the mass media, and that the center is an organization in urgent need of great change.

The committee found that CDER's organizational culture has both strengths and weaknesses. The positives are that science-based decision making is a clear priority that shapes CDER's culture, as does the staff's obvious awareness of the potential consequences of their decisions on the health of the public and individual patients. The negative features of the culture include a work environment that is not sufficiently supportive of staff (as evident in problems with morale and attrition), polarization between

BOX 3-1
Committee Information Gathering About CDER
Organizational Culture

To inform its deliberations, the committee held information-gathering sessions to hear from FDA and other stakeholders (see Appendix D). A small group of committee members and Institute of Medicine (IOM) project staff visited CDER on October 11, 2005, and February 22, 2006. From November 7, 2005, to May 2006, IOM staff with rotating committee representation of one or two members also held confidential discussions with over 30 current FDA staff, including personnel from the Office of New Drugs (OND) and the Office of Drug Safety (recently renamed Office of Surveillance and Epidemiology and referred to hereafter as ODS/OSE), FDA and CDER management, and several former FDA staff and leaders.*

The committee's high regard for the professionals who perform CDER's preapproval and postapproval functions under considerable time and resource constraints was reinforced by these conversations. As the committee gained greater understanding of CDER's work and functioning, committee members were able to identify or confirm a number of structural and related cultural challenges, including a troubling relationship between OND and ODS/OSE, insufficient management and leadership to address emerging problems and implement needed reforms, a lack of clear and consistent processes (for example, for identifying and addressing drug safety concerns both in the review process and in the postmarketing period, for determining the need for and nature of postmarketing, or phase 4, studies), overextended human and financial resources, and pressures added by the requirements of the current user-fee funding mechanism that funds about 50% of CDER's work (FDA, 2005b).

The major themes that emerged from the committee's conversations are consistent with those identified in government reports on FDA and CDER. The committee also found it helpful to refer to assessments of organizational problems in other government agencies that deal with risk and uncertainty, albeit in very different contexts, such as the National Aeronautics and Space Administration and the Federal Aviation Administration (GAO, 1996; Return to Flight Task Group, 2005).

---

*At the committee's request, the CDER Director sent a letter to all center staff urging them to contact IOM study staff if they wished to discuss issues related to their work and recent concerns.

the premarketing and postmarketing review staff, and evidence suggesting insufficient management attention to scientific disagreement and differences of opinion.

Change is needed because CDER's organizational problems may affect its ability to accomplish the mission of protecting and advancing the public's health; they clearly affect public perception of the agency's performance and credibility. Every organization has its share of dysfunctions, disgruntled staff members, and internal disputes, but the committee came away from various encounters with CDER staff and management with a deep concern about CDER's organizational health.

The committee approached this component of its work with special care, recognizing that structure and culture, as fundamental features of an organization, connect in complex and not easily discernible ways. Management literature shows that an organization's ability to fulfill its mission is considerably influenced by the health of its culture, the "social architecture" that determines whether excellence is promoted; whether the organization is adaptable, robust, and learning; and whether broad staff participation (in shaping the vision, making decisions, and so on) is prized and encouraged (Coffee, 1993; Heifetz and Laurie, 1998; Khademian, 2002). The committee was explicitly charged with assessing the structure and function of CDER, but because organizational function is linked to organizational culture, the committee had to consider CDER's culture and how it has been shaped by important changes in the policy, economic, and social environment; by structural factors, and the related policies and procedures that contribute to organizational dynamics; and by management. In the pages that follow, the committee describes the evidence and outlines the steps to be taken to align CDER's culture better with its mission "to make certain that safe and effective drugs are available to the American people."[1]

The External Environment

Organizational culture is rooted in the external environment, and this is particularly true of government agencies, which experience the environment as "a set of constraints, expectations, and pressures" (Khademian, 2002: 136). Some environmental and organizational challenges are peculiar to government agencies (Claver et al., 1999; O'Leary, 2006; Ostroff, 2006). For example, their leaders are chosen for attributes that do not necessarily include a track record of organizational leadership, an ability to transform complex organizations, or an in-depth knowledge of the leadership issues routinely faced by an agency, and their time in office is usually brief. Government agency operations are less flexible than those of their private-

---

[1]Source: http://www.fda.gov/cder/learn/CDERLearn/.

sector counterparts because of a wide array of laws and regulations and the requirement that they be responsive to the often conflicting expectations of multiple constituencies (Ostroff, 2006).

For FDA, and specifically CDER, the environment is shaped by many factors. First, the evolution of FDA's regulatory role has been shaped by the expectations of American society, as expressed through its national legislature, in its courts, and in the influence of its patient and consumer advocacy movements. The American public desires timely access to effective and safe therapies. Legislative attention to the regulation of drugs (and other products in FDA's purview, has resulted in the statute that dictates FDA's role: the Food, Drug, and Cosmetic (FD&C) Act of 1938 and its many subsequent amendments. Another influence on FDA's work is the economic and political agenda of a powerful and influential industry, whose concerns include the potential of regulation to dampen innovation. The health care delivery system (organizations, payors, pharmacies, etc.) and health care professionals who act as intermediaries between patients and the drug development and distribution system are another factor in FDA's environment. Patients must secure a prescription from a qualified health care provider, and health care providers can only prescribe drugs that are approved by FDA. FDA actions, including findings from postmarketing surveillance, inform drug formulary and reimbursement decisions by payors. Although FDA does not regulate drug pricing, and cost-effectiveness is not a consideration, these are important issues to the health care delivery system, given financial constraints and the diverse therapeutic needs of its patients. A final crucial dimension of FDA's external environment is the potential influence exercised by the top levels of the executive branch (the White House, the Office of Management and Budget) and the legislative branch. Congress plays an oversight function and provides a forum for the push and pull of legislative factions concerned with consumer safety and those inclined toward spurring economic competitiveness. Congressional concern about the public's safety may be one contributing factor to what the industry and other critics have seen as the agency's historically risk-averse stance in carrying out its regulatory duties. In their view, the agency has generally been more likely to err on the side of greater caution in approving drugs than to err on the side of faster approval, perhaps in response to the fact that congressional investigations generally focus on errors of commission (approving an unsafe drug) rather than omission (not approving a potentially good drug) (Cohn, 2003; Steenburg, 2006).

The multiple and often conflicting pressures of the external environment add to the complex nature of the agency's work (science-based decision making) and the enormous medical, social, and economic impact of its regulatory decisions. FDA has a dual mission: to protect public health "by assuring the safety, efficacy, and security of human . . . drugs" and to advance public health "by helping to speed innovations that make medicines . . . more effective, safer, and more affordable." Balancing speed and safety is not always easy. Many drugs are both life-saving, motivating timely approval and release to the marketplace, and life-threatening, requiring careful monitoring of safety and rapid action to address safety risks as appropriate. The challenge in regulating prescription drugs is to weigh the available evidence of efficacy and safety in the context of the prevalence and severity of specific disorders, and the availability, safety and efficacy of other approved therapies. Although FDA and the industry share an interest in the discovery and development of beneficial products that improve health,[2] the decisions of regulators may affect the regulated industry's success in the marketplace (House of Commons Health Committee, 2005a,b).

Two dimensions of the external environment deserve more detailed discussion in the context of this report. These include the relationship between FDA and the industry, which has been complicated by PDUFA, and FDA's relationships to Congress and to the White House.

The FDA–Industry Interface

It has become increasingly clear that the credibility of FDA is intertwined with that of the industry it regulates. If FDA is viewed as less trustworthy to make decisions that serve the public good, that may diminish the value and meaning of FDA approval, casting a shadow of doubt on FDA-approved products' reliability, quality, and most importantly, their safety and effectiveness. The concerns over drug safety described above have affected not only FDA's image, but that of the industry. In fact, the industry's integrity and its commitment to finding effective therapies for patients in need has been questioned (PricewaterhouseCoopers, 2005). Industry's credibility has been considerably affected by judicial action in response to non-compliance and by lawsuits related to how companies handled information about their products and in particular, whether they were adequately forthcoming about what they knew and when (Hensley et al., 2005; Kaiser Family Foundation, 2005; Wall Street Journal and Harris Interactive, 2005).

The user-fee funding mechanism established in 1992 to supplement congressional appropriations helped to expand and strengthen preapproval functions and the capabilities of the responsible CDER offices. PDUFA was renewed and revised in 1997 and 2002 and will be considered for reauthorization in 2007. The user-fee program has increased considerably the resources available for drug review (see Chapter 7) and made the review process more predictable and expeditious (see Box 3-2 and Appendix C).

---

[2]The Critical Path initiative is an example of FDA's interest in supporting innovation in drug discovery; it maps the way forward for applying cutting-edge science to drug discovery.

However, it has had some drawbacks, including increasing the agency's dependence on industry funding for its drug review activities, severely skewing CDER's focus to facilitating review and approval perhaps at the expense of other center activities, and creating an environment of intense pressure on its reviewers (Zelenay, 2005). A Department of Health and Human Services (DHHS) Office of the Inspector General (OIG) survey of CDER staff found that 40 percent of "respondents who had been at FDA at least 5 years indicated that the review process had worsened during their tenure in terms of allowing for in-depth, science-based reviews. Respondents cited lack of time as the main reason" (DHHS and OIG, 2003).

In discussions with FDA staff, the committee learned that the emphasis on timely review that is at the core of PDUFA and is linked with specific performance goals has added to reviewer workloads despite the increase in review staff. FDA must report to Congress annually about its success in reaching the performance goals. Some observers have charged that increased speed of review has led to decreased safety, in part because the time demands of PDUFA limit the ability of reviewers to examine safety signals as thoroughly as they might like (Sasich, 2000; Wolfe SM, 2006). Performance goals with reporting requirements for actions relating to review speed, but not for other actions, such as postmarketing safety monitoring and risk communication, may lead to the assigning of higher priority to those actions that have associated performance goals.

There has been some debate about PDUFA's effect on drug safety as demonstrated by drug withdrawals. Abraham and Davis (2005) found that in the period before enactment of PDUFA the United States had 50 percent fewer drug withdrawals than the United Kingdom largely because of the longer periods that the FDA took to review drug applications. They suggested that US efforts to speed approval may be compromising drug safety in the PDUFA era. However, drug withdrawals are very rare occurrences in general, and the total number of withdrawals in the last two decades of the 20th century represents a modest figure that may not be useful for generalization. For example, in reviewing 20 drug withdrawals in 1980–2004 (nearly half of which occurred before PDUFA was enacted), the Tufts Center for the Study of Drug Development found that "no trend emerges between speed of approval and withdrawal" (Tufts Center for the Study of Drug Development, 2005). Drug withdrawals are just one indicator of drug safety; the timeliness of a withdrawal may be more important than the fact of the withdrawal. Furthermore, drug withdrawals say nothing about the safety of drugs that remain on the market and continue to affect public health. Olson (2002) makes the point that drug withdrawal data are of limited value in drawing inferences about drug safety more generally and instead focuses on adverse drug reactions among all new chemical entities approved between 1990 and 1995. The Government Accountability Of-

---

BOX 3-2
A Short History of the Prescription Drug User Fee Act (PDUFA)

1992
Use revenues from user fees to achieve certain "performance goals"
• Primary focus: decrease review times
PDUFA I Commitments:
• Complete review of priority original new drug and biologic applications and efficacy supplements (90% in 6 months)
• Complete review of standard original new drug and biologic applications and efficacy supplements (90% in 12 months)
• Complete review of priority supplements (90% in 6 months)
• Complete review of standard supplements (90% in 12 months)
• Complete review of supplements that do not require review of clinical data (manufacturing supplements) (90% in 6 months)
• Complete review of resubmitted new drug and biologic applications (90% in 6 months)

1997
PDUFA II was reauthorized for 5 years (FY 1998–2002) as part of Title I of the Food and Drug Administration Modernization Act
• Primary focus: decrease review times and shorten development times
New PDUFA II commitments:
• Complete review of resubmitted efficacy supplements (90% in 6 months)
• Respond to industry requests for meetings (90% within 14 days)
• Meet with industry within set times (90% within 30, 60, or 75 days depending on type of meeting)
• Provide industry with meeting minutes (90% within 30 days)
• Communicate results of review of complete industry responses to FDA clinical holds (90% within 30 days)
• Resolve major disputes appealed by industry (90% within 30 days)
• Complete review of special protocols (90% within 45 days)

---

fice (GAO) analysis looked at withdrawals over 4-year intervals between 1985 and 2000, and found that the rate of withdrawals fluctuated from 4.39 percent in 1985–1988, to 1.96 percent in 1989–1992, to 1.56 percent in 1993–1996, to 5.34 percent in 1997–2000 (GAO, 2002). There were 15 drug withdrawals between 1985 and 2000, and in its response to GAO, FDA asserted that the variation in the withdrawal rate was probably related to the small number of withdrawals in any given year (GAO, 2002). The Berndt et al. (2005) analysis found that the proportion of approvals ulti-

- Electronic application receipt and review (in place by the end of FY 2002)

Changes in commitments
- Complete review of standard original new drug and biologic applications and efficacy supplements (90% in 10 months instead of 12 months)
- Complete review of manufacturing supplements that do not require review of clinical data (90% in 4 months instead of 6 months if prior approval is needed, otherwise 6 months)
- Complete review of resubmitted new drug and biologic applications (90% of class 1 in 2 months, and 90% of class 2 in 6 months instead of all in 6 months)

2002
PDUFA III was reauthorized for 5 years (FY 2003–2007) as part of Public Health Security and Bioterrorism Preparedness and Response Act
- Focus: expand interaction and communication in IND phase and during first cycle review
- Includes some funding for postmarket safety for 2–3 years after drug approval for drugs approved after 2002

New PDUFA III commitments:
- Discipline review letters for presubmitted "reviewable units" of new drug and biologic applications (90% in 6 months)
- Report of substantive deficiencies (or lack thereof) (90% within 15 days of filling date)

Changes to commitments:
- Complete review of resubmitted efficacy supplements (90% of class 1 in 2 months and 90% of class 2 in 6 months instead of all in 6 months)
- Electronic application receipt and review (enhanced by end of FY 2007)

SOURCES: FDA (1995, 2002, 2005e, 2006a).

mately leading to safety withdrawals prior to PDUFA and during PDUFA I and II were not statistically significantly different.

The user-fee system has exacerbated concerns about the relationship between FDA and the regulated industry by creating the appearance of conflict of interest in the regulators—critics assert that PDUFA gives sponsors inappropriate leverage or influence over regulation because FDA is obliged to please sponsors, now its "clients," in return for fees for service (Grassley et al., 2004; Harris, 2004; Wolfe S, 2006). Regulatory capture is a term used by regulatory scholars (such as Stigler, 1971) to describe successful industry pressure on regulators, and some observers actually believe that PDUFA has facilitated the capture of FDA. The core problem in the relationship between industry and FDA (leading FDA to consider industry a client) may lie in the power of the industry to shape the scope and nature of PDUFA goals (Olson, 2002; Carpenter et al., 2003; DHHS and FDA, 2005; Okie, 2005). In the negotiations between FDA and the industry, Congress has given the industry a considerable role in influencing what activities the user fees will fund, thus limiting regulatory discretion and independence. In particular, fee revenues only could be used to support activities designed to increase the speed and efficiency of the initial review process. Fee revenues could not be used to support postmarketing safety surveillance from 1992 to 2002. In the 2002 PDUFA reauthorization, a small amount of fee revenues (about 5 percent) was permitted to be used for postmarketing drug safety activities; however, restrictions on when these funds could be spent (only for drugs approved after 2002, and for up to 2 years after approval, or up to 3 years for "potentially serious drugs") limited their effectiveness (Zelenay, 2005). In Chapter 7, the committee discusses this troubling feature of PDUFA and suggests an alternative.

Concerns about inappropriate influence on regulatory decision making are not new, although it can be argued that PDUFA has made the connection between CDER performance and industry expectations much more explicit. In 1977, a government panel examined whether there was pressure on reviewers of new drugs to make regulatory recommendations favorable to the industry (DHEW[3] Review Panel on New Drug Regulation, 1977; DHEW, 1977). The panel concluded that the problem was largely linked to poor management rather than verifiable industry influence.

> The second basic issue explored by the Panel was whether industry exerts undue influence on FDA decisions. Many current and former FDA employees and consultants had testified to Congressional committees that industry pressure caused FDA officials to approve drugs that did not meet agency safety and effectiveness standards and that those who attempted to oppose industry demands were harshly and improperly treated by senior FDA officials. From detailed investigations of these allegations by its staff, the Panel concluded that there was no widespread use of improper influence by industry representatives. It did identify several instances in which FDA supervisors unfairly disciplined dissenting employees, but these lapses were found to result from poor management rather than improper efforts of industry to control agency decision-making [Dorsen and Miller, 1979:910].

---

[3]Department of Health, Education, and Welfare, predecessor of the DHHS.

The concerns raised or exacerbated by PDUFA have an additional dimension. The interests of industry and the public are sometimes at odds, and some critics fear that PDUFA may have increased FDA's responsiveness to one set of interests at the expense of the other set of interests, in some circumstances. It is important to note that FDA's various constituencies have mixed expectations. The public, as reflected in the goals of multiple consumer and patient advocacy groups, has a simultaneous desire for speed and safety. Although the public wants to preserve the consumer protections afforded by drug regulation in America, it also may demand earlier patient access to potentially life-saving therapies, as was so effectively exemplified in the successes of the AIDS treatment advocacy movement. The industry, while developing a product that serves the public good by providing reliable and effective therapies, has a superseding fiduciary duty to its shareholders—a duty that requires that it be profit-seeking and asset-conserving—so its expectations are for smooth review and approval processes and the fewest regulatory impediments. FDA itself is accountable to Congress, whose members represent the American people. The committee believes that FDA's most important constituency is the public and that commitment to the public good will ideally influence and check FDA's interactions with the industry.

Structural Factors, Policies, and Procedures

Structural Factors

External observers, from scientists to legislators, have noted that a key organizational challenge for CDER is the striking disparities between divisions responsible for premarket and postmarketing activities. There are disparities in the formal role, authority, resources, and relative institutional value conferred on the two groups of staff. Many of those issues have been confirmed by the 2006 GAO report on FDA's postmarket decision-making and oversight process. The committee is not arguing that the responsibilities, resources, and other features of OND and ODS/OSE must necessarily be equal in every respect. The committee did not attempt to undertake a point-by-point comparison of OND and ODS/OSE (roles, capabilities, resources currently and in a perfect world), but it does assert that the formal function and resources of ODS/OSE have not been commensurate with the importance of safety or with the tasks of monitoring postmarketing drug safety. Inadequate management, discussed later in this chapter, also may contribute to the gap between ODS/OSE and OND and to the sense of interoffice tension or, at best, disharmony between the two offices. To some critics, the most concerning outcomes of the disparities between the premarketing and postmarketing activities are that authority over postmarketing safety is solely in the hands of people who did the work of reviewing and approving a drug and that postmarketing safety activities appear to be secondary or subservient to the premarket processes and the task of approving drugs for marketing (Wolfe SM, 2006).

CDER's culture seems to have been influenced by how premarket and postmarketing functions have been divided historically. Randomized controlled trials are the gold standard for studies leading to drug approval. Epidemiologic, population-based studies are used after approval, when a drug is on the market and being used in real-life circumstances. Medical knowledge derives from both randomized clinical trials and epidemiologic studies (including observational studies that use automated health care databases), but the methods of the two approaches differ, as does the degree of confidence that can be accorded analytic results. Although the two approaches are complementary and can both be valuable depending on the nature of the medical problem addressed—for example, population-based studies provide different kinds of information that randomized controlled studies do not deliver before approval—recent depictions of the workings of CDER suggest that the disparate respect afforded to results of the different approaches adversely affects interactions when uncertainties about the data abound and the "call" regarding regulatory action is close. Most OND reviewers are physicians who are trained to analyze prospective, randomized controlled clinical trial data, whereas the ODS/OSE staff, including the safety evaluators and the epidemiologists, must typically work with uncontrolled or observational data. Most data bearing on safety issues generated and reviewed in the postmarketing period are from case reports and from epidemiologic studies. Recent controversies show that there is sometimes a marked difference of opinion between OND and ODS/OSE about the interpretation of such data. OND staff often view observational data as "soft" and unconvincing, whereas ODS/OSE staff see them as informative and carrying great weight in evaluating postmarketing safety questions.

The interdisciplinary tension is also an obstacle to full implementation of a lifecycle approach to drug regulation, in which the preapproval process actively and creatively involves anticipation of postapproval uncertainties and a plan for addressing them. That is a clear example of how structure and culture can connect. A structure that provides opportunities for crosscutting discussion and methods—an interdisciplinary "team approach"—would go a long way to encouraging a collaborative culture, in which differing viewpoints and types of expertise can make a contribution.

In the last decade, there have been four major restructuring efforts in the variously named office responsible for postmarketing safety and in CDER; most recently, steps have been taken to clarify and elevate the previously ad hoc role of ODS/OSE as part of a broader effort to "sustain a multidisciplinary, cross-center approach to drug safety" (Galson email to staff, May 15, 2006; see also Appendix A). Although those efforts may reflect CDER's desire to improve the effectiveness of its safety surveillance programs, the frequency of repositioning organizational "boxes" and changing unit names raises concern that such changes are more cosmetic than functionally effective responses to public dissatisfaction with the CDER's performance. Committee discussions with CDER staff and the history of reports documenting problems in CDER suggest that previous efforts at restructuring did not fundamentally alter the characteristics of or the relationship between OND and ODS/OSE or the morale and functioning of the center. Thus, the committee is not convinced that the recent changes will succeed without additional specific actions.

Policies and Procedures

The committee has reviewed the relevant CDER guidance documents and the numbered documents in the *Manual of Administrative Policies and Procedures* (individual documents are known as MAPPs)[4] to understand the current structure defining the roles of OND and ODS/ODE, and it reviewed various congressional and public proposals for restructuring (CDER et al., 2005; FDA, 2005d; Grassley, 2005; Johnson and US PIRG, 2005).[5] The committee has also discussed the technical or administrative details with the appropriate FDA staff and managers, and reviewed reports describing the many dimensions of drug regulation and its challenges (GAO, 2002, 2006; DHHS and OIG, 2003; Thaul, 2005).

CDER constitutes teams for New Drug Application (NDA) reviews (see Box 3-3). OND plays a formal lead role in most regulatory actions, and OND reviewers sign components of the approval package; OND managers (division directors, office directors, and the OND director) act in a final

---

[4]A description of MAPPs is available at http://www.fda.gov/cder/mapp.htm.

[5]CDER has issued several guidances and MAPPs related to the preparation of the review package; several of these are mandated by the PDUFA. FDA's guidance documents include the following disclaimer: "This guidance represents the Food and Drug Administration's (FDA's) current thinking on this topic. It does not create or confer any rights for or on any person and does not operate to bind FDA or the public. You can use an alternative approach if the approach satisfies the requirements of the applicable statutes and regulations. If you want to discuss an alternative approach, contact the FDA staff responsible for implementing this guidance. If you cannot identify the appropriate FDA staff, call the appropriate number listed on the title page of this guidance . . . FDA's guidance documents, including this guidance, do not establish legally enforceable responsibilities. Instead, Guidances describe the Agency's current thinking on a topic and should be viewed only as recommendations, unless specific regulatory or statutory requirements are cited. The use of the word 'should' in Agency guidances means that something is suggested or recommended, but not required." MAPPs, however, establish procedures to be used (with variations, as appropriate) by CDER staff.

BOX 3-3
Composition of the NDA Review Team

Review teams include a review project manager (RPM) and primary reviewers, who complete the discipline reviews, as needed, in the following disciplines:

- Medical/clinical*
- Pharmacology/toxicology
- Chemistry manufacturing, and controls
- Biometrics/statistical
- Clinical pharmacology and biopharmaceutics
- Clinical microbiology
- Bioresearch monitoring.

---

*CDER documents appear to use the terms "medical review" and "clinical review" interchangeably. It has been suggested that use of the phrase "clinical review" indicates that a primary reviewer need not necessarily be a physician, although most of them are. In this report we will use the more inclusive term "clinical review" or "clinical reviewer."

SOURCE: FDA (2005d).

---

decision-making capacity in most cases. Some members of the review team, such as statisticians, work in offices other than OND. The committee has learned that there is little integration of and a limited role for ODS/OSE staff in the premarket review process; they work in a consultative and supportive capacity and, with one exception, have no regulatory authority (CDER, 2005; GAO, 2006). Although postapproval responsibilities for ODS/OSE have been growing, resources have improved only modestly (since 2004, a growth from 94 to 132 full time equivalents dedicated to postmarketing safety), and its formal role has not expanded.

FDA's *Guidance for Review Staff and Industry: Good Review Management Principles and Practices for PDUFA Products* (GRMP) outlines in great detail the roles and responsibilities of the team leaders and reviewers drawn from other disciplines in CDER. It also addresses so-called consults from non-team members, such as staff from ODS/OSE, the Office of New Drug Chemistry, and the Division of Drug Marketing and Communication. The guidance document describes ODS/OSE staff as consultants, not as members of the review team, and their formal responsibilities, other than participating in consults, include participation in the preapproval safety conference and review of product labeling. The only formal authority given to ODS/OSE is to grant waivers to the industry sponsors of the postmarketing reporting requirements in 21 CFR 314.80.

The PDUFA deadlines, which affect mostly OND staff, may play a role in contributing to an organizational structure that limits ODS/OSE involvement. Review packages accompanying an NDA approval letter include what are called discipline reviews, often long documents written by CDER scientists reviewing material in a specific scientific discipline submitted by an applicant in support of the NDA. Discipline reviews and other documents related to the review of a drug, such as the approval letter, are made public on FDA's Web site only if an application is approved for marketing (see Chapter 4 for additional discussion). Review packages for products that are not approved are not made public. The clinical review is usually written by one OND staff person and includes summaries by the clinical reviewer of other discipline reviews.

A policy and procedure (MAPP 6010.3, see Box 3-4) (CDER, 2004a), the Clinical Review Template introduced in 2004, provides an opportunity for formal involvement of ODS/OSE medical officers in the review process. The purpose of the MAPP was to standardize the safety review components of an NDA and in particular the approach to postmarketing safety of the product (Racoosin, 2006). The MAPP suggests options for involvement of more than one OND clinical reviewer. If there is more than one, a lead reviewer is identified and has the responsibility for writing the overview and section 4.3, which describes how the review was prepared. Two options exist for the final review; one allows for multiple reviews by multiple authors incorporated into a single overview, and the other limits the review package to one final clinical review with sections prepared by multiple reviewers.

Although there is no formal public documentation of changes instituted by the MAPP, the committee's informal review of NDA packages approved before July 2004 suggests that the "Recommendation on Postmarketing Actions" introduced a substantial change in the clinical review template by creating a location in the review package for a review and recommendations on postmarketing actions pertaining to the drug to be approved. Based on a review of more recent NDA packages, it appears that the new template is being used by reviewers of new drugs, but the committee believes that that responsibility would be a reasonable and appropriate function for ODS/OSE medical officers.

Management

There have been many opportunities for CDER and FDA leadership to acknowledge to the committee and to others that there is a culture problem

---

BOX 3-4
Clinical Review Template—Postmarketing Actions

In July 2004 CDER issued MAPP 6010.3, the *Clinical Review Template* (CDER, 2004a), which established procedures for documenting the primary clinical review of NDAs. The clinical review is one of the discipline reviews prepared in response to an original or supplemental NDA (or Biologic License Application reviewed by CDER), amendments in response to action letters, and efficacy supplements. The MAPP describes the format of the discipline review and the responsibilities of the reviewers, other team members, and those in the supervisory chain. The review template includes 11 sections:

1. Executive Summary
2. Introduction and Background
3. Significant Findings from Other Review Disciplines
4. Data Sources, Review Strategy, and Data Integrity
5. Clinical Pharmacology
6. Integrated Review of Efficacy
7. Integrated Review of Safety
8. Additional Clinical Issues
9. Overall Assessment
10. Appendices
11. References

Section 9.3 of the template (part of Overall Assessment) is entitled "Recommendation on Postmarketing Actions" and includes subsections on "Risk Management Activity," "Required Phase 4 Commitments," and "Other Phase 4 Requests," and a review of and recommendations for the applicant's postmarketing risk management plan.

---

in CDER. However, although agency and center leaders generally mentioned the flurry of drug safety activities being undertaken, they did not seem to recognize the tensions and other strains within the center as anything more than a minor distraction. On the basis of its discussions with current and past FDA employees (both staff and management), and its review of several government reports and other relevant literature, the committee believes that CDER's organizational culture is characterized by problems in several important areas: a suboptimal work environment, a polarization between two major functions, an underestimation and poor handling of scientific disagreement and differences of opinion, a lack of consistency across divisions, and instability and politicization at the top (in the Office of the Commissioner). The committee believes that these issues may directly or indirectly affect CDER's handling of drug safety concerns.

A Suboptimal Work Environment

There is evidence of a persisting problem with retention, turnover, and morale in CDER. CDER's organizational culture does not seem to readily embrace the values of staff participation, inclusion, and empowerment that are generally thought to be essential to a healthy organization (Coffee, 1993). Relevant staff members are sometimes excluded from planning of administrative and program improvements and their initiative in proposing improvements is not well received (or "received" at all). Staff members are sometimes left out of discussion and decision making about the future of the center, new initiatives, etc.

Two government reports provide some information suggestive of potential difficulties in the CDER work environment. A GAO report (GAO, 2002) on the rate of safety withdrawals after enactment of PDUFA found that attrition among medical officers and other relevant FDA staff from 1998 to 2000 was noticeably greater than attrition in similar disciplines at the National Institutes of Health and the Centers for Disease Control and Prevention (10.5 percent vs. 5.5 and 4.7, respectively). Although one explanation for the turnover is that FDA staff leave for promising opportunities in industry (that arguably leads to a propagation of competent individuals with regulatory agency experience throughout industry), it is possible that turnover is indicative of a less-than-ideal organizational culture that requires attention. The GAO report attributed the turnover to reasons that included workload and decreased training opportunities. FDA data in a 2003 report on the drug review process showed that medical officers and pharmacologists had the highest attrition rates in CDER (DHHS and OIG, 2003).

The committee learned from its conversations with OND staff that their considerable workloads and time pressures exacerbated by PDUFA make it difficult for them to be as thorough as they would like in their assessments of safety after marketing. The committee's discussions with CDER staff resonated with the findings of previous assessments—reviewers of new drugs are often overwhelmed merely keeping up with the routine aspects of review, which leave little time to consider postmarketing safety plans thoughtfully, or to investigate (for example, with colleagues in other disciplines) safety signals that arise after approval (IOM Staff Notes, 2005–2006). In such circumstances, it is little wonder that professional development and internal interaction to facilitate communication and understanding among divisions and offices become luxuries. In 2005, a group of OND medical officers organized itself to identify possible causes of attrition and to make recommendations to CDER management about ways to improve retention (Medical Officer Retention Subcommittee, 2006). The group's recommendations included addressing OND reviewer workloads by hiring more staff, increasing division and office director awareness of reviewer needs, redefining the CDER vision, and in general transforming the CDER leadership philosophy. Members of that staff subcommittee expressed concern that the leadership philosophy in CDER did not encourage staff participation and input at all levels (Medical Officer Retention Subcommittee, 2006).

The failure of management to implement effective changes to address those important issues indicates that there is a problem. ODS/OSE and OND staff have reported being left out of regulatory meetings directly related to their work, and ODS/OSE staff have frequently been left out of relevant advisory committee meetings (GAO, 2006). There is evidence of a lack of consistent processes to facilitate and resolve safety issues identified by ODS/OSE and passed on to OND. The 2006 GAO report's finding that ODS/OSE consults and questions often went into a "black hole" and that initiating staff never received feedback is consistent with what this committee learned.

Some staff-generated ideas for process or culture improvements appeared to receive little or no attention from management. In its 2006 report, GAO noted that in December 2004, ODS epidemiologists requested a broadening of their role to include "presenting all relevant ODS data at advisory committee meetings" but management did not respond (GAO, 2006:22). To the best of the present committee's knowledge, CDER management also did not respond to the OND Medical Officer Retention Subcommittee's May 2005 proposal until June 2006. The committee was surprised to find out that although the Drug Safety Oversight Board (DSB) had been introduced to a variety of audiences (Congress, the public, etc.), some CDER staff seemed uninformed about what the board was expected to accomplish and how it could affect their work.

Management scholars have identified a strong attachment to the status quo in many organizations and a tendency to commit "sunk cost" errors by pursuing a course of action because so much has already been invested in it (Edmonson et al., 2005). A panel convened by the National Aeronautics and Space Administration after the Columbia disaster identified similar organizational tendencies, noting, for example, that "once the Agency is on record as committed to a specific achievement, it becomes unpalatable to back off of that target for fear of appearing to fail" and that there was an attitude of "comfort with existing beliefs" that justified a resistance to internal or external criticism and a stifling of dissenting views (Return to Flight Task Group, 2005; O'Leary, 2006). The perception that there are somewhat similar cultural attitudes in CDER is evident in the concerns of consumer advocates and academics and confirmed by the DHHS OIG and GAO reports that new drug reviewers feel pressured by the unstated expectations of the agency leadership (due to PDUFA goals and other reasons) to approve drugs and are unable to revise the regulatory approach to an already-approved drug.

Interoffice Polarization

The committee has seen evidence of a divide between the premarketing and postmarketing staff in CDER (generally represented by staff in OND and staff in ODS/OSE, respectively). ODS/OSE staff has been left out of regulatory discussions and advisory committee meetings (GAO, 2006; IOM Staff Notes, 2005–2006). The user-fee funding system may have also allowed (or at least exacerbated) the emergence of a major resource gap between OND and ODS/OSE (IOM, 2005; IOM Staff Notes, 2005–2006; Zelenay, 2005; GAO, 2006) (also see Chapter 7 for a more detailed discussion of the funding and staff imbalance). Although the committee did not explore the history of this divide, conversations with CDER leadership revealed disparities in how the two offices and their contributions to the agency's work are regarded. The 2006 GAO report has also confirmed the difference in status between the two offices. Given the high-profile concerns about drug safety, the fact that an office bearing the title of "Drug Safety" had a lower status than an office of "New Drugs," and agency spokespersons appeared dismissive of the work of staff in that office may have also exacerbated the perception of tension (Harris, 2006b). The committee is aware that there have been repeated attempts to reorganize or restructure CDER, both by moving boxes around a chart and by developing internal policies, procedures, and guidance documents (as described above), but culture problems have persisted.

The committee has seen little historical evidence of successful initiatives to strengthen ODS/OSE capabilities or to stabilize the office, which has experienced eight changes in leadership and four reorganizations in the past 10 years (GAO, 2006). Although the committee was encouraged by the appointment of a new permanent ODS/OSE director (after much turnover in that position [GAO, 2006]) and by evidence of planning to improve communication and collaboration between OND and ODS/OSE, it remains concerned that these attempts are "too little, too late."

The committee believes that management in CDER has not done enough to cultivate an atmosphere of mutual respect and appreciation across some of the disciplines. In interactions with CDER leadership, the committee formed the impression that ODS/OSE staff have been considered marginal players, compared with OND staff, in contributing to the work of ensuring drug safety. When the committee inquired about the apparent cultural divide in discussions with CDER leadership, it heard that ODS/OSE was not capable of a greater function in postmarketing safety because of a lack of qualified and trained staff, a lack of analytic sophistication, and inadequate understanding of the data and their weighing in the approval process. The committee also heard that problems between ODS/OSE and OND are simply a squabble, not warranting management attention. The GAO report (2006) appeared to touch a nerve when it interpreted ODS/OSE's role of consultant to OND as secondary, not well defined, and lacking clear responsibilities. In its response to GAO, FDA argued that the consultative role is important and that the GAO report did not recognize that; but the agency did little to explain specific steps it would take to clarify the role of ODS/OSE and to pay more than lip service to its contributions. The committee acknowledges that some recent changes have occurred in CDER. Some have been on ODS/OSE's own initiative—as the GAO report has acknowledged, the level of expertise and sophistication of analyses conducted by the office have evolved, and a promising new leader has been appointed to head the office (FDA News, 2005; GAO, 2006). As noted in Chapter 1 and in Appendix A, in the wake of highly publicized concern about the safety of some drugs approved by FDA, the agency and CDER announced the implementation of several strategies to improve attention to postmarketing safety and to strengthen the administrative processes that underlie drug safety work in FDA. Those strategies included two processes for dispute resolution at the staff level, and the establishment of the DSB for interdivisional difficulties (discussed below) (CDER, 2004b; CDER and FDA, 2005).

It does not appear that the various efforts to restructure CDER have improved interactions between review and postmarketing staff. The dispute resolution mechanism has yet to be used, and mass media reports about emerging drug safety concerns continue to give the appearance that the center is not managing those concerns adequately. On several occasions when the findings of safety staff have been cited in the mass media, agency spokespersons have downplayed or disparaged the information's quality or completeness, instead of assuring the public that the agency takes the concerns of its staff seriously and that staff collaborate to bring such important questions to resolution. New documents to guide CDER staff have not necessarily translated into greater clarity and effectiveness at the level of interoffice relationships and procedures; in fact, there is a continuing lack of established mechanisms for communicating about and following safety signals between offices. That attitude was apparent on numerous occasions when members of this committee spoke with FDA and CDER management who described ODS/OSE as lacking in needed expertise, sophistication, and depth of experience (IOM Staff Notes, 2005–2006). That disparity in management attitudes toward OND and ODS/OSE is also suggested by information provided in the 2006 GAO report, in the comments of FDA officials to the press, and in a recent response from the CDER director to an internal group's proposal to address medical officer attrition. May and June 2006 newspaper articles about the agency's handling of drug safety concerns about an antibiotic indicated that some postmarketing safety staff expressed concerns that were not addressed in a timely manner by CDER management. An FDA spokesperson described a safety reviewer's report of her concerns "a preliminary, raw assessment" and stated that "the final decision will be made by experts who have the full benefit of a large section of opinion and scientific fact" (Harris, 2006a).

Underestimation and Poor Handling of Scientific Disagreement and Differences of Opinion

Management's difficulties in addressing internal agency conflict and scientific disagreement transparently and competently, in communicating scientific uncertainty to diverse audiences effectively have played an important role in damaging the credibility of CDER and the FDA. As discussed in Chapter 4, the regulation of drugs rests on a foundation of incomplete but growing knowledge, and the risk-benefit assessment for every drug continues to evolve after approval, when use of the drug moves from the carefully controlled confines of clinical trials to the largely uncontrolled and much more complex circumstances of real-life prescribing and use. Legitimate scientific disagreement may occur at various points in the lifecycle of a drug. There may be disagreement about whether a reasonable threshold of certainty has been reached to justify approval (the absence of standard approaches to the risk-benefit assessment before approval is discussed in greater detail in Chapter 4). After approval, there may be scientific disagreement about the interpretation of adverse event signals (for example, there is no clear guidance on when a noise becomes a signal) and about what regulatory action is warranted.

The committee is concerned about information suggesting that scientific disagreement in the center is sometimes handled in ways that may create an inappropriate atmosphere of pressure or poor tolerance of disagreement. The 2003 DHHS OIG report of survey findings on 401 CDER reviewers (most in OND) stated that "18 percent of respondents indicated that they have felt pressure to approve or recommend approval for a drug, despite reservations about its safety, efficacy, or quality" (18 percent accounts for about 72 of 401 respondents to the survey). Although scientific disagreement is understandable and there are cases where a division or office director disagrees with a reviewer's recommendation on the basis of the science, having even one or two staff members who report pressure to approve or recommend approval is an entirely different and deeply troubling occurrence.[6]

In its visit and later discussions with FDA staff, the committee learned that differential valuation of disciplinary approaches affects the relationship between OND and ODS/OSE and contributes to a perception in each office that its counterpart does not have the full picture or does not give enough consideration to colleagues' different disciplinary perspectives. Although OND staff includes physicians, some of whom have training in statistics or epidemiology, their efforts are oriented substantially toward review of data from randomized controlled trials, and their experience with and confidence in epidemiologic studies may be slight. ODS/OSE staff, in contrast, have a greater level of comfort with epidemiologic approaches but less familiarity with randomized controlled trials and their analysis. But as mentioned above, the imbalance in formal role and authority between the new drug review staff and surveillance and epidemiology staff denotes subservience of the safety function, and a management devaluation of the latter discipline and approach.

The DSB, which consists of staff members of several CDER offices and representatives of other FDA centers and other government agencies is established to "improve public knowledge of emerging important drug safety concerns; strengthen internal drug safety management; foster practical policy development to improve consistency and timely resolution of important drug safety concerns; and *provide a standing venue for resolution of CDER organizational disputes*" (Cummins, 2006). Including members drawn from CDER offices not primarily responsible for any given product or issue, and from other federal agencies, is intended to provide some independent oversight regarding emerging issues while maintaining the ability to convene quickly without conflict-of-interest considerations or concern about the discussion of proprietary matters. Items for discussion can be brought to the DSB by a CDER division or by OND or ODS/OSE leaders. It is not

---

[6]In August 2006, the Union of Concerned Scientists (UCS) and Public Employees for Environmental Responsibility released their survey of FDA, which included the survey instrument used in the 2003 DHHS OIG survey. UCS findings echoed those reported by OIG in 2003, including the response to "Have you ever been pressured to approve or recommend approval for an NDA despite reservations about the safety, efficacy, or quality of the drug?" Of 217 CDER staff who responded to this question, nearly 19% (41) said "yes" (UCS, 2006a,b). After the UCS release, FDA Acting Commissioner Andrew von Eschenbach met with UCS staff, acknowledged his concern about the issues related to morale identified in the survey, and also vowed to work to create "an environment where there is free, open and vigorous debate and discussion" (UCS, 2006a,b). In the course of Senate committee questioning during the August 1, 2006, nomination hearing, Dr. von Eschenbach was asked about the UCS survey question regarding "pressure to approve . . . despite reservations." The acting commissioner stated that "no one should ever alter the data or the scientific facts" (von Eschenbach, 2006).

clear whether DSB can on its own initiative address an issue of which it has become aware if it is not formally referred to them. The DSB emerged as part of the agency's response to congressional and public concern over highly publicized drug safety problems. Because many critics called for independent external oversight of drug safety, the creation of the board was believed by some to be a solution to address that particular concern (FDA, 2005c). The composition of the board caused confusion and gave rise to criticism that the board as constituted was not independent. That confusion was furthered by FDA's silence on the board's actual (and potentially useful) function, and the underlying public and legislative concern about independence was left unaddressed. Because the DSB has been in operation for only a short time, it is too early to judge its effectiveness, but some of its drug safety problem resolution, management, and policy functions seem to constitute a sensible approach. DSB is analogous to industry practices of bringing together leaders of different groups in a company to consult with a group facing a difficult problem. However, the committee believes that the external communication function of the board seems to be a vastly different and equally important set of concerns that should be handled by a different entity in CDER (see Chapter 6). That would allow the DSB to focus its energies and resources on addressing the internal management of drug safety issues.

There has been additional confusion about the apparent overlap between the Drug Safety and Risk Management Advisory Committee (DSaRM) and DSB. CDER management has described the latter as a "venue for resolving CDER organizational drug safety disputes" and "discussing [the] need for AC [advisory committee] meetings about emerging safety information" whereas DSaRM has been described as a way to obtain public input and facilitate discussion to inform CDER decision making. The committee believes that DSaRM fulfills the function of the sought-after independent, external safety advisory and review body, in contrast with DSB, which is intended to bring serious and complex internal safety issues to resolution.

Inconsistency

Many interactions in CDER appear to be idiosyncratic and personality-driven. The committee understands that there is great variation within and among drug classes and from one product to another and that flexibility is desired. However, there seem to be subjects on which consistency would be beneficial, for example, methods of risk-benefit analysis, preapproval decisions on postmarketing studies, handling of disagreements between offices, ODS/OSE participation in the review process, monitoring of drug safety signals after approval, responding to drug safety signals, communication of important risks to the public, and followup of postmarketing study commitments. Some best practices have not been disseminated throughout CDER.

For example, one division's model for ensuring internal safety capacity by establishing its own safety team of epidemiologists has attracted interest in CDER and from drug safety advocates but has not yet been replicated in any other division (the committee has heard that this model may be expanded to other divisions).[7]

Instability and Politicization at the Top

The absence of stable leadership at the commissioner level and lack of consistent oversight of CDER by the commissioner may have contributed to overarching management problems in CDER. Although the day-to-day work of CDER is not immediately affected by what is happening in the commissioner's office, the recurring absence of a confirmed commissioner has implications for the agency. First, the absence of stable leadership has meant much more than going without an agency figurehead. As discussed above, the external environment places great pressure on FDA and its centers, and the agency's top leadership plays a crucial role in setting the course for the agency and in mediating the effects of external pressures by representing the agency in interactions with other government agencies, Congress, the industry, and the public. An acting commissioner does not carry the same weight symbolically, and lacks the authority to articulate agency positions. PDUFA reauthorization talks in 2002 were reportedly slowed down by the lack of a commissioner (Validation Times, 2002). An individual in an acting capacity also may be unable to act decisively; such a person would likely defer making any difficult decisions or setting a new course for the agency. Furthermore, staff may be unlikely to take such a leader seriously because an acting position is by its very definition temporary (Miller, 2006; Ross, 2006). In cases when an acting commissioner is also the president's nominee facing the prospect of challenging Senate hearings, making decisions on high-profile issues could potentially complicate the road to confirmation. As appointing and confirming a permanent commissioner is delayed, FDA staff and the public may also conclude that their government does not consider a commissioner's position important, and that may have demoralizing consequences on staff and affect the agency's credibility (Kaufman, 2004b; Alonso-Zaldivar, 2006).

Industry leaders have asserted that the lack of a leader leads to an increase in agency caution and a decrease in predictability in the eyes of companies and investors (Young, 2005). In 2002, the Biotechnology Industry Organization (BIO) petitioned President George W. Bush to appoint

---

[7]That is the Neuropyschiatry Drug Products Division was recently split into two, a Neurology Products Division and a Psychiatry Products Division. The safety team currently resides in the Division of Neurology Products but supports both divisions.

a commissioner, arguing that the industry and the nation needed "strong leadership from an FDA commissioner with vision and experience in science, medicine and administration" (BIO, 2002). In the same year, the PhRMA president and CEO reported that the industry was challenged by the absence of agency leadership and that PDUFA negotiations were slowed down by the absence of a commissioner (National Journal's Congress Daily, 2002; Validation Times, 2002). Former commissioner Jane Henney stated that in the absence of leadership, "industry loses because it needs predictable and strong signals about the review process, the consumers need to make sure somebody is in charge and the FDA staff needs somebody who can take the heat if necessary" (Kaufman, 2004a). In 2002, FDA staff were questioned in a congressional hearing without the support of a Senate-confirmed commissioner (Kaufman, 2004a). In the 2005 Senate committee session on the nomination of the then Acting Commissioner, Senator Enzi cited a letter from the Senate committee to the president urging the nomination of a commissioner "to provide the agency with greater clarity and certainty in its mission," and stated that a "fully confirmed Commissioner is essential to ensuring that these medical breakthroughs can be brought to the market safely and effectively. Consumers deserve to have a fully functional FDA that can oversee the industry with confidence and authority and harness the technical achievements that can improve and save lives" (Senate Executive Session, July 18, 2005).

Management literature has made it clear that organizations, including government agencies, cannot function well without effective leadership to set them and keep them on course to achieve their mission (GAO, 1996). In the last 30 years, FDA has had eight commissioners and seven acting commissioners (including the current acting commissioner) or, when the post was vacant, an acting principal deputy commissioner. The eight commissioners have served an average of 2.5 years with a range of 2 months to 6.3 years (FDA, 2006b). That instability is thought to have contributed to CDER's problems. CDER is the largest center in the agency, the center director reports to the commissioner, and the center's decisions and their repercussions are highly visible and sometimes controversial, as was the case with the Plan B over-the-counter switch application (GAO, 2005). The committee believes that turnover and instability in the commissioner's office leave the agency without effective leadership or the potential to emphasize safety as having high priority in the work of the agency. Without stable leadership strongly and visibly committed to drug safety, all other efforts to improve the effectiveness of the agency or position it effectively for the future will be seriously, if not fatally, compromised. A priority for the agency should be to regain the trust of the public while positioning itself for the future.

The controversy over the emergency contraceptive Plan B has further highlighted the power of the commissioner. In this area, the political environment interfaces with issues of leadership. Plan B, a prescription emergency contraception drug, was approved in 1999. In 2002, FDA staff met twice to discuss and prepare for the sponsor's expected application for a switch of Plan B from prescription to over-the-counter (OTC) status. In April 2003, the sponsor submitted its supplemental NDA for the OTC switch, and FDA set a PDUFA goal date of February 2004 (for a total of 10 months, a typical timeline for a standard review) to reach a decision on the application. A joint meeting of the two relevant advisory committees—those for non-prescription drugs and for reproductive health drugs—concluded with a vote that overwhelmingly favored an OTC switch (GAO, 2005). However, the agency denied the application, raising questions about the basis for that decision making. In the end, it became clear that the ultimate decision was made in the Office of the Commissioner for reasons that were not clearly linked with a scientific rationale. The perception of political considerations overruling scientific judgment, even just in a single case, inevitably raises concerns about the legitimacy of decision making in every case.

Proposed Solutions to CDER's Organizational Dysfunction

Management

On the basis of its review of relevant government reports, conversations with present and former FDA staff and managers, and its examination of CDER guidance and policies and procedures documents, the committee finds that CDER's organizational culture is under great strain and that change is needed to ensure that the center can fulfill its components of the FDA mission. The last several years of newspaper articles about FDA and CDER specifically and relevant public opinion polls have shown a decline in FDA's credibility with the public, some scientists and academics, and others. Over the years, there have been multiple initiatives, taskforces, and panels on CDER's work and multiple government reports identifying problems and recommending solutions. The fact that many substantial changes have not been made may be a primary symptom of management failure, a lack of leadership, and of a lack of appropriate oversight by Congress.

According to management research, organizational cultures that are constructive or healthy are more effective in accomplishing their mission. But cultural change may take many years to implement and requires sustained and comprehensive effort (GAO, 1996; Khademian, 2002). Assessments of federal agency management have found that when federal executives reorganize agencies, organizational culture is rarely a focus of attention—it is often an afterthought or considered a nicety irrelevant to the complex and technically challenging work of many government agencies (Khademian, 2002).[8] In that regard, FDA is no different. The consistent neglect of cultural problems in the organization betrays a lack of recognition of the importance of healthy culture. Even if FDA and CDER leaders do not see themselves as managers who stifle dissent or exclude participation from staff, that perception clearly exists (affecting agency credibility), and problems with retention and morale confirm it.

Agency Leadership

Healthy organizations require effective and stable leadership. The committee believes that there is an urgent need for a full-time, confirmed FDA commissioner who will be visible and forceful in creating a culture of safety by facilitating a systematic, science-based approach to continually assessing and acting on risk-benefit during the lifecycle of every drug (pre- and post-approval). The commissioner's role is also to provide effective oversight of CDER, particularly given the strong external pressures on the center's work. Many observers from industry and from the scientific community have expressed concern in recent years that the commission position has remained unfilled or filled by deputy commissioners functioning as acting commissioner for long periods of time.

The committee recognizes that the daily work of FDA staff may not be strongly affected by what happens in the office of the commissioner, but there is fairly widespread agreement, described above, that the absence of a commissioner has been a problem because without a legitimate, Senate-confirmed leader, it is harder for the agency to define and achieve its strategic vision.

The committee wishes to emphasize that in making the following recommendations, it does not imply that politics can or should be removed from a top scientific position, such as the FDA commissioner. However, it is important to the credibility of a science-based regulatory agency that scientific evidence, not solely political considerations, prevail in cases where high-profile regulatory decisions must be made. The Plan B decision described above may have undermined the agency's credibility, as evidence

---

[8]In 1996, Congress asked GAO to determine whether performance problems at the Federal Aviation Administration were related to its organizational culture. GAO found that the culture impeded the agency's work. Characteristics highlighted included a system of bureaucratic incentives that rewarded staff who preserved the status quo and punished those who identified problems (GAO, 1996). Assessments of government agency performance and examples from the management literature have shown repeatedly that organizational cultures that stifle dissent, exclude staff from decisions about the organization's vision, and allow cultural problems to linger unaddressed are not healthy cultures, and those problems interfere with their ability to achieve their goals (Weick and Sutcliffe, 2001; Heifetz and Laurie, 1998; Khademian, 2002; Return to Flight Task Group, 2005; O'Leary R, 2006).

emerged that the basis for decision making was not scientific, but other types of considerations (Bridges, 2006; Rockoff, 2006; Washington Drug Letter, 2006).

Finally, the committee believes that a fixed-term appointment for the FDA commissioner may help to lessen turnover. Reports from GAO and from the National Academy of Sciences (NAS) have found that turnover in government agency leadership is linked with a focus on short-term goals and uncertain accountability and that fixed terms for presidential appointments help to ensure stability and strengthen an agency's leadership (GAO, 1996; GAO, 2003). Currently, presidential appointment with Senate confirmation positions for fixed terms include: surgeon general of the Public Health Service, 4 years; director of the National Science Foundation (NSF), 6 years; commissioner of the Bureau of Labor Statistics, 4 years; under secretary for health in the Department of Veterans Affairs (also the Chief Executive Officer of the Veterans Health Administration), 4 years; commissioner of the Social Security Administration, 6 years; and commissioners of the Federal Communications Commission, 5 years. Another NAS committee that recommended a 6-year term for the National Institutes of Health (NIH) director concluded that the NSF director's 6-year term "has been a good model for creating a system of accountability and periodic review that has the possibility of transcending changes in administration" (NRC, 2003).

Fixed terms can vary in length, be renewable or not, and have more or less strict terms of removal, depending on the degree of insulation desired. In all cases, to be constitutional, the president must retain the power of removal—incumbents of term appointments should be accountable and subject to removal by the president. On the one hand, establishing a term appointment and specifying the reasons for which an appointee may be removed changes the terms of removal to some extent. It creates a presumption that individuals in these positions should stay rather than be automatically removed with every change in administration, and it requires an administration to give good reasons for such a removal. On the other hand, the use of terms also indicates that there should be periodic turnover—not for partisan reasons but to ensure new blood and fresh ideas.

> **3.1: The committee recommends that the FD&C Act be amended to require that the FDA Commissioner currently appointed by the President with the advice and consent of the Senate also be appointed for a 6-year term of office. The Commissioner should be an individual with appropriate expertise to head a science-based agency, demonstrated capacity to lead and inspire, and a proven commitment to public health, scientific integrity, transparency, and communication. The President may remove the Commissioner from**

office only for reasons of inefficiency, neglect of duty, or malfeasance in office.

Given the influence of the social, policy, and economic environment on CDER's work and its major structural and management challenges, the committee believes that a confirmed commissioner will need support to effect organizational change, particularly with respect to CDER. The committee believes that a mechanism to support the commissioner is necessary because transforming an organization's culture requires relevant leadership and management expertise and sustained effort.

3.2: The committee recommends that an external Management Advisory Board be appointed by the Secretary of HHS to advise the FDA commissioner in shepherding CDER (and the agency as a whole) to implement and sustain the changes necessary to transform the center's culture—by improving morale and retention of professional staff, strengthening transparency, restoring credibility, and creating a culture of safety based upon a lifecycle approach to risk-benefit.

Although the committee is not aware of entities analogous to what it is recommending, it is worth noting that NIH has an Advisory Committee to the Director, which advises the agency head on major plans and policies, including those related to resource allocation, program development, and "administrative regulation and policy" (NIH, 2006). The external Management Advisory Board to the FDA commissioner would operate under Federal Advisory Committee Act rules. The secretary of HHS should consult with an independent organization in identifying candidates to ensure that the board's composition is appropriate for the task, including familiarity with the regulatory system for drug development and FDA's role in it and proven experience in successfully managing culture or organizational change.[9] (Ideally, conflict-of-interest concerns would be addressed by ensuring that a majority of board membership should have no substantial personal financial interest in the pharmaceutical industry, and board members should not be selected from current pharmaceutical industry representatives.) Board

---

[9]Two examples of independent advice in identifying members of Federal Advisory Committees: DHHS consults with the NAS on the composition of the National Vaccine Advisory Committee, and the Consumer Product Safety Commission appoints a Chronic Hazard Advisory Panel of independent scientific experts from nominations submitted by the president of the NAS.

members would serve staggered 3-year terms that may be renewed once. The board would meet no less frequently than twice a year.

The Management Advisory Board would assist FDA and CDER in their efforts to understand how organizational culture in the center is shaped by the environment, by a legacy of structural imbalance, and by management problems. The committee has learned that a variety of promising steps have been taken to improve interactions among offices, evaluate and improve internal processes, and even familiarize disciplines with one another. However, given CDER's long history of reorganizations, external studies, and fitful change initiatives, the committee is not optimistic that current efforts will be sustained without the absolute commitment of managers and of center and agency leaders to act on many different levels, with broad staff participation and input and in an atmosphere of openness, and to be "relentless" in creating, seizing, and sustaining opportunities for change (Khademian, 2002:126). The committee believes that it is imperative that the director of CDER, with support from the commissioner and the assistance of the Management Advisory Board, take immediate steps to strengthen leadership, organization, and function to create and visibly champion a culture of drug safety in the center.

3.3: The committee recommends the Secretary of HHS direct the FDA commissioner and Director of CDER, with the assistance of the Management Advisory Board, to develop a comprehensive strategy for sustained cultural change that positions the agency to fulfill its mission, including protecting the health of the public.

As part of the strategy for cultural change, the director of CDER should establish an effective organizational development capability in CDER by forming a staff working group consisting of people who represent diverse disciplines, roles, and viewpoints and including one or two staff members with organizational development expertise. The group would work with and support the center director in providing meaningful opportunities for two-way communication with staff, identifying and addressing culture problems, and nurturing a culture that values disagreement and thinking outside the box.

Structural Factors

The imbalance in authority, formal role, and resources between OND and ODS/OSE constitutes a major obstacle to a healthy organizational culture in CDER. On the basis of the rationale described above, the committee sets forth its recommendation to address the cultural challenges exacerbated by the existing structure.

The aforementioned development of MAPPs as the primary strategy to manage how OND and ODS/OSE interact and to document differences of professional opinion may indicate that using procedural modifications to mollify critics is easier than engaging in the hard work of transforming a culture to embrace scientific disagreement and dissent and handle them in a constructive and transparent manner. Organizational literature shows that the bureaucratic cultures of public organizations are frequently rigid, authoritarian, and oriented toward obeying orders rather than toward innovation and independent thought (Kets de Vries and Miller, 1986; Claver et al., 1999; Khademian, 2002; O'Leary, 2006). That could explain why it is so easy to turn to policy and procedure development. However, it is important to note that the inflexibility and conformity that characterizes some government agencies are at least in part created by the requirements of Congress and the Office of Management and Budget. As described above, creating a healthy organizational culture in CDER depends on more than the efforts of management and staff—the external environment, including the top levels of the executive branch and relevant congressional committees.

The tension between the approaches of CDER professionals who focus largely on the premarketing period of a drug's lifecycle and those who deal with the postmarketing period is not unusual (consider, for example, areas of scholarship where the practitioners of quantitative and qualitative methods come in conflict). However, the friction has often been unconstructive, particularly when the goal is to achieve close integration of the two approaches, and to facilitate an atmosphere of mutual respect and appreciation between the two sets of disciplines involved. Facilitating such a shift, from an uneasy relationship to a collaborative and constructive one, requires skilled management and leadership.

The committee believes that a public health orientation and a lifecycle approach to understanding and minimizing the risks posed by drugs is best served by better and formal integration of the OND and ODS/OSE perspectives. The committee understands that new drug review and approval are undertaken with a matrix team approach, however it notes with concern the lack of formal participation of ODS/OSE in the review team. That might reflect a sentiment in CDER that ODS/OSE has only incidental contributions to make to the intellectual basis of new drug review and to recommendations about postapproval regulatory actions. A strengthened ODS/OSE would have much to contribute.

The committee believes that in keeping with the goal of an integrated lifecycle approach to considering drug safety, mechanisms for anticipating potential postmarketing safety issues at the time of approval can be formalized and strengthened. Although OND retains authority over approval decisions, the committee believes that ODS/OSE's role in the approval process needs to be formalized, specifically in the area of postmarketing safety.

3.4: The committee recommends that CDER appoint an OSE staff member to each New Drug Application review team and assign joint authority to OND and OSE for postapproval regulatory actions related to safety.

To formalize the changes recommended above, CDER's GRMP should be modified as appropriate. The ODS/OSE team member should be responsible for formal review of and comments on the clinical reviewer's "Integrated Review of Safety" (Section 7 in the *Clinical Review Template*) and for authoring the "Recommendation for Postmarketing Actions" (Section 9.3 in the *Clinical Review Template*).

Through their active and formal participation in the NDA review process, ODS/OSE staff members would develop a fuller appreciation of the risks as well as the benefits associated with a drug, which some have stated they do not now have because of their exclusive focus on postmarketing safety. That appreciation would strengthen their evaluation and advice on postmarketing safety actions, which have been described as too risk-averse and lacking in understanding of the efficacy data and clinical context, that is, the benefits of the drug to individual patients. In addition, active participation could lead to better communication and understanding between the clinical reviewers and the epidemiologists, who have been described as "speaking different languages." The committee believes that following this recommendation would help to break down cultural barriers between OND and ODS/OSE as staff work together on integrated review teams with the common goal of evaluating and ensuring drug safety and efficacy over a product's lifecycle. However, bringing the two types of staff together in teams is not sufficient to facilitate mutual understanding and appreciation. Additional efforts are needed to apply this ethos to all interactions between pre- and postmarketing, and OND and ODS/OSE staff. The committee was pleased to learn about plans in ODS/OSE to conduct a class to orient OND colleagues to the approaches and methodologies employed by ODS/OSE epidemiologists. The committee hopes that the leadership of the center will initiate other such efforts and sustain them.

The goal of a more integrative, lifecycle approach to drug risk and benefit is to have a preapproval process in which there is more active discussion about using clinical trial data to move drugs out quickly for high-need populations while coupling the process with far greater attention to a comprehensive plan for addressing uncertainties or emerging risks when used after marketing in lower-need populations. Incorporating a lifecycle approach to risk and benefit into various aspects of CDER organizational culture and communicating that fact to all stakeholders could help bring speed and safety into optimal balance.

The committee is aware that consumer advocates, legislators, and others have asserted that the only solution to what, in their view, appear to be intractable problems in CDER with regard to ensuring drug safety and efficacy would be to create a separate center in FDA (or even a separate agency) to work on postmarketing safety. The committee acknowledges the legitimacy of the concerns that underlie such proposals, and it recognizes that if the full complement of recommendations made in this report fails to restore public trust in CDER's (and FDA's) credibility, competence, and appearance of independence, the secretary of DHHS and Congress may have no alternative but to mandate substantial structural changes in the agency. The committee believes, however, that if the recommendations made in this report are implemented fully and change is sustained, other, more drastic measures would be unnecessary. Safety and efficacy must always be in balance, and the ideal organizational solution is a team approach to assessing both. Achieving a balanced approach to the assessment of risks and benefits would be greatly complicated, or even compromised, if two separate organizations were working in isolation from one another. Premarket reviewers develop extensive knowledge based on years of experience of monitoring and reviewing the results of the premarket studies, and the system would stand to lose a great deal if that knowledge were excluded from postmarketing safety considerations.

External Environment

As described above, the environment that shapes the culture of CDER and FDA is the product of societal expectations, legislative imperatives, and economic forces. PDUFA represents a convergence of these factors.

Although PDUFA has led to increases in the speed of review and has facilitated patient access to innovative drugs, it has also altered the environment in CDER, increased the pressure on reviewers to meet review deadlines, and perhaps even affected the agency's relationship with sponsors. The presence of PDUFA performance goals for review timeliness has increased agency accountability to Congress and sponsors and has contributed to the success of this reform in increasing review speed over time. However, the existing PDUFA goals relate only to the speed of approval or non-approval decisions and do not also reflect goals related to safety. If PDUFA is reauthorized in 2007, the committee believes that the goals on which FDA reports to Congress need to include actionable performance goals for drug safety activities in the premarket and postmarketing periods to ensure that important agency functions receive sufficient resources. That would also help to demonstrate that timeliness and safety are valued equally, just as risks and benefits must be assessed together. There are now no explicit safety-related goals that drive CDER's work, whether or not associated with PDUFA funding. Introducing new safety goals would be consistent with the lifecycle approach to regulation.

The committee offers a series of suggested goals to assist CDER in thinking about ways to couple accountability for timeliness and safety. Such goals will ideally be quantifiable. Whether or not PDUFA is reauthorized the committee believes it is important to measure and report on achieving safety goals.

> **3.5: To restore appropriate balance between the FDA's dual goals of speeding access to innovative drugs and ensuring drug safety over the product's lifecycle, the committee recommends that Congress should introduce specific safety-related performance goals in the Prescription Drug User Fee Act IV in 2007.**

Those goals, independent of funding source, could include the following (organized topically):

Expertise in preapproval evaluation:
- Target participation rate for ODS/OSE staff involvement in drug review teams: for priority original NDA and biologic license application submissions 60 percent year 1, 70 percent year 2, 80 percent year 3, 90 percent year 4, and 100 percent year 5; for standard original NDA and BLA submissions 40 percent year 1, 50 percent year 2, 60 percent year 3, 70 percent year 4, and 80 percent year 5.
- Report annually to Congress on the number of new molecular entities (NMEs) for which data were evaluated by external advisory committees, and the proportion of all NME NDAs that that number represents.

Monitoring of adverse drug reactions and Adverse Event Reporting System (AERS):
- Prepare a summary analysis of the adverse drug reaction reports received for a newly approved drug, which identifies any new risks not previously identified, potential new risks, or known risks reported in unusual number not previously identified within 18 months of drug launch or after exposure of 10,000 persons, whichever is later. Reports should be publicly available and posted on the agency's Web site.
- Conduct regular (biweekly) screening of the AERS database, especially 15-day reports, to identify new safety signals.
- Ensure that public access to AERS reports is updated every 6 months.

Postmarketing study commitments:

- Review the entire backlog of postmarketing commitments to determine which commitments require revision or should be eliminated and report to Congress on these determinations. Of commitments that remain, those without start dates should have start dates associated with them to prevent perpetual "pending" status (12 months from PDUFA IV initiation) (also see Chapter 5 for a discussion of postmarketing, or Phase IV, commitments).
- Report completion rates (by company) for (i) postmarketing studies requested prior to approval and (ii) postmarketing studies requested when a drug is already on the market and the number of delinquent studies (past the original projected completion date) in each category.
- Report on enforcement actions taken to ensure timely completion of postmarketing study commitments (for commitments that are currently required, such as those associated with accelerated approval, and for other commitments FDA will be able to require and enforce after implementation of recommendations made in Chapter 5).
- Review and propose action, if warranted, on completed postmarketing studies (within 60 days from submission of the study for actions deemed urgent, 120 days for less urgent actions).

Postmarketing risk communication activities and risk management:

- In the annual PDUFA performance report to Congress, include the timeliness of implementing regulatory actions[10] (from the date of the agency's initial proposed action to the date of the actual labeling change) and the number of such changes.
- In the annual PDUFA performance report to Congress, include the number of patient information sheets developed for new drugs and the proportion of new drugs approved in that year for which patient information sheets are developed. (The committee recognizes that DrugWatch and other activities of the Drug Safety Oversight Board are still under development. The final outcome could affect the relevance and usefulness of this suggestion.)
- Review an applicant's implementation of risk management plans and make the report available on the agency's Web site.
- Review and act on drug advertisements and promotional materials submitted to the agency (within 90 days in year 1, 60 days in year 2, 30 days in year 3 and beyond).

---

[10]Including labeling changes, black boxes, and measures leading to drug withdrawal (see Chapter 5 for discussion and recommendations on strengthening FDA's authority).

Performance management:

- Convene an open forum 12–18 months before renewals of the PDUFA to solicit public and industry comments on proposed and existing safety goals for FDA.
- In the annual PDUFA performance report to Congress, include the status of meeting of all agency safety goals.

Discussion among all stakeholders is needed to consider what goals would be the most valuable from a public health perspective.

REFERENCES

Abraham J, Davis C. 2005. A comparative analysis of drug safety withdrawals in the UK and the US (1971-1992): implications for current regulatory thinking and policy. *Soc Sci Med* 61(5):881-892.

Alonso-Zaldivar R. 2006. *Without Clear Leadership, the FDA Is Falling Short.* [Online]. Available: http://seattletimes.nwsource.com/html/health/2002968229_fda03.html [accessed June 5, 2006].

Berndt ER, Gottschalk AHB, Strobeck MW. 2005 (June). *Opportunities for Improving the Drug Development Process: Results From a Survey of Industry and the FDA.* National Bureau of Economic Research (NBER), Working Paper 11425.

BIO (Biotechnology Industry Organization). 2002 (May 21). *FDA Commissioner.* Letter to the Honorable George W. Bush.

Bridges A. 2006. *Plan B Pill Snarls FDA Nominee Hearings.* [Online]. Available: http://www.nexis.com [accessed August 1, 2006].

Carpenter D, Chernew M, Smith DG, Fendrick AM. 2003. Approval times for new drugs: does the source of funding for FDA staff matter? *Health Aff (Millwood) Suppl Web Exclusives* W3-618-624.

CDER (Center for Drug Evaluation and Research). 2004a. *Clinical Review Template, MAPP 6010.3.* [Online]. Available: http://www.fda.gov/cder/mapp/6010.3.pdf [accessed May 19, 2006].

CDER. 2004b. *Documenting Differing Professional Opinions and Dispute Resolution—Pilot Program, MAPP 4151.2.* [Online]. Available: http://www.fda.gov/cder/mapp/4151.2.pdf [accessed June 20, 2005].

CDER. 2005. *Review Management: Risk Management Plan Activities in OND and ODS, MAPP 6700.1.* [Online]. Available: http://www.fda.gov/cder/mapp/6700.1.pdf [accessed November 14, 2005].

CDER and FDA. 2005. *Drug Safety Oversight Board Membership Center for Drug Evaluation and Research.* [Online]. Available: http://www.pharmtech.com/pharmtech/article/article-Detail.jsp?id=163473 [accessed June 29, 2005].

CDER, FDA, DHHS. 2005. *Reviewer Guidance: Conducting a Clinical Safety Review of a New Product Application and Preparing a Report on the Review.* [Online]. Available: http://www.fda.gov/cder/guidance/3580fnl.pdf [accessed December 30, 2005].

Claver E, Llopis J, Gasco JL, Molina H, Conca FJ. 1999. Public administration: from bureaucratic culture to citizen-oriented culture. *Int J Pub Sector Man* 12(5):455-464.

Coffee JN. 1993. *A Comparative Study of Organization Culture Change in Federal Agencies' Success Patterns of Long-Term Efforts.* Los Angeles: University of Southern California.

Cohn J. 2003. *Politics, Profits & Pharma.* [Online]. Available: http://www.pbs.org/wgbh/pages/frontline/shows/prescription/politics/ [accessed September 14, 2006].

Consumers Union. 2005. *FDA Board Told Proposed Drug Safety Reforms Are Inadequate; Major Changes Needed.* [Online]. Available: http://www.consumersunion.org/pub/2005/04/002149print.html [accessed June 30, 2006].

Crawford LM. 2004. *FDA Statement: FDA Acts to Strengthen the Safety Program for Marketed Drugs.* [Online]. Available: http://www.fda.gov/bbs/topics/news/2004/NEW01131.html [accessed February 23, 2005].

Cummins SK. 2006 (February 10). *New Drug Safety Initiatives & the Drug Safety Oversight Board.* PowerPoint presentation to the Drug Safety and Risk Management Advisory Committee, Gaithersburg, MD: Food and Drug Administration, Center for Drug Evaluation and Research.

DHEW (Department of Health Review Panel on New Drug Regulation). 1977. *Final Report.* Dorsen N, Weiner N, Astin AV, Cohen MN, Cornelius CE, Hamilton RW, Rall DP, Eds. Washington, DC.

DHHS (Department of Health and Human Services), FDA (Food and Drug Administration). 2005 (November 14). Prescription Drug User Fee Act (PDUFA) FDA and Stakeholders Public Meeting Transcript. Bethesda, MD.

DHHS, OIG (Office of Inspector General). 2003. *FDA's Review Process for New Drug Applications: A Management Review.* OEI-01-01-00590. Washington, DC: DHHS/OIG.

Dorsen N, Miller JM. 1979. The drug regulation process and the challenge of regulatory reform. *Ann Intern Med* 91(6):908-913.

Edmondson AC, Roberto MA, Bohmer RMJ, Ferlins EM, Feldman LR. 2005. The recovery window: organizational learning following ambiguous threats. In: Farjoun M, Starbuck W, Eds. *Organization at the Limits: NASA and the Columbia Disaster.* Blackwell. Pp. 220-245.

FDA (Food and Drug Administration). 1995. *Appendix A: PDUFA Performance Goals, FY 1993–FY 1997.* [Online]. Available: http://www.fda.gov/ope/pdufa/report95/appenda.html [accessed June 21, 2006].

FDA. 2002. *Enclosure: PDUFA Reauthorization Performance Goals and Procedures.* [Online]. Available: http://www.fda.gov/oc/pdufaIIIGoals.html [accessed June 21, 2006].

FDA. 2005a. *Guidance for Industry: Development and Use of Risk Minimization Action Plans.* March 2005. Rockville, MD: FDA.

FDA. 2005b. *White Paper, Prescription Drug User Fee Act (PDUFA): Adding Resources and Improving Performance in FDA Review of New Drug Applications.* [Online]. Available: http://www.fda.gov/oc/pdufa/PDUFAWhitePaper.pdf [accessed December 5, 2005].

FDA. 2005c. *FDA Fact Sheet: FDA Improvement in Drug Safety Monitoring.* [Online]. Available: http://www.fda.gov/oc/factsheets/drugsafety.html [accessed February 23, 2005].

FDA. 2005d (April). *Guidance for Review Staff and Industry Good Review Management Principles and Practices for PDUFA Products.* Rockville, MD: FDA.

FDA. 2005e. *Enclosure: PDUFA Reauthorization Performance Goals and Procedures.* [Online]. Available: http://www.fda.gov/cder/news/pdufagoals.htm [accessed July 3, 2006].

FDA. 2006a. *Catalysts for Enactment of PDUFA.* [Online]. Available: http://www.fda.gov/ohrms/dockets/dockets/05n0410/05n-0410-ts00010-gottleib.ppt [accessed July 11, 2006].

FDA. 2006b. *Commissioners and Their Predecessors.* [Online]. Available: http://www.fda.gov/oc/commissioners/default.htm [accessed July 12, 2006].

FDA NEWS. 2005 (October 19). *FDA Names New Director of Drug Safety, Goals for Center for Drug Reorganization Announced.* [Online]. Available: http://www.fda.gov/bbs/topics/news/2005/new01245.html [accessed October 20, 2005].

Fontanarosa PB, Rennie D, DeAngelis CD. 2004. Postmarketing surveillance—lack of vigilance, lack of trust. *JAMA* 292(21):2647-2650.

GAO (Government Accountability Office). 1996. *Aviation Acquisition: A Comprehensive*

Strategy Is Needed for Cultural Change at FAA. GAO/RCED-96-159. Washington, DC: GAO.

GAO. 2002. *Food and Drug Administration: Effect of User Fees on Drug Approval Times, Withdrawals, and Other Agency Activities.* GAO-02-958. Washington, DC: GAO.

GAO. 2003. *Air Traffic Control FAA's Modernization Efforts—Past, Present, and Future. Statement of Gerald L. Dillingham, Director, Physical Infrastructure Issues.* GAO-04-227T. Washington, DC: GAO.

GAO. 2005. *Decision Process to Deny Initial Application for Over-the-Counter Marketing of Emergency Contraceptive Drug Plan B Was Unusual.* GAO-06-109. Washington, DC: GAO.

GAO. 2006. *Drug Safety: Improvement Needed in FDA's Postmarket Decision-Making and Oversight Process.* GAO-06-402. Washington, DC: GAO.

Grassley C. 2005. A bill to amend the Federal Food, Drug, and Cosmetic Act with respect to drug safety, and for other purposes. S.930. 109th Cong., 1st Sess. April 27, 2005.

Grassley C, Baucus M, Graham D, Singh G, Psaty B, Kweder S, Gilmartin R. 2004. *FDA, Merck and Vioxx: Putting Patient Safety First?* Statements at the November 18, 2004 hearing before the United States Senate Committee on Finance, United States Senate.

Harris G. 2004. *At F.D.A., Strong Drug Ties and Less Monitoring.* [Online]. Available: http://www.nytimes.com/2004/12/06/health/06fda.html [accessed December 6, 2004].

Harris G. 2005. *F.D.A. Moves Toward More Openness with the Public.* [Online]. Available: http://query.nytimes.com/gst/fullpage.html?sec=health&res=9A0CEFDE1E3AF933A157 51C0A9639C8B63 [accessed July 17, 2006].

Harris G. 2006a. *Halt Is Urged for Trials of Antibiotic in Children.* [Online]. Available: http://www.nytimes.com/2006/06/08/science/08drug.html [accessed June 8, 2006].

Harris G. 2006b. *Approval of Antibiotic Worried Safety Officials.* [Online]. Available: http://www.nytimes.com/2006/07/19/health/19fda.html [accessed July 21, 2006].

Heifetz RA, Laurie DL. 1998. The work of leadership. Harvard Business Review on leadership. *Harvard Business School Press.* Pp. 171-199.

Henderson D. 2005 (December 6). Whistleblower's case casts further shadows on FDA's ties with drug makers. *The Boston Globe.*

Hendrick B. 2006 (July 21). Respiratory drugs' safety questioned. *The Atlanta Journal-Constitution.* p. 8A.

Hensley S, Davies P, Martinez B. 2005. *Vioxx Verdict Stokes Backlash That Hit FDA, Manufacturers.* [Online]. Available at: http://online.wsj.com/article/0,,SB112467370587619279-email,00.html [accessed October 10, 2005].

House of Commons Health Committee. 2005a. *The Influence of the Pharmaceutical Industry Fourth Report of Session 2004–05 Volume I.* London: The Stationery Office Limited.

House of Commons Health Committee. 2005b. *The Influence of the Pharmaceutical Industry Fourth Report of Session 2004–05 Volume II.* London: The Stationery Office Limited.

IOM (Institute of Medicine). 2005 (July 20). Transcript, *Meeting Two of the IOM Committee on the Assessment of the US Drug Safety System.* Washington, DC: IOM.

Johnson L, US PIRG (United States Public Interest Research Group). 2005 (July 19). *Presentation at Meeting Two of the IOM Committee on the Assessment of the US Drug Safety System.* Washington, DC: Institute of Medicine.

Kaiser Family Foundation. 2005. *Kaiser HealthPoll Report Views on Prescription Drugs and the Pharmaceutical Industry.* [Online]. Available: http://www.kff.org/healthpollreport/feb_2005/upload/full_report.pdf [accessed September 22, 2005].

Kaufman. 2004a (December 19). FDA's reliance on unconfirmed chiefs is faulted. *Washington Post,* p. A01.

Kaufman M. 2004b. *White House Defends FDA as Drug Safety Debate Looms.* [Online]. Available: http://www.washingtonpost.com/wp-dyn/articles/A11900-2004Dec19.html [accessed December 20, 2004].

Kets de Vries MFR, Miller D. 1986. Personality, culture, and organization. *Acad Manage Rev* 11(2):266-279.

Khademian A. 2002. *Working with Culture, the Way the Job Gets Done in Public Programs.* Washington, DC: CQ Press.

Mathews AW. 2004 (November 10). Did FDA staff minimize vioxx's red flags? *Wall Street Journal.*

Medical Officer Retention Subcommittee. 2006. *Medical Officer Retention Subcommittee Recommendations and Response from S. Galson.* Personal Communication: E-mail to Stratton K (Institute of Medicine Staff) from Henderson D (Food and Drug Administration Staff). June 2, 2006.

Miller HI. 2006. *Drug Safety: Image vs. Reality.* [Online]. Available: http://www.washingtontimes. com/commentary/20060321_093254_5884r_page2.htm [accessed May 25, 2006].

National Journal's Congress Daily. 2002. Drug group focuses on renewing user fee legislation. *National Journal Group.*

NIH (National Institutes of Health). 2006. *Charter of the Advisory Committee to the Director.* [Online]. Available: http://www.nih.gov/about/director/acd/acdcharter.htm [accessed September 16, 2006].

NRC (National Research Council). 2003. *Enhancing the Vitality of the National Institutes of Health: Organizational Change to Meet New Challenges.* Washington, DC: The National Academies Press.

O'Leary R. 2006. *The Ethics of Dissent: Managing Guerrilla Government.* Washington, DC: Congressional Quarterly Inc.

Okie S. 2005. What ails the FDA? *N Engl J Med* 352(11):1063-1066.

Olson MK. 2002. How have user fees affected the FDA? *Regulation* Spring:20-25.

Ostroff F. 2006 (May). *Change in Management in Government.* Harvard Business Review.

PricewaterhouseCoopers' Health Research Institute. 2005. *Recapturing the Vision: Integrity Driven Performance in the Pharmaceutical Industry.* [Online]. Available: http://www. pwc.com/extweb/pwcpublications.nsf/docid/EE74BACB6DE454768525702A00630CFF [accessed March 10, 2006].

Racoosin JA. 2006 (January 17). *Pre-Marketing Assessment of Drug Safety.* PowerPoint presentation, presented at the Institute of Medicine Workshop on Advancing the Methods and Application of Risk-Benefit Assessment of Medicines, Washington, DC. Institute of Medicine Committee on the Assessment of the US Drug Safety System.

Ray WA, Stein CM. 2006. Reform of drug regulation—beyond an independent drug-safety board. *N Engl J Med* 354(2):194-201.

Return to Flight Task Group. 2005. *Final Report of the Return to Flight Task Group: Assessing the Implementation of the Columbia Accident Investigation Board Return-to-Flight Recommendations.*

Rockoff JD. 2006. *FDA Chief Took Over Plan B: In Deposition, Crawford Says He Bypassed Usual Approval Process.* [Online]. Available: http://www.baltimoresun.com/news/nation-world/bal-te.planb25may25,0,1214374.story?coll=bal-nationworld-headlines [accessed May 30, 2006].

Ross W. 2006. FDA at 100: alumni take its temperature: as the Food and Drug Administration prepares to celebrate its centenary. *Med Mark & Media* 41(5):52-56.

Sasich LD, Public Citizen's Health Research Group. 2006. *Comments Before the Food and Drug Administration's Public Meeting on the Prescription Drug User Fee Act (PDUFA).* [Online]. Available: http://www.citizen.org/publications/release.cfm?ID=6737 [accessed September 16, 2006].

Senate Executive Session. 2005. *Nomination of Lester M. Crawford to be Commissioner of Food and Drugs, Department of Health and Human Services. S8403.*

Steenburg C. 2006. The Food and Drug Administration's use of postmarketing (Phase IV) study requirements: exception to the rule? *Food Drug Law J* 61(2):1-91.

Stigler G. 1971. The theory of economic regulation. *Bell J Econ Manage Sci* 2:2-21.

Thaul S. 2005. *Drug Safety and Effectiveness: Issues and Action Options After FDA Approval.* [Online]. Available: http://www.law.umaryland.edu/marshall/crsreports/crsdocuments/RL3279703082005.pdf [accessed June 27, 2005].

Tufts Center for the Study of Drug Development. 2005. Drug safety withdrawals in the US not linked to speed of FDA approval. Tufts Center for the Study of Drug Development. *Tufts CSDD Impact Report* 7(5):1-4.

UCS (Union of Concerned Scientists). 2006a. *Acting FDA Director Pledges to Address Abuse of Science.* [Online]. Available: http://www.ucsusa.org/news/press_release/acting-fda-director-pledges.html [accessed August 9, 2006].

UCS. 2006b. *FDA Scientists Pressured to Exclude, Alter Findings; Scientists Fear Retaliation for Voicing Safety Concerns.* [Online]. Available: http://www.ucsusa.org/news/press_release/fda-scientists-pressured.html [accessed July 24, 2006].

Validation Times. 2002 (January 1). PhRMA opposes user fees for further FDA enforcement. *Validation Times* 4(1).

von Eschenbach A. 2006. *Nomination Hearing.* Statement at the Aug. 1, 2006 Hearing of the Committee on Senate Committee on Health, Education, Labor, and Pensions.

Wall Street Journal and Harris Interactive. 2005. *The Public Has Doubts About the Pharmaceutical Industry's Willingness to Publish Safety Information About Their Drugs in a Timely Manner.* [Online]. Available: http://www.harrisinteractive.com/news/printerfriend/index.asp?NewsID=882 [accessed March 10, 2006].

Wall Street Journal and Harris Interactive. 2006. *The FDA's Reputation with the General Public Is Under Assault.* [Online]. Available: http://www.harrisinteractive.com/news/newsletters/wsjhealthnews/WSJOnline_HI_Health-CarePoll2006vol5_iss09.pdf. accessed [September 16, 2006].

Washington Drug Letter. 2006. *Crawford Reverses Stance on Plan B Testimony.* [Online]. Available: http://www.nexis.com [accessed July 26, 2006].

Weick KE, Sutcliffe KM. 2001. *Managing the Unexpected: Assuring High Performance in and Age of Complexity.* San Francisco, CA: Jossey-Bass.

Wolfe S. 2006. *Public Citizen: The 100th Anniversary of the FDA: The Sleeping Watchdog Whose Master Is Increasingly the Regulated Industries.* [Online]. Available: http://www.pharmalive.com/News/index.cfm?articleid=353196&categoryid=54 [accessed July 11, 2006].

Wolfe SM. 2006 (January 19). *Statement before the IOM Committee on the Assessment of the US Drug Safety System.* Washington, DC: Institute of Medicine.

Young JH. 2005 (January 25). *DoD Pharmacy Programs.* PowerPoint presentation at the TRICARE Conference: Fit for Life, Healthy Force, Healthy Families, Washington, DC.

Zelenay JL. 2005. The Prescription Drug User Fee Act: is a faster Food and Drug Administration always a better Food and Drug Administration? *Food Drug Law J* 60(2):261-338.

4

The Science of Safety

The deliberation and decisions of a science-based regulatory agency depend on the quality of the scientific data that it obtains and reviews to make valid scientific judgments. The science underlying drug development is complex and multidisciplinary. As Chapter 2 describes briefly, the early phases of drug development involve basic in vitro and in vivo research to characterize general attributes of a drug. The staff of the Food and Drug Administration (FDA) Center for Drug Evaluation and Research (CDER), particularly in Office of New Drugs (OND) review divisions, works with the industry sponsor of a drug to guide the design and the collection and analysis of those data. The FDA Critical Path Initiative is designed to foster the development of innovative scientific approaches to drug discovery and development. (Critical Path also includes some effort to develop methods for predicting safety problems better, for example, biomarkers of QT prolongation and indicators of liver toxicity; see Chapter 1.) This report of the Committee on the Assessment of the US Drug Safety System focuses on data generated and reviewed further along the development spectrum, so Critical Path will not be addressed in detail, but the committee recognizes Critical Path's importance and the potential for better tools for the prediction and early detection of the safety of pharmaceuticals as biomedical knowledge increases (FDA, 2004). Enthusiastic as the committee is about the potential of new biology and personalized medicine to contribute to the development and use of safe drugs, the promise of the "right drug for the right person at the right time" is not likely to be realized for most patients for some time.

There will always be a need for clinical trials and postmarket, population-based studies to fully understand the risks and benefits associated with drugs, especially to identify rare or unsuspected safety problems. Controlled phase 4 studies will remain important for verifying that drugs approved on the basis of limited exposures and surrogate end points actually have health benefits and for assessing whether common adverse events can be attributed to a drug when such events (such as heart attacks in older adults) emerge as a potential safety signal. This chapter underscores the importance of generating strong science to support regulatory decision-making about the risks and benefits associated with drugs and the importance of ensuring that the decisions made throughout a drug's lifecycle are credible and transparent.

GENERATING THE SCIENCE

Understanding Risk and Benefit for Approval Decisions

As has been described in Chapter 2, a New Drug Application (NDA) and the reviews of an NDA by CDER staff contain thousands of pages of information about the effects of a drug. CDER clinical reviewers are expertly trained to analyze the efficacy and safety data from clinical trials. Individual case reports of adverse events from the trials are reviewed, as are comparisons of event rates of many safety outcomes in the overall product database, including those in uncontrolled safety studies. The reviewers also consider the statistical methods used by the company to generate the results. CDER has issued many guidances and documents of policies and procedures outlining the best ways to review and analyze such data (DHHS et al., 2005; FDA, 2005c). Clinical trials are designed to test hypotheses that are the agreed-on bases for determining efficacy. Trials designed to test hypotheses about serious safety outcomes would in most cases require many more subjects than are needed for an efficacy endpoint. For some conditions, the efficacy outcomes may be surrogate endpoints, which are expected to capture the information about efficacy but are usually not informative about safety.

Safety information can emerge from clinical trials, but rare events may not surface at all; if they do, it is at a rate so low that one cannot distinguish a drug-caused event from one expected by chance (background incidence). Safety information is usually limited to reports of common adverse events, the relation of which to drug exposure can be assessed by comparing rates between study treatment groups, or adverse events already predicted by results of animal studies or in connection with other drugs in the same class. Safety information also includes abnormalities in clinical laboratory test values seen during preapproval trials that may portend occasional clinically significant events. That set of suspected adverse events serves as a starting point for decisions about postmarket surveillance and drug safety research. The safety profile of a new molecular entity (NME) is especially uncertain, because of a lack of information on similar drugs already on the market.

Murglitazar, a drug for diabetes that activates both alpha- and gamma-peroxisome proliferator-activated receptors, was reviewed by FDA for approval during the committee's work. In the preapproval trials, compared with the other arms of the trials (some compared the drug with a placebo, others with another diabetes medicine), murglitazar improved sensitivity to insulin and the control of blood lipids in patients with type 2 diabetes. Those efficacy outcomes are examples of surrogate endpoints because they are expected to predict the occurrence of cardiovascular events. In the same preapproval trials, however, patients randomized to murglitazar had a significantly higher incidence of the combined outcomes of death, heart attack, stroke, and heart failure. The reason for the discrepancy between surrogate endpoints and health outcomes is not clear, but the case of murglitazar illustrates the importance of verifying the assumed health benefits of new drugs and of conducting more complete risk-benefit analyses (Nissen et al., 2005).

As described in Chapters 2 and 3, OND clinical reviewers are primarily responsible for assessing the safety information in an NDA, and interactions and involvement of the Office of Drug Safety/Office of Surveillance and Epidemiology (ODS/OSE)[1] staff vary among OND offices. A recent time-accounting exercise by CDER reports that OND devotes 51 percent of total scientific and technical staff effort on safety-related activities (FDA, 2005a). Despite that large investment of time and effort, the safety profile of a drug at the time of NDA review is necessarily uncertain at the time of approval. The only certainty at the time of approval is that the CDER official who signed the approval letter has not identified safety problems that in his or her best judgment outweigh the potential benefit of the drug for the specific indication and population studied. However, to expect that premarket studies or FDA review of these studies can reveal all the information about the risks and benefits of new drugs that is needed to make optimal treatment decisions would occasion unreasonable delay in approval.

Reducing Uncertainty About Risk and Benefit After Approval

As described in other sections of this report, important new information about a drug's effectiveness[2] accumulates after approval, although effectiveness is extremely diffcult to assess outside the context of a randomized trial. The committee has chosen to describe the major components essential to as-

---

[1]In May 2006, CDER renamed the Office of Drug Safety (ODS) the Office of Surveillance and Epidemiology (OSE). The committee will refer to this office as ODS/OSE in the report in recognition that some statements refer to actions of the office in the past and some statements refer to the present.

[2]Efficacy refers to effects in controlled clinical trials; effectiveness refers to effects in the "real world."

sessment of drug safety after approval as the **generation** of hypotheses based on early safety signals, the **strengthening** of safety signals, the conduct of **confirmatory** studies to identify and quantify new or hypothesized risks and benefits, the **evaluation of risk management programs** to minimize known safety risks, and the **continuing evaluation of risks and benefits** in light of new risk or new benefit information to ensure that the known benefits of a drug continue to outweigh the known risks. The committee concludes that although CDER is involved in a variety of activities to generate and assess postmarket safety information, the current approach is not as comprehensive and systematic as is needed to serve drug safety and public health objectives optimally. The committee offers specific recommendations to CDER and other federal departments and agencies for improving postapproval assessment of drug-related risks and benefits.

Signal Generation

Although some safety signals are generated in laboratory tests and clinical trials conducted in the preapproval setting or from known or suspected biologic actions of a drug, the primary method by which FDA documents new adverse events in the postmarket setting is monitoring of suspected adverse drug reaction reports entered into the Adverse Event Reporting System (AERS). AERS combines the voluntary adverse drug reaction reports from MedWatch, such as direct reports from healthcare practitioners and consumers, and the required reports from manufacturers—15-day expedited reports of serious[3] and unexpected adverse events and manufacturer periodic reports. The information provided by this part-voluntary, part-mandatory system of reporting forms the basis of detection of many safety signals and has been useful in identifying rare adverse events.

Spontaneous AERSs have many limitations, but they offer the possibility of identifying rare serious adverse events in a timely manner among all persons across the entire region to which the system applies. For example, if there is a one-in-a-million serious adverse event applicable to those exposed to a drug used in 10 million people per year in the United States, it might never be observed in a database of several hundred thousand, or even several million people in which the number exposed to the drug might be only a few thousand per year. But in the entire United States it is not so unlikely that at least one such event would get reported. Even a small number of reports of events that are commonly caused by drug exposure, such as liver or kidney failure, aplastic anemia, anaphylaxis, Stevens-Johnson syndrome,

---

[3]A serious adverse event is any untoward medical occurrence that at any dose: results in death, is life-threatening, requires or prolongs inpatient hospitalization, results in persistent or significant disability or incapacity, is a congenital anomaly or birth defect (CFR 312.32).

and so on, can constitute an important safety signal. Spontaneous reporting is subject to certain limitations, including underreporting, the influence of bias in reporting, lack of denominator data, and difficulties in attribution of association between reported event and drug exposure.

Little has been done to optimize the usage of AERS for drug safety signal detection until recently. The work of DuMouchel and others raised the real possibility of doing automated searches of AERS to identify possible associations worthy of further followup. These "data mining" techniques greatly increase the value of AERS data, and that of other spontaneous reporting systems. Developing more rigorous systems in which to investigate AERS signals or any other possible risks of interest is warranted and long overdue; such systems have the potential to improve the ability to develop safety information in a more rapid and more reliable manner. The Centers for Education and Research on Therapeutics (CERTs) are assessing the potential use of health care databases for enhanced identification of adverse drug events. But the addition of new tools such as the use of health care databases does not mean we should abandon the old, especially now that we have methods to substantially enhance the value of these older tools.

In 2004, FDA received 422,889 reports of suspected drug-related adverse events. Of those reports, 21,493 were MedWatch reports directly from individuals (about 15 percent of which came directly from consumers), 162,107 were manufacturer 15-day (expedited) reports, 89,960 were reports of serious events included in manufacturer periodic reports, and 149,329 were reports of other events included in manufacturer periodic reports. As described in Chapter 2, safety evaluators in ODS/OSE review case reports in their drug-class portfolios. That is necessarily very time-consuming. Electronic submission of adverse event (AE) reports makes the system more efficient and timely, although it is reported that only half of the AE reports are submitted electronically, so the AERS contractor must spend time in performing data entry before the information can be reviewed by the safety evaluators.

A safety evaluator receives about 650 electronic reports per month. Review of AE reports can sometimes identify rare or unusual events that require additional research to understand. The following are some drugs for which AEs were identified through AERS: terfenadine (torsade de pointes and sudden death), cisapride (torsade de pointes and sudden death), troglitazone (hepatic failure), infliximab (tuberculosis and opportunistic infections), and cerivastatin (rhabdomyolysis) (Wysowski and Swartz, 2005). Statistical approaches available for the analysis and display of AERS data (such as the WebVDME program) have received only limited use by CDER until recently. CDER staff have recently described how the use of a Bayesian statistical analysis would have confirmed the cerivastatin, rhabdomyolysis, and renal failure association after 6 months of postapproval use if it had been available (Szarfman et al., 2002). Other systematic methods of screening for AEs have also received little attention, although their use appears to be increasing. The committee is aware of the criticisms of AERS, but the committee believes that the planned update known as AERS-2 will useful. The committee supports a focused improvement in how CDER uses passive-surveillance reports as a tool in drug safety research.

> **4.1:** **The committee recommends that in order to improve the generation of new safety signals and hypotheses, CDER (a) conduct a systematic, scientific review of the AERS system,[4] (b) identify and implement changes in key factors[5] that could lead to a more efficient system, and (c) systematically implement statistical-surveillance methods on a regular and routine basis for the automated generation of new safety signals.**

The committee does not intend that review of AE reports, whether submitted by manufacturers as mandatory under federal regulation or submitted by patients or their providers through the MedWatch program, be the primary tool used by CDER for postmarket safety analysis. The committee does not support making AE reporting mandatory. Enforcing mandatory reporting is difficult and the committee's goal is to have better reporting and better use of what is reported, not to increase the workload of CDER safety evaluators with unhelpful information. The passive reporting system in place today is capable of, and has made, important contributions, and the committee hopes that CDER will work to make the current system more efficient. In the next section, the committee offers recommendations for tools that will supplement and complement the AERS system and provide better data for regulatory and public health purposes.

Signal Strengthening and Testing

The development and implementation of a lifecycle approach to the evaluation of the risks and benefits related to drugs will require expanded efforts in signal strengthening and signal testing in the postmarket setting. Once safety evaluators in ODS/OSE or clinical reviewers see sufficient numbers of similar case reports, they have to decide whether apparent signals are real—that is indicative of a problem—or just "noise" in the system. That determination should begin with the application of available tools, such as sector maps and empirical Bayes reporting ratios for analyzing spontane-

---

[4]The committee is aware that CDER is beginning to undertake an information-technology upgrade of AERS.

[5]Such as data sources, coding, quantity, quality of reports, and best use of CDER staff.

ous reports and should continue with more active methods of evaluating signals.

Sometimes, the need for signal-strengthening studies is anticipated at the time of approval. Just before approval, CDER negotiates about phase 4 studies that the company commits to conducting. Chapter 2 includes information about the number of those studies that are not completed. An exception to the inability of CDER to compel the studies is the case in which a drug is approved under accelerated approval. Postmarketing studies range from simple pharmacokinetic studies through analysis of data in administrative databases to controlled trials. The current approach, leaving the negotiations of plans for postmarket studies to the late stages of the pre-approval process, is not optimal and may lead to studies that are not well designed. That is one of the reasons why a large proportion of postmarket commitments are not started or completed. Another factor that could contribute to suboptimal design is uncertainty of OND clinical reviewers about the types and designs of postmarket studies that might be developed, particularly observational studies. It is unusual for CDER to bring in outside experts for independent review and advice about the hypotheses and design of phase 4 studies committed to at the time of approval, but such advice might be useful. As described in Chapter 2, input from advisory committees is often not sought because of committee meeting schedules.

A strong postmarket safety system requires a wide array of data resources that permit continuing evaluations. Some may be directed at tracking patterns of drug use, the indications for the use of a drug in the population, and a general description of the types and frequencies of various AEs. Others may be directed at signal generation. For instance, as electronic medical-records databases are further developed, it may be possible to incorporate real-time reporting of AEs that can be made available to FDA for analysis. Such an effort would require considerable development.

Signals or hypotheses about safety issues may arise from other sources, including known or suspected biologic drug effects that become evident through animal and human studies. Once a potential signal is identified, followup studies are likely to involve the use of a variety of study designs and data sources, including large electronic administrative databases. ODS/OSE has four task-order contracts[6] for access to administrative databases for epidemiologic research. The contractor sites are the HMO Research Network, Ingenix Inc., the Kaiser Foundation Research Institute, and Vanderbilt University (Seligman, 2005). Cumulatively, those organizations cover 23.5 million people, and each has characteristics that make it particularly useful. For example, the Vanderbilt site uses Medicaid data from Tennessee and Washington and thereby obtains information about high-risk and eth-

---

[6]This program had previously been funded through a cooperative agreement mechanism.

nically diverse populations. The Ingenix site has access to some laboratory data in addition to claims data, and the HMO Research Network and the Kaiser Foundation Research Institute sites have access to electronic medical records. Study designs for the contracted studies often are presented to the Drug Safety and Risk Management Advisory Committee or involve other outside experts through the special government employee mechanism for review and comment as a form of scientific peer review.

The funding for the cooperative agreement program is severely limited and the program has always been small. In 1985, the funding level was $1.2 million; since then, resources have varied. Despite inflation in the interim, funding for FDA drug safety cooperative agreements reached a low of $900,000 in 2000 (personal communication, Gerald Dal Pan, FDA, March 30, 2006). In fiscal year (FY) 2006, funding for FDA drug safety contracts totals only $1.6 million, and it is scheduled to decrease to $900,000 in FY 2007. According to an ODS annual report, the contract program in 2004 supported five feasibility[7] studies and three in-depth studies, but in FY 2006 the program will have sponsored feasibility studies for two drug safety questions and will not have sufficient funds to execute one high-priority in-depth study fully—on the cardiovascular risks posed by drugs prescribed for attention deficit hyperactivity disorder (ADHD) (IOM Staff Notes, 2005–2006). In contrast, a similar program funded by the Centers for Disease Control and Prevention (CDC) to study safety problems associated with vaccines, the Vaccine Safety Datalink (VSD), included data on more than 7 million people covered by eight managed-care organizations. CDC supported the VSD with $13 million and eight full-time staff persons in FY 2004 (Davis, 2004).

FDA also works with the CERTs that have access to large healthcare databases, including the HMO Research Network and the Department of Veterans Affairs (VA). CDER has internal access to the General Practice Research Database (GPRD)[8] and to proprietary databases[9] that house extensive information on drug use. Access to the GPRD was expected to provide valuable information to CDER for drug safety purposes, but ODS/OSE has struggled to get sufficient computer resources and staff trained to use it. Four full-time safety evaluators now work with those databases, and two staff epidemiologists work part-time with them in their research.[10] CDER staff presented their first findings from the GPRD at the 2006 summer meeting of the International Society of Pharmacoepidemiology.

---

[7]A feasibility study involves preliminary assessments of whether a database contains sufficient exposures or outcomes in appropriate populations to answer the study question.

[8]A computerized database of longitudinal medical records from primary care practices in the United Kingdom and a source of data for many epidemiologic studies around the world.

[9]Verispan, LLC; IMS Health; and Premier.

[10]Personal Communication, G. Dal Pan, FDA (ODS/OSE), 2006.

VA serves an enrolled population of 7.7 million veterans, their family members, and survivors through its more than 1,300 sites of care, including 154 medical centers. The presence of automated databases and a prescription drug benefit makes VA a promising setting for postmarket drug studies. There are some examples of the use of data from the VA system for studies of the prevalence of AEs (Nebeker et al., 2005) and case-control studies of possible adverse effects of drugs (Shannon et al., 2005). VA and CDER would like to work together to use this resource more broadly, but resource limitations prevent more extensive collaboration. VA populations are included in the research of a few of the CERTs (CERTS, 2006; UI Health Care News, 2006).

There is near-unanimous agreement that the Medicare Modernization Act and the Medicare Part D benefit offer potential new resources for postmarketing drug studies. As of January 2006, an estimated 43 million people on Medicare were eligible to sign up for prescription drug coverage through Part D plans, and the Department of Health and Human Services (DHHS) indicates that 19.7 million beneficiaries were enrolled as of April, 2006 (Kaiser Family Foundation, 2006). Because the elderly are frequent users of multiple medications for concomitant diseases, data from Medicare Part D could play an important role in postmarket drug studies, particularly given the opportunity to create linkages among pharmacy, outpatient, inpatient, physician office, and emergency-department claims. FDA has endorsed a proposal, lacking in detail, to establish a postmarketing surveillance system for prescription drugs that would use billing data and health care information collected from Medicare beneficiaries (Kaiser Family Foundation, 2005). Through the Agency for Healthcare Research and Quality (AHRQ) Developing Evidence to Inform Decisions about Effectiveness (DEcIDE) Network, investigators are developing a methodologic toolbox and data-analytic framework for using population-based claims and administrative data sources in pharmacoepidemiologic and pharmacovigilance research (DHHS and AHRQ, 2006).

This kind of research is labor-intensive, and specialized knowledge is required to use some of the databases. A small number of ODS/OSE epidemiologists and safety evaluators are trained to use the databases directly or to collaborate with other researchers to design and analyze data, and they have limited time to conduct research because of their other responsibilities (such as responding to OND consults, working to develop needed CDER guidances, and preparing for meetings).

The advantages of research using health care databases include the ability to conduct studies of uncommon diseases or understudied populations with respect to drug exposures, minimization of study costs, reduction in the time required to complete a study, and the opportunity to study large numbers of patients. Those systems can also provide valuable information on the background incidence of AEs, which is helpful in understanding the significance of findings in passive-surveillance systems. The disadvantages include missing data and misclassification of key data on outcomes (Hripcsak et al., 2003), drug use, or potential confounding factors. Information on severity of illness or functional status is often uniformly missing (Jackson et al., 2006) and selection bias cannot be prevented from influencing results. The large samples in administrative databases can provide considerable power to assess associations; however, precise but biased estimates of risk are not generally useful. Other disadvantages are difficulties in gaining access to primary medical records (and access to patients themselves), either entirely or on more than just a sample basis; dependence on diagnostic coding systems, which can be problematic for some conditions or topics; and drug-formulary restrictions in some health plans that limit the ability to study newer drugs if they are not on the formulary. Finally, much of the useful clinical information, such as descriptions of adverse reactions, exists only in narrative form, which makes automated analysis difficult (Jollis et al., 1993). There are strategies for correcting for some of the limitations of the databases (such as chart review to find missing data or to improve the accuracy of information), but they are sometimes resource-intensive. Consideration must be given to the strengths and limitations of the data in setting priorities within the program and between research methods for addressing a specific safety problem.

In some instances, active surveillance to generate safety signals and resolve other knowledge gaps is useful. Active surveillance is the regular, periodic collection of case reports from health care providers or facilities. CDER has been involved in developing a limited number of active-surveillance strategies. One example is an emergency room-based surveillance project for drug-induced injury, the National Electronic Injury Surveillance System–Cooperative Drug Adverse Event Surveillance System (NEISS–CADES), jointly funded by the Consumer Product Safety Commission, CDC, and FDA. FDA recently issued a request for information that stated its interest in this regard. In addition, FDA has cosponsored pilot development of a drug-based surveillance system that explores the feasibility of using data-mining techniques to identify safety signals in automated claims databases (DHHS, 2005). NEISS-CADES was used very recently to document AEs associated with stimulant medications used for ADHD (Cohen et al., 2006).

4.2: The committee recommends that in order to facilitate the formulation and testing of drug safety hypotheses, CDER (a) increase their intramural and extramural programs that access and study data from large automated healthcare databases and (b) include in these programs studies on drug utilization patterns and background incidence rates for adverse events of interest, and (c) develop and implement active surveillance of specific drugs and diseases as needed in a variety of settings.

Other federal partners in the drug safety system (VA and the Centers for Medicare and Medicaid Services, CMS, in particular) also use automated databases and should work with CDER, as appropriate, to accomplish the goal of improved formulation and testing of drug safety hypotheses for the entire drug safety system. As will be described in Chapter 7, CDER and its federal partners in the drug safety system will need increased resources to accomplish these goals.

Confirmatory Studies

Passive surveillance, epidemiologic research with administrative databases, and active surveillance can be used to answer many drug safety questions. When they do not provide definitive answers, they can sometimes provide guidance for the development of further studies or provide sufficient information to narrow the uncertainty about drug-related risks and benefits and guide regulatory actions and the decisions of patients and providers. In some instances, full-scale observational studies or clinical trials will be required to answer key questions, particularly if the outcome of interest is common in the patients taking a drug. Such studies are often expensive and time-consuming, but they provide valuable information that less rigorous studies cannot provide. For example, the Women's Health Initiative (WHI) and the Antihypertensive and Lipid-Lowering Treatment to Prevent Heart Attack Trial (ALLHAT) cost an estimated $725 million and $125 million, respectively, but provided valuable evidence about efficacy and safety.

Although $125 million seems like a lot of money, 28.4 percent of the adult population, or about 65 million men and women, of the United States have high blood pressure (Fields et al., 2004), and more than half of them are taking medications for it (Hajjar and Kotchen, 2003). The annual costs of two of the blood-pressure medications used in ALLHAT are about $547 for amlodipine (a calcium-channel blocker) and $83 for chlorthalidone (a low-dose diuretic) (The Medical Letter, 2004). Demonstration that low-cost and older drugs, such as diuretics, are the most effective first-line treatment for high blood pressure can improve health outcomes and save money. ALLHAT also helped to resolve uncertainty about the safety profile of the calcium-channel blockers.

There is no realistic mechanism to ensure that important phase 4 clinical trials are done. As discussed in Chapter 2, some phase 4 studies to be conducted by the drug sponsor are agreed on at the time of drug approval, but for various reasons, many of those studies are never completed. FDA has no authority to compel the completion of these studies, and industry could be reluctant to conduct them because of high costs and the possibility that unfavorable results would negatively influence market share.

A significant impediment to the successful completion of studies is that they are typically negotiated between CDER and the industry very late in the approval process. The study designs can be inadequate, and there is little opportunity given time constraints imposed by the Prescription Drug User Fee Act (PDUFA), for CDER to bring in outside experts when they are needed to help with study design. Experts who are in the pool of potential special government employees (including advisory committee members) can be consulted, but they must be screened for conflicts of interest, and only one can be brought in at a time to comply with the Federal Advisory Committee Act. Although there may be legitimate reasons for abandoning some of the phase 4 study commitments, many could be useful, especially with study-design improvement.

Once a drug is approved, unless the industry sponsor is looking for a new indication for the drug, CDER has no leverage to require further studies by the company. Pharmaceutical companies continue to conduct clinical trials of their drugs, and there is an emerging recognition that these are often marketing-driven and their designs may be inadequate for any reliable assessment of safety or efficacy (Psaty et al., 2006), may underreport AEs, may lead to selective publication of favorable results and non-publication of studies whose findings are unfavorable for marketing (Psaty and Rennie, 2006), and therefore can be misleading. The concept of these "seeding" trials, performed primarily for marketing purposes, is not new (Kessler et al., 1994).

CDER does not have the resources to fund large randomized clinical trials, nor was it ever intended to do so. The drug safety system is currently dependent on the industry, the National Institutes of Health (NIH), or foundations to fund such studies. Other groups have a strong interest in reducing the uncertainty about therapeutic risks and benefits—health care payers, for example—but they have not typically conducted large and expensive phase 4 trials. No entity is responsible for helping to set priorities among the drug safety and drug efficacy questions that need to be examined, particularly with resource-intensive controlled trials. Some studies are necessary for answering questions for regulatory purposes (such as whether risks outweigh benefits and what regulatory action should be taken); others are important for public health purposes and are not likely to be funded by industry (such as head-to-head trials of drugs approved for the same indication).

The potential cost of large safety trials has been a concern for many. A model for "large, simple trials" was established in the United Kingdom in the 1970s; a series of increasingly large randomized trials was conducted to examine regimens for treatments to prevent cardiovascular mortality in those at elevated risk. Those trials were conducted with very modest budgets. Although the costing of trials in the United Kingdom and the United States is admittedly very different due to differences in the way health care and biomedical research are supported in the two countries, there may be ways to conduct trials in the United States with substantially smaller budgets than has been assumed. The increasing computerization of medical data and move toward electronic medical records may facilitate the implementation of more efficient trials with fewer personnel needs. Research into methods for conducting simpler, less expensive trials that might be suitable for answering straightforward but important safety questions is warranted, and represents a logical area for FDA scientific involvement, even leadership.

4.3: The committee recommends that the Secretary of HHS, working with the Secretaries of Veterans Affairs and Defense, develop a public-private partnership with drug sponsors, public and private insurers, for-profit and not-for-profit health care provider organizations, consumer groups, and large pharmaceutical companies to prioritize, plan, and organize funding for confirmatory drug safety and efficacy studies of public health importance. Congress should capitalize the public share of this partnership.

The program for confirmatory studies should focus on the conduct of large, long-term phase 4 clinical trials to evaluate the health risks and benefits associated with chronic-disease medications approved on the basis of short-term trials of surrogate endpoints—such as blood pressure and lipid and hemoglobin A1c concentrations—and on comparative safety and effectiveness studies. The public-private partnership could also consider studies of cost-effectiveness, particularly comparative cost-effectiveness, which is unlikely to be studied by industry and would be very important for those members of the public-private partnership who are insurers and provider organizations, including the VA, CMS, and Department of Defense (DoD). The randomized clinical trial is the optimal method of assessing the efficacy and safety of a drug therapy, but there are other approaches, including analyses of physical or electronic medical records, patients, and specimens identified in the large automated databases and analyses of data from observational studies.

DHHS agencies with an interest in drug safety include FDA, NIH, AHRQ, CDC, and CMS. VA already partners in a limited way with FDA in some drug safety studies, and both agencies express an interest in expanding that collaboration. With a system of 7.7 million veterans and over 100 million prescriptions filled every year and with excellent electronic records, VA would provide valuable data as well as insight and expertise to this partnership. The committee is not aware of any collaborations with DoD on such studies,[11] but DoD provides health care coverage to over 9 million persons and has excellent epidemiologic research capacity, easily accessible research subjects, and a national interest in the safest and most effective use of drugs for troop readiness and cost containment for the largest health care system in the country. That is why the committee included DoD in the partnership. NIH has supported many important such trials, and the committee expects it will continue to do so. Each agency in the collaboration will need staff dedicated to this work in addition to information-technology upgrades and administrative support.

Discussions about needed confirmatory studies should include regulatory findings and related advisory committee input, should address major study-design issues, and should lead to studies that supplement and complement those being done by industry sponsors as part of their postmarket study commitments. The committee urges industry to use the expertise of the proposed public-private partnership for comment on the design of studies and for oversight of study conduct and analysis of results. Proposals for all confirmatory drug safety studies, whether funded or conducted by public or private entities, should be subject to a peer-review process modeled after NIH study sections to ensure scientific excellence.

An important outcome of the partnership should be that federal agencies provide FDA access to all administrative databases[12] (under conditions consistent with the protection of patient privacy) managed by the federal government for purposes related to postmarketing surveillance, safety monitoring and analysis, and risk-benefit assessment of approved drugs.

Funding for the studies planned by the partnership would come from different sources, including congressional appropriations, depending on the questions to be addressed. Some studies planned under this partnership would have been conducted absent the partnership; therefore, the resources needed are not all additional costs to the system. It is hoped that the partnership would help prioritize questions and advise on important study design issues. The partnership might also facilitate collaborations that otherwise would not occur. The committee believes that industry bears the responsibility for paying for clinical trials and other observational studies which support a product's approval and its safe and effective use (e.g., specific

---

[11]DoD and other agencies have collaborated in planning and analyzing complementary studies of the safety of the smallpox and anthrax vaccines.

[12]This could be accomplished by training CDER staff to use the databases directly or to work with staff in the other agencies. In either arrangement, new staff will be needed to implement this recommendation. Access to the databases could be obtained through an interagency task force (either existing or to be created) including representatives of FDA, representatives of federal agencies that manage medical databases, and other members to coordinate and ensure effective use by FDA of such medical databases for postmarketing drug safety.

postmarket study commitments) and that both government and industry, in collaboration with others, bear the responsibility for funding other clinical trials or observational studies performed for broader public health objectives rather than specific regulatory purposes. Industry also has a social responsibility to make sure that its products are safe and effective, so it should contribute to these trials of public health importance. The secretary of DHHS should provide funding for the administrative management of the partnership, but funds for the research will need to come from a variety of sources. CDER will need support from the FDA commissioner and from the secretary of DHHS to use the information from the studies for the best regulatory policy-making. The committee understands that priority-setting and collaboration will not be easy, but they are necessary for advances in drug safety.

Risk Minimization Action Plans

As described above, some drug safety problems are suspected, some are unknown and unsuspected, and others are known at the time of approval. Risk management is an iterative process that encompasses the assessment of risks and benefits, the minimization of risks, and the maximization of benefits. The committee views with concern the CDER statement that the "cornerstone" of risk management encompasses "efforts to make FDA-approved professional labeling clearer, more concise, and better focused on information of clinical relevance" (FDA, 2005b). There is widespread acknowledgment that product labeling has not been a very effective means of communication to prescribers about risk management.

PDUFA III required FDA to issue guidances to industry on risk management. The preceding sections of this chapter describe tools to assess and clarify drug risks and benefits. Risk minimization is the effort to minimize risks already identified. Risk minimization action plans (RiskMAPs) constitute a relatively new approach to minimizing known risks of a drug beyond the standard industry responsibilities related to routine risks, such as labeling and reporting of AEs. According to the guidance entitled "Guidance for Industry, Development and Use of Risk Minimization Action Plans," "RiskMAP means a strategic safety program designed to meet specific goals and objectives in minimizing known risks of a product while preserving its benefits. A RiskMAP targets one or more safety-related health outcomes or goals and uses one or more tools to achieve those goals" (FDA, 2005b). The guidance describes the following possible RiskMAP tools:

- Targeted education and outreach to communicate risks and appropriate safety behaviors to healthcare practitioners or patients.

- Reminder systems, processes, or forms to foster reduced-risk prescribing and use.
- Performance-linked access systems that guide prescribing, dispensing,
  and use to target the population and conditions of use most likely to
  confer benefits and to minimize particular risks.

NDAs for NMEs are required to include RiskMAPs, but at the time of
approval most non-NMEs will not need RiskMAPs. Known risks can be addressed through standard industry and CDER activities. Information about
possible risks can be sufficiently uncertain that appropriate minimization
strategies are not obvious.

RiskMAPs can also be developed or modified after marketing. Every
RiskMAP should be viewed as a "living document" that evolves throughout
the lifecycle of a drug. One of the best examples is the case of isotretinoin, a
teratogenic drug indicated for severe cystic acne. The risk minimization activities for this drug have increased in complexity. The Pregnancy Prevention
Program (PPP) was established in 1988 in an attempt to prevent exposure of
pregnant women to isotretinoin. The PPP asked female users of isotretinoin
to enroll voluntarily in a survey administered by Boston University's Sloane
Epidemiology Unit and enrolled 45 percent of women of reproductive age
who were using the drug. Of these women, 36 percent did not have any type
of pregnancy test before beginning treatment, and about 900 pregnancies
occurred among enrollees during 1989–1998 (No Author, 2000). A new
program, SMART (System to Manage Accutane Related Teratogenicity),
was implemented in 2002 (Levine A, 2002; Honein et al., 2004). SMART
retained the voluntary registration of PPP and

- Added a requirement for two negative pregnancy tests before the
  first prescription with the second pregnancy test occurring during
  menses.
- Added qualification stickers on each prescription to confirm that the
  patient had agreed to use contraception and had signed an informed
  consent about the teratogenic risks posed by isotretinoin and to
  verify that the physician had confirmed the negative pregnancy tests
  and had counseled the patient about participation in the voluntary
  followup survey.
- Added a requirement that prescriptions not be filled without a qualification sticker.
- Added a requirement that prescriptions not be filled more than 7 days
  later than the qualification date on the sticker.
- Added a restriction that limited all prescriptions to a 30-day
  supply.
- Disallowed automatic refills and telephoned-in prescriptions.

• Increased incentives for survey participation.

The first-year evaluation of SMART found that 127 pregnancies were reported among isotretinoin users in the year before SMART (April 1, 2001, to March 31, 2002) and 120 during SMART's first year (April 1, 2002, to March 31, 2003) (Avigan and DalPan, 2004; Pitts and Karwoski, 2004; Ackermann Shiff et al., 2006).

The ineffectiveness of SMART led to a more aggressive approach. iPLEDGE, the risk management program instituted in March 2006, drew praise for its comprehensiveness but criticism that the complicated responsibilities for patients, prescribing physicians, and dispensing pharmacists would discourage use. Key components of iPLEDGE are registration of patients and pharmacists, documentation by female patients of child-bearing potential of two forms of contraception and a laboratory-confirmed negative pregnancy test, verification by the pharmacist that the prescription is valid, and distribution of a medication guide.

RiskMAPs are a fairly new development, and an FDA guidance acknowledges the need for evaluation of plan performance (FDA, 2005b). PDUFA III gave ODS/OSE a role in the review and evaluation of risk management plans. The PDUFA III goals call for ODS/OSE participation in pre-NDA meetings and pre-biologic license application meetings to discuss preliminary risk management plans and proposed observational studies and, in the period 2–3 years after approval, to evaluate risk management plans after implementation.

4.4: The committee recommends that CDER assure the performance of timely and scientifically-valid evaluations (whether done internally or by industry sponsors) of Risk Minimization Action Plans (RiskMAPs). This review should include determining whether an individual RiskMAP is effective and overall evaluations of the strategies used and the processes of CDER staff and industry sponsors for planning and implementing RiskMaps. Evaluations should consider burdens and consequences in addition to design and effectiveness.

Risk-Benefit Analyses Throughout the Lifecycle

The regulatory decision to approve a drug requires the determination that the benefits of the drug outweigh the risks associated with it when used for the indication for which the drug is approved. That is, the drug must demonstrate a favorable risk-benefit profile. As a country we have chosen to place a significant degree of decision-making about the availability and potential use of medicines in the hands of a science-based regulatory body.

The FDA is the first gatekeeper regarding access to drugs in exercising approval authority. Some drugs, perhaps even many, will not and should not be permitted to be used by patients who expect their medicines to be safe and effective. Some believe that drugs should be made much more freely available on the market for anyone who wishes to use them, particularly if the patient has a fatal disease for which they are willing to take the chance that a drug will have little benefit and possibly many serious risks (Burroughs and Walker, 2006). For many of these situations, accelerated approval was developed as a mechanism to make selected promising drugs available early in their evaluation.[13] However, it is widely accepted that the FDA has the authority to determine whether the risk-benefit profile for a drug is appropriate to release the drug on the market. Whether the "bar" for approval is too high or too low for particular drugs has not been the focus of this committee's efforts. In practice, once a drug is approved, health care providers and patients make many decisions about use of a drug. In this section we discuss ways that the regulator can make those decisions easier, by being more explicit about what is known and not known about the sum total of a drug's benefits and its risks.

As described elsewhere in this report, there are many uncertainties at the time of approval. Eliminating all those uncertainties prior to approval would require an unreasonable number of premarketing studies and would have serious implications not only for pharmaceutical companies in terms of research and development but also for patients awaiting new and important medicines. What regulators and drug sponsors know about the drug at approval will change over time. Some of that new information will pertain to the benefits of potential new indications for the drug and other new information will pertain to the risks or adverse effects of the drug. For example, the results of additional studies completed during a drug's postapproval period can alter our understanding and perception of the risk-benefit profile and result in new actions on the part of FDA, clinicians, and the public.

FDA reviews a drug for benefits and risks from the perspective of its intended use (the indication in a population), but in most instances, the drug will not have been evaluated for so-called off-label use. Spontaneous reports of adverse events may indicate a potential safety problem and warrant a safety study. Safety and effectiveness data from studies on uses other than the approved indication are gathered if the sponsoring company is studying the drug in clinical trials for a supplemental NDA for a new indication or if sufficient off-label use occurs. Formal studies of safety and/or effectiveness can also be undertaken. There is a "rolling" or incremental increase in information about the risk-benefit of most drugs after licensure and the

---

[13]Other mechanisms to increase access to drugs include compassionate use protocols and enrollment in clinical trials.

committee is interested in formalizing the accumulation, integration, and communication of that increased and improved knowledge.

In both the preapproval and the postmarketing setting, the risk-benefit analysis that currently goes into regulatory decisions appears to be ad hoc, informal, and qualitative. For preapproval, review divisions work relatively autonomously under general guidance on how to review applications in the absence of clear guidelines about how to make the final decision regarding approval (FDA, 2005c). Some variability is necessary, due to the very nature of the drugs themselves. Considerations regarding the balance of efficacy and safety for a new drug to treat a fatal condition are different from those for the tenth drug in a therapeutic category to treat minor symptoms. However, variability in how review divisions operate is of concern to industry (Tilson et al., 2006) and to CDER. CDER leaders have expressed interest in standardizing their means of analyzing risk and benefit and in doing so, when possible, in an integrated way. A recent study by Boston Consulting Group performed for Pharmaceutical Research and Manufacturers of America (PhRMA) confirms that CDER lacks standard approaches to this important responsibility (Tollman, 2006). Consistency in the approval process will benefit the drug sponsors in preparing their NDA packages and in planning postmarket study commitments.

In addition, increased efforts at risk-benefit analysis will help support postapproval decision making by regulators, drug sponsors, physicians, and patients. More robust risk-benefit analyses can provide quantitative estimates that may be useful to clinicians and patients in deciding whether to use a medicine. For example, a recent publication summarizing safety outcomes from the WHI used a relatively simple table to present results from that study (see Table 4-1). The WHI was three large clinical trials in one, and the major interventions were hormone replacement therapy, low-fat diets, and calcium plus vitamin D. The main outcomes for the comparison of estrogen plus progestin with placebo are summarized in the table (Women's Group for the Women's Health Initiative Investigators, 2002). When all types of outcomes are treated as equal, hormone replacement therapy is associated with an overall increase in adverse health events of about 20 per 10,000 women per year. Women will vary in their baseline risk of these types of disease conditions; however, they will also vary in the preferences for avoiding one type of disease condition or another as well as in their views about the value of symptomatic relief from menopausal symptoms. The information from the WHI trial provides patients and physicians with a useful empirical basis for the discussion of risks and benefits relating to the use of combined hormone therapy. Moreover, risk-benefit analyses can help to identify what key questions remain to be answered and thus generate the most important issues or hypotheses that require additional study.

Integrated comprehensive quantitative assessments and weighing of

TABLE 4-1 One-Year Increase or Decrease in the Number of Major Health Outcomes Among 10,000 Women Taking Estrogen Plus Progestin Compared with Women Taking Placebo

Event Type	Number*
Coronary heart disease	+7
Stroke	+8
Pulmonary embolus	+8
Invasive breast cancer	+8
Colorectal cancer	−6
Hip fracture	−5
Total	+20

*A plus sign means that, compared with placebo, there were more events in the women taking hormone therapy, and a minus sign means that there are fewer events in the women taking hormone therapy.

SOURCE: Adapted from Women's Group for the Women's Health Initiative Investigators (2002).

risks and benefits are far from perfect. Some misleading analyses (with resulting inappropriate regulatory or clinical decision making) are likely because of imperfect information. Nevertheless, the potential advantages of having a systematic approach to risk-benefit analysis for prescription drugs include increasing consistency of approach to approval decisions among the review divisions; a growing common understanding about the criteria for approval and other regulatory actions; increased transparency for the industry, health care providers, patients, and researchers; increased credibility of FDA and CDER; and direct assessments of comparable drugs. Ideally, the weighing of a product's risks and benefits will be both transparent and reproducible.

The barriers to moving pharmaceutical risk-benefit assessment toward a more systematic and scientific endeavor include those related to data and to methods. Data are a primary rate-limiting factor in the evaluation of risks and benefits. Information on a drug's risks and benefits comes from preclinical and clinical studies, but it is phase 3 clinical trials that provide the bulk of the data used to make risk-benefit determinations at the time of approval. Risk or safety assessment is limited by what is missing. Most important for risk assessment is the lack of information that would enable estimation of event rates, their comparison across treatment groups, and evaluation of causality. Findings from preapproval clinical trials may suggest safety signals, but the numbers of events tend to be small and may not lend themselves to precise statistical analyses. The trials lack the ability, both because of their size and because of the relative homogeneity of the typical clinical trial population, to yield confident statements about the plausible range of risks that would affect the populations who would actually take the drug if it were approved. Therefore, when a safety signal is apparent but uncertain, in some cases additional studies should be designed to reduce the uncertainty about potential risk. Benefit data may also be limited by what is missing, namely, information on health benefits if the approval was based on surrogate endpoints rather than health outcomes. Also typically lacking is information on risk-benefit relationships in important subgroups of patients (such as those with severe disease or comorbidities), or large numbers of patients exposed to the drug for long durations, or results of other treatments (head-to-head trials), and on long-term health outcomes.

Regarding methods, a growing set of tools can be used to attempt to quantify the value of research. Because the results of a research program are intrinsically uncertain, the tools are based on a "value of information" approach that identifies the value of research as the expected value of the improvements in outcomes that would be generated by a research project (Meltzer, 2001; Claxton et al., 2005b). The techniques to guide research priorities are beginning to be used in other countries to assess when additional research on a drug should be required as part of a regulatory decision. For example, in the United Kingdom the National Institute for Health and Clinical Excellence has begun to explore the use of the approaches to evaluate research priorities (Claxton et al., 2005a). Quantitative measures of treatment benefits and the application of risk-benefit analysis should consider such factors as the seriousness of a disease, its chronicity, and the effect of a drug on quality of life or the disease process.

Metrics that have been used to measure benefits include absolute differences in event rates, mortality, number of lives saved, and quality-adjusted life years (QALYs) (the relative differences are not nearly as helpful as the absolute ones in this setting). Quantifying benefits in terms of those metrics is difficult or impossible if efficacy is assessed only in terms of surrogate endpoints. Risks can be summarized in terms of incidence, risk difference, excess risk, severity, and duration. Rates and risks are quantitative, but only the more common events that occur with enough frequency in premarket clinical trials can be incorporated into the metrics with any precision. As the comittee learned in its workshop (see Appendix D for the workshop agenda), the science and the acceptance of approaches to simultaneously and explicitly considering multiple benefits and risks for pharmaceuticals and their preferences is evolving (Weiss Smith, 2006).

4.5: The committee recommends that CDER develop and continually improve a systematic approach to risk-benefit analysis for use throughout the FDA in the preapproval and postapproval settings. The systematic approach should have the following characteristics:

- Use the most rigorous possible scientific methods to provide guidance about what information should be collected and how that information should be analyzed and used for decision making.
- Help assure that the studies required to conduct risk-benefit analyses are properly designed to answer key public health questions and completed in a timely fashion.
- Make the product of these analyses available to patients, physicians, policy makers, and researchers in terms that will aid their decision making. Information on the specific consequences (such as treatment benefits and adverse effects) of therapeutic options, and the level of uncertainty about those consequences should be provided for all drugs.
- Provide when possible population-level measures of effectiveness and cost-effectiveness using standard measures that aggregate across domains of health (such as QALYs) to help inform approval and coverage decisions.[14]
- Calculate when possible the expected value of research to guide recommendations about when to perform additional studies.
- Provide guidance about what new data are needed and how those data should be analyzed.
- Be updated as new information becomes available.
- Be described in publicly available documents that are appropriate for all stakeholders.

The benefits of the effort will be harmonization of the work of different review divisions, a growing understanding of the criteria for approval and other regulatory actions, and increased transparency for the industry, healthcare providers, patients, and researchers. The committee believes that with the tools described above, the evidence base on the risks and benefits associated with drugs will be more complete and will serve the health of the public better. In addition to generation and evaluation of data, the drug safety system must be viewed by the public and the prescribing community as credible. The next section describes some concrete steps that will reassure the public that the science on which FDA makes regulatory decisions about risks is credible.

CREDIBILITY OF THE SCIENCE

As has already been discussed extensively, uncertainty about benefits and risks is common throughout much of a drug's lifecycle. Once safety

---

[14]FDA does not make coverage decisions or consider cost-effectiveness, but other partners in the drug safety system do, and this information will be valuable.

signals begin to emerge, unless observational studies or controlled trials are done to examine safety endpoints, difficult judgments about the meaning of data that are less than perfect data must be made. As Chapter 3 describes, CDER's functioning is stressed when there is disagreement about the best course of action in the face of uncertainty. It is important that CDER staff— and industry sponsors, healthcare providers, and patients—believe that the best decisions possible have been made. Confidence in the judgments depends on the expertise of those informing the decisions, their wisdom and leadership ability, and the transparency of the information itself.

Expertise in the Center for Drug Evaluation and Research

The committee has made several recommendations to expand the data on drug risks and benefits to improve decisions. However, appropriate expertise must be brought to bear to plan research and use the resulting data. That expertise comes from the CDER staff and their advisory committees and other non-governmental experts. The committee believes that there is a need to expand the available expertise to take on the new responsibilities described in recommendations made in this report. CDER will need more expert staff, deeper expertise in the staff it already has, and different kinds of expertise.

4.6: The committee recommends that CDER build internal epidemiologic and informatics capacity in order to improve the post-market assessment of drugs. In recognition of the human resource limitations in the current employment market to meet this role, a combination of advancing professional skills through continuing education and support for academic training programs is needed.

Informatics experts should track progress on the national health-information infrastructure, look for opportunities to gather information about drug safety and efficacy after approval, coordinate partnerships with external groups to study the use of electronic health records for AE surveillance, participate in FDA's already strong role in setting national standards and track the development of tools for data analysis in industry and academe, and encourage the incorporation of the tools into FDA practice where appropriate.

Expanded epidemiologic expertise will allow ODS/OSE to apply more sophisticated methods in extracting information from the case reports from the passive-surveillance system and information from administrative databases. ODS/OSE staff could serve as principal investigators for some research projects in the expanded epidemiology-contracts program; this could help in recruitment and retention of staff. In addition, the increased sophistication regarding epidemiologic methods could lead to more productive and respectful interactions with other CDER staff, advisory committee members, and industry scientists. The recommendation in the preceding chapter that would give ODS/OSE staff more responsibilities in both preapproval and postapproval settings will require increased capacity in numbers of staff and in the expertise that ODS/OSE staff contribute.

However, expanding epidemiologic capacity in CDER staff may be challenging. Few academic centers are capable of providing appropriate training in pharmacoepidemiology. That has led to a national dearth of adequately trained personnel in drug safety and risk management (Lo Re and Strom, 2006). A recent commentary from the International Society of Pharmaco-epidemiologists echoes the concern for Europe as well (ISPE, 2006).

Options for improving training in drug safety and risk management have recently been proposed to the committee (Lo Re and Strom, 2006). The federal government has never offered career-development awards in pharmacoepidemiology, except to those whose interests matched the interests of categorical institutes of NIH, which allowed them to apply to those institutes for mentored career development awards, such as the K01, K08, and K23 Awards. The only federal funding now available for training in pharmacoepidemiology is in the CERTs program (see below). The National Institute of General Medical Sciences is about to award its first pharmaco-epidemiology training grant in its clinical pharmacology training program. However, it will contain only two slots per year—this is far too few to meet the needs of FDA alone, much less those of the field in general.

Increasing the epidemiologic capacity of CDER, focusing on ODS/OSE but also in OND if desired, could take the form of hiring new staff with training in epidemiology in addition to their professional medical, nursing, or pharmacy training or could be accomplished through targeted programs of training of existing ODS/OSE staff. That could range from short courses, to the support of degree programs at either the master's or the doctoral level, to a formal training program, such as the Epidemic Intelligence Service program at CDC.[15] A first step in laying out the options for increasing training opportunities could be a committee of ODS/OSE and OND staff with input from epidemiologists from CDC, NIH, AHRQ, and other FDA centers. Priority should be given to training programs with direct links to advancing the scientific work that underpins CDER's regulatory mission.

With expanded expertise and resources, CDER could be a more effective steward of postmarket safety and a more credible scientific partner with industry and academe by actively participating in defining important

---

[15]The committee has not done an independent assessment of how those options are used but understands that they are all viable options.

research questions and designing appropriate studies. More details about increasing CDER resources is presented in Chapter 7.

Increasing the scientific sophistication of the CDER staff should not take place in isolation. The goal is to support good science-based regulatory decision-making, and a corollary goal is to support the research infrastructure of the agency. There is a small research program in CDER and in other FDA centers, but history shows a slow decline in that capacity. The committee notes with satisfaction the recent decision of the FDA Science Board to look into ways to expand the research capacity in FDA.

FDA depends on research conducted by the regulated industry and by academic scientists who are financially dependent on the industry. The committee believes that the scientific reviewers in CDER would be well served by having opportunities to engage in scientific research that complement but do not conflict with their regulatory duties. There is little opportunity in CDER for OND and ODS/OSE reviewers (and possibly other offices as well) to engage in research (DHHS and OIG, 2003). For example, the ODS annual report for 2004 states that ODS staff were coauthors of three papers in the peer-reviewed literature (all of which were with coinvestigators in the cooperative agreement program). The FDA Center for Biologics Evaluation and Research, CDER's sister center, has a long history of research publication in many areas, including postmarket surveillance, as do epidemiologists at CDC, and the committee urges that CDER encourage such efforts.

The progenitor of FDA, the Bureau of Chemistry established in the Department of Agriculture in 1906, created at its inception the Food Research Laboratory to underscore its commitment to science-based regulation, and for over 50 years special advisory committees to the department secretary or the FDA commissioner have repeatedly affirmed the central importance of intramural scientific research to the functioning of the agency (see Box 4-1).

Since 1955, at least six committees have consistently asserted the centrality of high-quality scientific research to the regulatory missions of FDA and called for major changes in the organization and management of the agency's scientific endeavors.

In response to those committees' recommendations, FDA has established (and then disestablished) multiple new research organizations (centers, bureaus, and at least one institute) and repeatedly recreated the senior management position of scientific director under various names. History indicates that those repetitive efforts all failed, and although the reasons for failure are not self-evident, the record points to the common problem of discordance among well-intentioned scientific aspirations, ever-increasing regulatory mandates and complexities, and annual budgets that were chronically insufficient to accommodate the desired objectives.

The admonition of the 1991 advisory committee that the agency "avoid

---

BOX 4-1
History of Reports Regarding Research at FDA

In 1955, the report of the Citizen's Advisory Committee on the Food and Drug Administration to the secretary of health, education, and welfare, stated: "Research is the heart of any scientific operation. Although the FDA is primarily a regulatory agency, it must engage in research of the sort that leads to more accurate scientific methods for determining whether a food or drug is safe. Such research in scientific methodology, and perhaps a limited amount of what might be termed 'random research,' can do much to upgrade the professional competence, elevate the morale of scientific workers, and contribute to the general effectiveness of the FDA."

In May 1991, the final report of the Advisory Committee on the Food and Drug Administration, convened by the secretary of health and human services asserted: "In an era of rapid technological advancement, the FDA must reaffirm its commitment to research as an integral component of its activities. The FDA's intramural and extramural research projects must be linked to the Agency's primary functions . . . High levels of scientific expertise are required to review product applications and to respond to public health crises . . . FDA scientists who are actively engaged in research help build a vital foundation of Agency understanding and expertise. Without that foundation, the Agency's ability to address emerging regulatory problems is hampered. It is essential that the FDA avoid being blind-sided by rapid advances in biomedical science and technology."

For more information see: Science Board to the Food and Drug Administration. 1955. Appendix D, An Abbreviated History of at Least Four Decades of Efforts to Upgrade the Quality of Science in the FDA.

---

being blind-sided by rapid advances" in biomedical and other sciences and technologies resonates with the present committee, which reaffirms the importance of a robust program of intramural scientific research to inform FDA's regulatory deliberations and actions. Such an intramural program would provide an excellent interface with the agency's relatively modest investments in extramural research conducted by CERTs and other contractors. The committee applauds those extramural investments and does not intend that they be threatened by the recommended strengthening of the intramural research program. On the contrary, the committee believes that there is an abundance of extraordinary research opportunities that could substantially enhance the agency's regulatory processes with respect to both the efficacy and the safety of new therapeutics. Many of the opportunities involve the creation and application of new algorithms and methods to improve the processes of preclinical and clinical drug development and new processes to enable effective safety and efficacy monitoring and evaluation over the entire lifecycle of a therapeutic. If FDA is to take advantage of the many research opportunities, research must be recognized as critical to its core mission and be adequately funded. Opportunities for research bring opportunities for real and perceived conflicts of interest, and the committee urges that these be watched carefully. The committee urges that the research opportunities be linked explicitly to FDA's regulatory mission. The committee affirms that a strong program of intramural scientific research provides an essential foundation for sound, science-based regulatory policy and performance.

4.7: The committee recommends that the Commissioner of FDA demonstrate commitment to building the Agency's scientific research capacity by:

a. Appointing a Chief Scientist in the office of the Commissioner with responsibility for overseeing, coordinating, and ensuring the quality and regulatory focus of the agency's intramural research programs.
b. Designating the FDA's Science Board as the extramural advisory committee to the Chief Scientist.
c. Including research capacity in the Agency's mission statement.
d. Applying resources to support intramural research approved by the Chief Scientist.
e. Ensuring that adequate funding to support the intramural research program is requested in the Agency's annual budget request to Congress.

Advisory Committees

Chapter 2 describes some basic characteristics of FDA drug-product advisory committees. Those experts and their input constitute an important resource for FDA in tackling particularly difficult or challenging questions related to its regulated products. Scientific advances, changing technology, and the increasing complexity of new drug products have necessitated the establishment of a strong advisory committee system. Through its advisory committees, FDA can seek advice experts from outside the agency who serve as "special government employees". The system enables FDA to tap into critical expertise at major research institutions.

Advisory committees are used as a source of independent advice about questions raised by the agency regarding new drugs in the review process, safety or efficacy issues that emerge after drug approval, methodological approaches in study design, conduct or analysis, and policy issues. Committees may be asked to comment on whether there are sufficient data to support product approval. They may be asked to comment on some aspect of safety, effectiveness, or clinical development peculiar to a product. They may also be asked to recommend whether additional studies are needed for some products or whether changes should be made to a drug's label in response to new risk information. Typically, after presentations by the sponsor, agency representatives, and a public comment period, advisors will vote on the questions posed to them. Advisory committee recommendations are not binding, but the agency usually abides by them.[16]

FDA uses its advisory committees selectively because of time and cost considerations. Typically, advisory committees are involved in decisions involving new or complex technologies or issues that involve some element of controversy. Advisory committees tackle issues that do not have simple answers. Soliciting the advice of an advisory committee is usually at the discretion of the division director of one of FDA's five product centers.

Advisory committees promote several goals of the agency. They contribute to the quality of agency decisions and ensure that important public health decisions are based on informed and expert advice. They also increase the transparency of those decisions in that the transcripts of all meetings and the material presented at the meetings are made public, and the meetings receive much mass-media attention. The use of such critical outside expertise to inform agency decision-making lends credibility to the agency's decisions. In addition, because advisory committees always include a consumer or patient representative to provide insight or feedback about the public's or patient's perspective, those meetings are among the few opportunities for the public to play an active role in FDA decisions. Participation in the public comment period is another such opportunity.

The present system has served the agency well, but several factors have made the use of advisory committees more challenging. Review deadlines adopted as part of PDUFA have made it increasingly difficult for the agency to convene advisory committees for questions related to product approval. With review deadlines for priority-rated drugs set at 6 months (10 months for standard-rated drugs), the agency is hard pressed to complete its review, formulate its questions for the advisory committee, and then schedule the meeting within a timeframe that permits these 6-month deadlines to be met. Such committees typically must be scheduled 2 months in advance, so regulators cannot fully anticipate the questions or problems that they will encounter in the review process (DHHS and OIG, 2003; IOM Staff Notes,

---

[16]It is precisely the practice of following advisory committee recommendations that makes the Plan B controversy so notable.

2005–2006). The problem is mainly one of logistics, timing, and complying with the regulations for using special government employees, including the process for considering conflict of interest.

Some in the agency have suggested that the review deadlines have forced them to plan for advisory committee input too early in the process, before the questions to be presented have been fully developed and the appropriate expertise is fully recognized, and hence reduced the effectiveness of this important agency resource. Data also show that from 1998 to 2001 there was a 50 percent reduction in the agency's use of advisory committees for approved NMEs and priority drugs (DHHS and OIG, 2003). NMEs and in particular priority-rated drugs are the most innovative and complex new drug products and have been shown to be associated with increased drug risks (Olson, 2004). Although reduction in product submissions has contributed in part to the decline in use of advisory committees, FDA managers indicate that they have little time to hold advisory committee meetings within the current review deadlines (DHHS and OIG, 2003:11–12). The reduction in the use of the committees has important implications for the agency. Reduction in input from informed independent experts may reduce the quality of the decisions and thereby lead to a reduction in public confidence in the agency. Reduction in use of advisory committees also reduces the public's role in FDA decisions and reduces the transparency and perhaps the credibility of the regulatory decisions in the public's mind.

4.8: The committee recommends that FDA have its advisory committees review all NMEs either prior to approval or soon after approval to advise in the process of ensuring drug safety and efficacy or managing drug risks.

The committee recognizes that it might be impossible for all NMEs to be reviewed by an advisory committee before approval, because of the time constraints described elsewhere. However, it believes that such review is important and allows for review of the drug after approval if preapproval review is not possible. If FDA is granted the authorities that the committee believes it should have (as described in Chapter 5), there will ample opportunity for useful input even after approval. Careful review of phase 4 study designs by advisory committees and/or by the public-private partnership should obviate concerns that giving CDER more control over phase 4 studies could be wasteful and inefficient. The goal is for better-designed studies that will be conducted and answer needed questions.

The committee has concerns about the composition of product-specific advisory committees. Traditionally a statistician serves on these committees, but other than Drug Safety and Risk Management (DSaRM) Committee, there is no guidance related to epidemiology or other public health expertise.

Because consideration of risk and benefit often depends on understanding the population perspective and review of observational studies and because drug safety problems are not reviewed only by DSaRM, the committee would like to ensure that the recommendations of advisory committees are based on a broad spectrum of disciplinary expertise.

> **4.9: The committee recommends that all FDA drug product advisory committees, and any other peer review effort such as mentioned above for CDER-reviewed product safety, include a pharmacoepidemiologist or an individual with comparable public health expertise in studying the safety of medical products.**

In addition to concerns about advisory committee expertise and appropriate review, the committee shares concerns about the appearance of independence of advisory committees as it is affected by financial relationships of members with pharmaceutical or other private interests. In making the determination of whether a financial interest poses a conflict, FDA applies the terms of two statutes, 18 U.S.C. § 208, and 21 U.S.C. § 505(n). Under both, FDA may grant a waiver of any conflict of interest provided that some criteria are met. In addition, both statutes provide for public disclosure of financial interest information when a waiver has been granted (see 18 U.S.C. § 208(d)(1) and 21 U.S.C. § 355(n)(4)).

The guidance "FDA Guidance on Conflict of Interest for Advisory Committee Members, Consultants and Experts" describes the type and amount of information that is considered in deciding whether a financial interest presents a potential conflict of interest that needs to be merely disclosed or needs to be reviewed by the ethics staff for consideration of a waiver regarding a topic to be discussed by the advisory committee whose meeting the special government employee is attending (FDA, 2000). Table 4-2 describes key information considered as a level of financial interest that is transmitted to the ethics staff in a memo but does not require a waiver although it is disclosed to the public. For interests that exceed such levels, FDA uses a "sliding scale" to decide whether levels of conflict of interest are acceptable. Levels are different for participation in a "general matter"[17]

---

[17]A particular matter of general applicability is a matter that is focused on the interests of a discrete and identifiable class of persons but does not involve specific parties. For example, a guidance document that affects an entire class of products and all similarly situated manufacturers is a matter of general applicability. In addition, the use of a potential product solely as a model or example for general discussion whose results will apply to a class of products may be a matter of general applicability.

TABLE 4-2 Conflicts of Interest That Lead to a "Cover Memo" Only (Disclosure Required, but Waiver)

Type of Conflict of Interest	Party Matters	General Matters	Any Matter
Stocks and Investments	Stock value is less than or equal to $5,000 in aggregate *(5 CFR 2640.202(a) de minimis exemption)*	Stock value is less than or equal to $25,000 per entity/$50,000 in aggregate *(5 CFR 2640.202(b) de minimis exemption)*	
Primary Employment	SGE is a federal employee and his agency, not his organizational component, is conducting research on the product under review—funding from the sponsor is less than $500,000/per year	Matters will not have a special or distinct effect on the SGE or employer, the committee's decision may affect SGE/employer only as a part of a class of product manufacturers (5 CFR 2640.203 (g) *exemption for non-Federal employment interests of SGEs on advisory committees)* SGE is a federal employee, and his agency is conducting research for one or more firms with an interest in the general matter before the committee	

continued

TABLE 4-2 Continued

Type of Conflict of Interest	Party Matters	General Matters	Any Matter
Consultant/ Advisor	SGE receives less than $10,000 per source per year and consulting on unrelated issue in the past or completed within the past 12 months (all monies paid)	SGE receives less than $10,000 per source per year and consulting on related or unrelated issue completed within the past 12 months (all monies paid)	
	SGE receives between $10,000 and $50,000 per source per year and consulting on unrelated issue in the past or completed within the past 12 months (all monies paid)	SGE receives between $10,000 and $50,000 per source per year and consulting on related or unrelated issue completed within the past 12 months (all monies paid)	
		SGE receives more than $50,000 per source per year and consulting on related or unrelated issue completed within the past 12 months (all monies paid)	

TABLE 4-2 Continued

Type of Conflict of Interest	Party Matters	General Matters	Any Matter
Contracts/ Grants/ CRADAs	Remuneration is less than $100,000 per source per year to institution/$10,000 per source per year as salary support to the SGE and work on unrelated product is currently active or completed within the past 12 months	Remuneration is less than $100,000 per source per year to institution/$10,000 per source per year as salary support to the SGE and work on unrelated matter is current or completed within the past 12 months	
		Remuneration is less than $100,000 per source per year to institution/$10,000 per source per year as salary support to the SGE and work on related matter has been completed over a year ago	
		Remuneration is between $100,000–$300,000 per source/year to institution/$10,000–$15,000 per source/year as salary support to the SGE and work on unrelated matter is current or completed within past 12 months	
Patents/ Royalties/ Trademarks	SGE receives less than $15,000 in royalties per affected source annually and SGE has a patent on an unrelated product, licensed by a competing firm, and receives royalties		
Expert Witness		Remuneration is less than $5,000 per affected source per year and SGE makes no statement for or against any product of a sponsor or competitor	

continued

TABLE 4-2 Continued

Type of Conflict of Interest	Party Matters	General Matters	Any Matter
Teaching/ Speaking/ Writing			SGE receives less than $5,000 per source per year and topic is unrelated to the particular matter and SGE receives no compensation
			SGE receives less than $5,000 per source per year and topic is unrelated and SGE is compensated
			SGE receives less than $5,000 per source per year and topic is related but SGE receives no compensation (including travel)
			SGE receives less than $5,000 per source per year and topic is related but not specific to the matter under discussion by the committee and SGE is compensated

TABLE 4-2 Continued

Type of Conflict of Interest	Party Matters	General Matters	Any Matter
Department Heads— Contracts/ Grants/ CRADAs	Remuneration is less than $300,000 per source per year to SGE's department and work on unrelated matter is current or has been completed within the past 12 months	Remuneration is less than $300,000 per source per year to SGE's department and work on unrelated matter is current or has been completed within the past 12 months	
	Remuneration is less than $300,000 per source per year to SGE's department and work on related matter has been completed within the past 12 months and SGE had only an administrative role	Remuneration is less than $300,000 per source per year to SGE's department and work on related matter has been completed within the past 12 months, and SGE had only an administrative role	
	Remuneration is between $300,000–$600,000 per source per year to SGE's department and work on an unrelated matter is current or has been completed within the past 12 months	Remuneration is between $300,000–$600,000 per source per year to SGE's department and work on unrelated matter is current or has been completed within the past 12 months	
		Remuneration is between $300,000–$600,000 per source per year to SGE's department and work on related matter has been completed within the past 12 months and SGE had only an administrative role	
Exceptions for Institutional Directors	The interests reported are unrelated to the product at issue or to the competing products (up to $750,000 per source per year)		

and in a "party matter."[18] Higher levels of conflicting financial interests require review by the DHHS ethics office and are balanced against the need for a member's expertise and unique contributions. Waivers can be granted for the participation of members who have more than minimal financial conflicts. That information is disclosed on the FDA Web site and is read at the start of each advisory committee meeting. No policies limit the number of advisory committee members receiving waivers who are allowed to vote on any specific matter.

A recent analysis of over 200 CDER advisory committee meetings held between 2001 and 2004 shows a weak association between the presence of advisory committee members with conflicts of interest and the outcome of votes to approve or not approve a drug for marketing (Lurie et al., 2006), which supports a perception in some that advisory committee functioning is less than independent. However, Lurie et al. acknowledge that "excluding advisory committee members and voting consultants with conflicts would not have altered the overall vote outcome at any meeting studied." FDA responded to the article with additional analyses of the data reviewed by Lurie[19] concluding ". . . advisory committee members and consultants with financial ties to pharmaceutical companies tend to vote against the financial interest of those companies" (FDA, 2006). The committee notes that concerns about voting patterns by waivered advisory committee members presume that a vote by someone with a waivered conflict of interest is a "wrong" or "incorrect" vote, but concludes that there is no evidence to suggest that this is necessarily so.

Although some have proposed that there be a zero-tolerance policy regarding conflict of interest on FDA advisory committees (H.R.2744 Sec. 795), others express concern that such a policy could lead to severely underinformed advisory committees or leave a very small pool of potential advisory committee members. The committee recognizes that many leaders in academic medicine with experience designing and conducting clinical trials receive research support from the pharmaceutical industry and that they conduct their research in an unbiased manner. The committee also recognizes that researchers who consult for industry gain important insights that are needed in the review process. However, not all researchers with some of the relevant expertise necessary for these advisory committees have current or recent industry funding (of consultancies or the conduct of clinical

---

[18]A particular matter involving specific parties focuses on a specific product application or other matter affecting a specific manufacturer and its competing products or manufacturers (such as NDA, PMA, PLA or BLA, or efficacy supplement for a new indication). That is, it focuses uniquely and distinctly on a given product/manufacturer.

[19]Including votes by advisory committee members with conflicts of interest related to relationships with companies that would be considered competitors to the drug whose approval was being voted upon.

trials). NIH, for example, funds clinical trials, and investigators associated with those would bring necessary practical expertise to a drug products advisory committee. The committee also recognizes that financial conflicts are not the only conflicts that could influence votes. It is hard to screen out or to waive positions of intellectual bias (Stossel and Shaywitz, 2006). The committee supports narrowing the policies in place today but acknowledges the difficulties of convening sufficient experts for the numerous advisory committees that review drug products. The committee supports a position of nonwaivable limits, but not a zero-tolerance policy, for financial conflicts of interest on FDA drug-product advisory committees.

4.10: The committee recommends FDA establish a requirement that a substantial majority of the members of each advisory committee be free of significant financial involvement with companies whose interests may be affected by the committee's deliberations. The committee supports 60 percent as a reasonable definition of substantial majority and believes that a reasonable definition of free of significant financial involvement are those involvements that currently require only disclosure and do not require a waiver (see Table 4.2 for a summary). The committee urges that FDA issue waivers for the participation of the other 40 percent of advisory committee members very sparingly. The committee also urges that FDA routinely analyze the effect of their conflict-of-interest policies in protecting the objectivity and quality of committee activities. The committee further urges that each posting of an advisory committee transcript be accompanied by a list of waivers granted and that FDA publish a yearly summary of the number of waivers granted per advisory committee.

Most members of advisory committees work in academic institutions, particularly medical schools and teaching hospitals, and policies of those institutions can help to protect the integrity of those who serve. That is particularly important because the pool of experts in pharmaceutical policy who are free of financial conflicts appears to be shrinking. Pharmaceutical support of research and other academic and medical activities is widespread—a fact that the committee views with some concern. In that vein, it would be helpful if all universities and nonprofit academic healthcare institutions promulgate and enforce rigorous conflict-of-interest policies governing academe-industry relationships on the part of their faculty and their institutional leaders. At a minimum, such policies should require disclosure in all publications, speaking engagements, and consultations with government of any relationships with the pharmaceutical and device industries. Policies should also conform with recommendations concerning conflicts of interest developed by the Association of American Medical Colleges. All universities and nonprofit academic health care institutions should have standing conflict-of-interest review committees that are independent of their technology-transfer functions and are staffed by professionals who are experienced in managing conflicts of interest.

Transparency

All stakeholders in the drug safety system have a legitimate interest in understanding the data on which drug availability in the marketplace depends. Not all people are interested in firsthand knowledge of the science and depend on the decisions of others (such as their physicians and regulator) to assure them that drugs they take are safe and effective. Others wish to have more knowledge of the data. Many data are made public in some form, at some time, and at some place on the FDA or another government or industry Web site, but the process is not systematic, comprehensive, or well organized. The committee believes strongly in the importance of increasing the availability to the public and to researchers of information about drug risks and benefits, whether specific study results or analyses of concerns by agency staff, and it provides several recommendations related to clinical trial registration and results reporting, Web-site posting of all NDA-review packages, and timely public release of all CDER summaries of emerging data relevant to the safety and effectiveness of a drug after approval.

As described in Chapters 2 and 3, information related to the efficacy of drugs approved for use in the United States is examined in extensive detail in the reviews prepared by CDER staff. Most of those review packages are posted on FDA's Web site and summarize a significant amount of data supporting the approval of the drug, yet these postings do not include the entirety of what is known about a drug. A sponsor's NDA is not made public (even in redacted form to protect proprietary interests), and FDA reviews of an NDA are not made public if approval is not granted. Those reviews of unapproved NDAs could provide valuable information about a drug if the application is a supplemental NDA or if it is for a new member of a class of products already on the market. Although pharmaceutical companies are required to submit to FDA information about all studies conducted under an IND, results of studies that are not submitted as part of a sponsor's application package for approval or are finished after approval are not necessarily disclosed to the public. There is no way to know the results of clinical trials involving a drug if those results are not submitted to the FDA as part of an NDA or other review package or are not published in the scientific literature.

Several important efforts in recent years are aimed at increasing the availability of at least a minimum of information about current or completed clinical trials. A recent Institute of Medicine (IOM) workshop provided a summary of the major initiatives by DHHS, the pharmaceutical industry, international medical journal editors, and the World Health Organization (WHO) (IOM, 2006). The requirement in the Food and Drug Administration Modernization Act of 1997 (FDAMA) that the federal government develop a way to register clinical trials of drugs intended to treat serious or life-threatening diseases led to the creation of ClinicalTrials.gov in the National Library of Medicine. Section 113 of FDAMA specifically requires companies to register a trial conducted under an investigational NDA if it is for a drug to treat a serious or life-threatening disease or condition and is a trial to test effectiveness (42 U.S.C. 282(j)(3)(A)). The trial must be registered no later than 21 days after enrollment is opened. Companies can register nonrequired trials in the databank as well. As of July 1, 2006, more than 30,000 trials have been registered on the site. PhRMA encourages its members to do so voluntarily for all hypothesis-testing[20] studies required for the condition being studied.

This registry, which in recent years has won broad acceptance by industry, requires the completion of 20 data fields, developed by the WHO as a "minimum required dataset" for full registration, and provides regularly updated information about federally and privately supported clinical research in human volunteers. The minimum required dataset provides information about a trial's purpose and the therapeutic agent being tested, its primary and secondary hypotheses and prespecified endpoint(s), who may participate, locations, and contact information for more details. It does not, however, include the results of the trials, nor does the registry program have the resources to do so.

In 2002, pharmaceutical companies that are members of PhRMA committed to voluntary disclosure of the results of hypothesis-testing clinical trials for marketed and investigational drugs; and in 2004, PhRMA launched the Web site ClinicalStudyResults.org for this purpose. A review of the site shows great variability in the ease of accessibility and completeness of the information. In addition, in the past few years many drug sponsors have created their own "registries" on company Web sites, which list their clinical trials, and may list summaries of trial results. These voluntary commitments may signify good intentions for increasing transparency, but the history leading to their introduction may, on the other hand, suggest that they may rather represent efforts to avoid mandatory disclosure of results.

---

[20] "Also known as "confirmatory" clinical studies, hypothesis-testing studies are always well-controlled and are intended to provide meaningful results by examining pre-stated questions (i.e., hypotheses) using predefined statistically valid plans for data analysis, thereby allowing firm conclusions to be drawn to support product claims. Hypothesis-testing studies may occur at any stage of drug development and include all phase III studies, some earlier-phase studies, and many studies of marketed products" (Clinicalstudyresults.org, 2006).

4.11: To ensure that trial registration is mandatory, systematic, standardized, and complete, and that the registration site is able to accommodate the reporting of trial results, **the committee recommends that Congress require industry sponsors to register in a timely manner at clinicaltrials.gov, at a minimum, all phase 2 through 4 clinical trials, wherever they may have been conducted, if data from the trials are intended to be submitted to the FDA as part of an NDA, sNDA, or to fulfill a postmarket commitment. The committee further recommends that this requirement include the posting of a structured field summary of the efficacy and safety results of the studies.** The committee does not offer specific details regarding this summary, preferring that NIH and FDA, in consultation with the pharmaceutical industry, should work together to agree on a reasonable plan.[21] However, the committee suggests that mandatory fields could include, but are not limited to, (1) primary hypothesis, (2) experimental design, (3) primary predefined outcome measure(s), (4) planned and actual sample size per treatment arm, (5) number and type of serious AEs, (6) overview of results, and (7) risk-benefit summary. The company should have the responsibility of submitting the structured field summary to the FDA, who should review it for completeness and accuracy. The information should then be posted either on an easily accessible Web site at FDA with linkage to the trial's registration on clinicaltrials.gov, or posted directly on the latter.

For those clinical trials covered by this recommendation, every completed trial would have to comply with this mechanism of results reporting, regardless of trial outcomes. For every covered trial that is stopped before prespecified completion, the sponsor would have to submit a summary describing the reasons for termination (Drug Safety Management Board action, economic considerations, etc.) to FDA/NIH for review and posting. The committee did not attempt to resolve what to do about postmarket studies conducted by investigators independent of industry. If these studies are federally funded, the funding agency could require as a condition of award that the lead investigators prepare and submit the structured summary to clinicaltrials.gov after publication of the study. Enforcement mechanisms for studies not conducted under federal grant/contract support are less clear. The committee believes that to ensure that results to be posted

---

[21]Because the committee is not suggesting that raw data be posted, this recommendation should provoke no concerns regarding patient privacy. The committee recognizes that this recommendation will require significant additional resources to NIH, which runs clinicaltrials. gov, and to FDA, for their role in developing the results format and vetting the submissions.

that are not vetted by the FDA are described completely, accurately, and in an unbiased manner, clinicaltrials.gov would have to establish some form of editorial review process. The National Library of Medicine, which runs clinicaltrials.gov, will need to be provided the necessary authorization and resources to accommodate results posting.

The format of clinical trial registration and results reporting should be done in a way that harmonizes with emerging international standards (such as those specified by WHO, for example, the minimum required dataset for registration, and the requirements for results reporting, in the ICH E3 Summary of Clinical Trial Results). The committee notes with interest the recent WHO call for registration of all interventional trials. The committee strongly urges the Congress to consider the status and benefits of harmonization with international standards when drafting legislative language to implement this recommendation.

The committee also encourages further steps to make drug safety and effectiveness information available to the public. The committee believes that CDER is the appropriate body to assume the responsibility for sharing important safety and efficacy information promptly and dependably with patients, providers, and researchers. One important source of this information at the time of approval is the NDA review package.

In response to the Electronic Freedom of Information Act Amendments of 1996, which were designed to broaden public access to government documents in electronic form, CDER posts NDA review packages[22] on its Web site (at the "drugs@fda" portion of the site http://www.accessdata.fda.gov/scripts/cder/drugsatfda/). As of April 2006, review packages for NMEs approved from 1998 to the middle of February 2006 and non-NMEs approved in 1998–2001 are posted. There is a backlog for posting review packages for non-NMEs approved after 2001.[23] All other NDA approval documents (that is, for drugs approved before 1998 and for all supplements) are posted on completion of a Freedom of Information Act (FOIA) request for that information (D. Henderson, personal communication).

4.12: The committee recommends that FDA post all NDA review packages on the agency's Web site. Regardless of whether they were disclosed in response to a FOIA request, FDA should post all supplemental-NDA review packages and continue to work to post reviews for drugs approved before 1998 in a timely manner and as

---

[22]Review packages are described in Chapters 2 and 3 and refer to the set of documents prepared by CDER staff. These packages provide the summary judgment that leads to decisions regarding approval.

[23]Of 531 non-NME NDA approvals since 2001, 397 had been posted on the Web as of March 31, 2006, as had all the non-NME NDAs approved in 1998–2001.

resources allow. High priority should be given to posting all review materials related to any product for which there are emerging safety concerns, particularly if they have been discussed at an advisory committee meeting.

OND and ODS/OSE staff prepare reviews or summaries of RiskMAPs and other postmarket safety information and, if discussed at an advisory committee meeting, these reviews are made public in accordance with the Federal Advisory Committee Act; however, reports of general ODS/OSE consultations are not, as a rule, made public. In 2005, ODS/OSE completed 439 reviews of postmarket safety issues (generated in ODS/OSE or as a result of consultations for OND). Materials from advisory committees are found on a portion of the CDER Web site distinct from that where the NDA reviews are posted. There is no one place where every public document regarding a specific drug is posted.

The committee recognizes that public disclosure of every internal document discussing a potential safety problem has drawbacks. Any one document likely describes only one aspect of a complicated topic. Full disclosure of those documents in real time could be confusing to the public and does not necessarily contribute to reducing the uncertainty about the risks and benefits associated with a drug. However, there is a marked imbalance between the disclosure of data accumulated before approval (the CDER discipline reviews) and disclosure of data summarized and presented after approval. The synthesis by CDER of postmarketing information that is made public about risks and benefits is minimal. The committee believes that CDER has a role to play in putting forth the views of the regulatory agency about emerging information and should not leave that task in the hands of the pharmaceutical industry or the academic community.[24] Periodic and regular review by CDER of risk and benefit information is consistent with a lifecycle approach to drug regulation.

4:13: The committee recommends that the CDER review teams regularly and systematically analyze all postmarket study results and make public their assessment of the significance of the results with regard to the integration of risk and benefit information.

Drug regulation must follow scientific advances; as science progresses, so must regulation. The role of the regulator is not to impede the develop-

---

[24]Product safety specialists from the Center for Biologics Evaluation and Research routinely develop reviews of the postmarket safety experience with a new vaccine within 2–3 years of the time the vaccine is licensed. These reviews are published in journals and are available on the FDA Web site's VAERS (Vaccine Adverse Event System) page.

ment of innovative medicines, but to ensure that needed drugs are available to patients and that risk-benefit information is accurate and widely available. The regulator must be the gatekeeper of the scientific foundation on which regulatory decisions are made. CDER must have the best data to review and an expert scientific staff to review them. Patients and their physicians must be assured that the scientific foundation on which CDER regulates drugs is credible.

REFERENCES

Ackermann Shiff S, Mundkur C, Shamp J. 2006. *iPLEDGE: Isotretinoin Pregnancy Risk Management Program.* [Online]. Available: http://www.fda.gov/ohrms/dockets/ac/06/slides/2006-4202S2_05-Sponsor.ppt# [accessed June 22, 2006].

Avigan M, DalPan G. 2004. *Overview of First Year Evaluation of the Isotretinoin Risk Management Program.* [Online]. Available: http://www.fda.gov/ohrms/dockets/AC/04/briefing/4017B1-06a%20FDA%20Backgrounder-ODS%20Sec%20C%20Tab%202.doc [accessed July 10, 2006].

Burroughs F, Walker S, Abigail Alliance for Better Access to Developmental Drugs. 2006 (January 19). *PowerPoint presentation to the IOM Committee on the Assessment of the US Drug Safety System.* Washington, DC: Institute of Medicine.

CERTS (Centers for Education & Research on Therapeutics). 2006. *Ongoing Projects.* [Online]. Available: http://certs.hhs.gov/projects/ongoing.html [accessed September 14, 2006].

Claxton K, Cohen JT, Neumann PJ. 2005a. When is evidence sufficient? *Health Aff (Millwood)* 24(1):93-101.

Claxton K, Eggington S, Ginnelly L, Griffin S, McCabe C, Philips Z, Tappenden P, Wailoo A. 2005b. *A Pilot Study of Value of Information Analysis to Support Research Recommendations for the National Institute for Clinical Excellence.* [Online]. Available: http://www.york.ac.uk/inst/che/pdf/claxtonnice.pdf [accessed June 22, 2006].

Clinicalstudyresults.org. 2006. *Glossary.* [Online]. Available: http://www.clinicalstudyresults.org/glossary/#hypothesis [accessed August 14, 2006].

Cohen AL, Jhung MA, Budnitz DS. 2006. Stimulant medications and attention deficit-hyperactivity disorder. *N Engl J Med* 354(21):2294-2295.

Davis R. 2004 (August 23). *Vaccine Safety Datalink: Overview.* Presentation to the Committee on Review of NIP's Research Procedures and Data Sharing Program. Washington, DC: Insitute of Medicine.

DHHS (Department of Health and Human Services). 2005. *Request for Information on Active Surveillance Programs in the United States for the Identification of Clinically Serious Adverse Events Associated with Medical Products.* RFIHHSF200601. Rockville, MD: DHHS, FBO (Federal Business Opportunities).

DHHS, AHRQ (Agency for Healthcare Research and Quality). 2006. *Medicare Prescription Drug Data Development: Methods for Improving Patient Safety and Pharmacovigilance Using Observational Data.* [Online]. Available: http://effectivehealthcare.ahrq.gov/decide/decide.cfm?topic=12 [accessed September, 14 2006].

DHHS, FDA (Food and Drug Administration), CDER (Center for Drug Evaluation and Research). 2005. *FDA's Communication of Drug Safety Information: Transcript, December 8, 2005.* [Online]. Available: http://www.fda.gov/cder/meeting/RiskComm2005/1208fda.pdf [accessed February 13, 2006].

DHHS, OIG (Office of Inspector General). 2003. *FDA's Review Process for New Drug Applications: A Management Review.* OEI-01-01-00590. Washington, DC: HHS, OIG.

FDA (Food and Drug Administration). 2000. *FDA Guidance on Conflict of Interest for Advisory Committee Members, Consultants and Experts Table of Contents.* [Online]. Available: http://www.fda.gov/oc/advisory/conflictofinterest/guidance.html [accessed July 13, 2006].

FDA. 2004. *Innovation Stagnation: Challenge and Opportunity on the Critical Path to New Medical Products.* [Online]. Available: http://www.fda.gov/oc/initiatives/criticalpath/whitepaper.pdf [accessed October 10, 2005].

FDA. 2005a. *Center for Drug Evaluation and Research-Activities and Level of Effort Devoted to Drug Safety.* Submitted to the Institute of Medicine Committee on the Assessment of the US Drug Safety System by the Food and Drug Administration.

FDA. 2005b. *Guidance for Industry: Development and Use of Risk Minimization Action Plans.* March 2005. Rockville, MD: FDA.

FDA. 2005c. *Reviewer Guidance: Conducting a Clinical Safety Review of a New Product Application and Preparing a Report on the Review, Good Review Practices.* February 2005. Rockville, MD: FDA.

FDA. 2006. *Comment on "Financial Conflict of Interest Disclosure and Voting Patterns at Food and Drug Administration Drug Advisory Committee Meetings."* [Online]. Available: http://www.fda.gov/oc/advisory/analysis.html [accessed March 13, 2006].

Fields LE, Burt VL, Cutler JA, Hughes J, Roccella EJ, Sorlie P. 2004. The burden of adult hypertension in the United States 1999 to 2000: a rising tide. *Hypertension* 44(4):398-404.

Hajjar I, Kotchen TA. 2003. Trends in prevalence, awareness, treatment, and control of hypertension in the United States, 1988–2000. *JAMA* 290(2):199-206.

Honein MA, Moore CA, Erickson JD. 2004. Can we ensure the safe use of known human teratogens? Introduction of generic isotretinoin in the US as an example. *Drug Saf* 27(14):1069-1080.

Hripcsak G, Bakken S, Stetson PD, Patel VL. 2003. Mining complex clinical data for patient safety research: a framework for event discovery. *J Biomed Inform* 36(1-2):120-130.

IOM. 2006. *Developing a National Registry of Pharmacologic and Biologic Clinical Trials: Workshop Report.* Washington, DC: The National Academies Press.

ISPE (International Society for Pharmacoepidemiology). 2006. *Response to: "European Commission Public Consultation: An Assessment of the Community System of Pharmacovigilance."* [Online]. Available: http://www.pharmacoepi.org/resources/ispe_response_6-29-06.pdf [accessed July 14, 2006].

Jackson LA, Nelson JC, Benson P, Neuzil KM, Reid RJ, Psaty BM, Heckbert SR, Larson EB, Weiss NS. 2006. Functional status is a confounder of the association of influenza vaccine and risk of all cause mortality in seniors. *Int J Epidemiol* 35(2):345-352.

Jollis JG, Ancukiewicz M, DeLong ER, Pryor DB, Muhlbaier LH, Mark DB. 1993. Discordance of databases designed for claims payment versus clinical information systems. Implications for outcomes research. *Ann Intern Med* 119(8):844-850.

Kaiser Family Foundation (Daily Health Policy Report). 2005. *Medicare | FDA Says It Supports Tracking Medication Safety Using Medicare Drug Benefit Data.* [Online]. Available: http://www.kaisernetwork.org/daily_reports/rep_index.cfm?hint=3&DR_ID=30734 [accessed September 14, 2006].

Kaiser Family Foundation. 2006. *Medicare: Prescription Drug Coverage Among Medicare Beneficiaries.* [Online]. Available: http://www.kff.org/medicare/upload/7453.pdf [accessed August 28, 2006].

Kessler DA, Rose JL, Temple RJ, Schapiro R, Griffin JP. 1994. Therapeutic-class wars—drug promotion in a competitive marketplace. *N Engl J Med* 331(20):1350-1353.

Levine A. 2002. FDA enforcement: how it works. In: Pina KR, Pines WL, Eds. *A Practical Guide to Food and Drug Law and Regulation.* 2nd Ed. Washington, DC: Food and Drug Law Institute. Pp. 271-298.

Lo Re V, Strom B. 2006. *The Role of Academia and the Research Community in Assisting FDA and the Drug Safety System.* Paper commissioned by the Institute of Medicine Committee on the Assessment of the US Drug Safety System, Washington, DC.

Lurie P, Almeida CM, Stine N, Stine AR, Wolfe SM. 2006. Financial conflict of interest disclosure and voting patterns at Food and Drug Administration Drug Advisory Committee meetings. *JAMA* 295(16):1921-1928.

The Medical Letter. 2004. Initial therapy of hypertension. *Med Lett Drugs Ther* 46(1186): 53-55.

Meltzer D. 2001. Addressing uncertainty in medical cost-effectiveness analysis implications of expected utility maximization for methods to perform sensitivity analysis and the use of cost-effectiveness analysis to set priorities for medical research. *J Health Econ* 20(1):109-129.

Nebeker JR, Hoffman JM, Weir CR, Bennett CL, Hurdle JF. 2005. High rates of adverse drug events in a highly computerized hospital. *Arch Intern Med* 165(10):1111-1116.

Nissen SE, Wolski K, Topol EJ. 2005. Effect of muraglitazar on death and major adverse cardiovascular events in patients with type 2 diabetes mellitus. *JAMA* 294(20):2581-2586.

No Author. 2000. Accutane-exposed pregnancies—California, 1999. *MMWR* 49(2):28-31.

Olson MK. 2004. Are novel drugs more risky for patients than less novel drugs? *J Health Econ* 23(6):1135-1158.

Pitts M, Karwoski CB. 2004 (February 2). *Letter to Seligman P and Trontell A, Office of Drug Safety, Food and Drug Administration.* Subject: PID D030417; Drug: Isotretinoin; Topic: Pregnancy Exposure.

Psaty BM, Rennie D. 2006. Clinical trial investigators and their prescribing patterns: another dimension to the relationship between physician investigators and the pharmaceutical industry. *JAMA* 295(23):2787-2790.

Psaty BM, Weiss NS, Furberg CD. 2006. Recent trials in hypertension: compelling science or commercial speech? *JAMA* 295(14):1704-1706.

Seligman P. 2005 (July 20). *Assessing Drug Safety.* Presentation to the Committee on the Institute of Medicine Committee on the Assessment of the US Drug Safety System. Washington, DC: IOM.

Shannon J, Tewoderos S, Garzotto M, Beer TM, Derenick R, Palma A, Farris PE. 2005. Statins and prostate cancer risk: a case-control study. *Am J Epidemiol* 162(4):318-325.

Stossel T, Shaywitz D. 2006 (July 2). What's wrong with money in science? *The Washington Post.* P. B03.

Szarfman A, Machado SG, O'Neill RT. 2002. Use of screening algorithms and computer systems to efficiently signal higher-than-expected combinations of drugs and events in the US FDA's spontaneous reports database. *Drug Saf* 25(6):381-392.

Tilson H, Gibson B, Suh R. 2006. *FDA and the Drug Safety System: The Role of the Pharmaceutical Industry.* Paper commissioned by the Institute of Medicine Committee on the Assessment of the US Drug Safety System. Washington, DC.

Tollman P. 2006 (May 30). *How Do We Currently Assess Risk/Benefit Ratios for Pharmaceuticals? Advantages and Drawbacks of the Current System.* Presentation to the Institute of Medicine Drug Forum: Understanding the Benefits and Risks of Pharmaceuticals. Washington, DC: IOM.

UI Health Care News. 2006. *UI Center to Focus on Therapeutics Use, Efectiveness Among Elderly.* [Online]. Available: http://www.uihealthcare.com/news/news/2006/07/03certs.html [accessed September 14, 2006].

Weiss Smith S. *Summary of Issues: January 17, 2006, IOM Workshop.* Paper commissioned by the Institute of Medicine Committee on the Assessment of the US Drug Safety System. Washington, DC.

Women's Group for the Women's Health Initiative Investigators. 2002. Risk and benefits of estrogen plus progestin in healthy postmenopausal women. Principal results from the Women's Health Initiative Randomized Controlled Trail. *JAMA* 288(3):321-333.

Wysowski DK, Swartz L. 2005. Adverse drug event surveillance and drug withdrawals in the United States, 1969–2002: the importance of reporting suspected reactions. *Arch Intern Med* 165(12):1363-1369.

5

Regulatory Authorities for Drug Safety

Major components of the Food and Drug Administration (FDA) statutory authority have evolved in response to drug-related public health crises and in response to a changing environment. The social and health care environment has changed and continues to evolve—health care providers and patients expect timely access to effective drugs, the user-fee program established in 1992 has increased the pace of drug review and approval, the practice of medicine and the use of drugs have changed, and the information available to the public from advertising and the Internet and from commercial and government or nonprofit sources has transformed consumer knowledge and the patient's role in health care (see Chapter 1 for more information). In view of those changes, the agency's regulatory authority must be reconsidered and strengthened to ensure that it is equal to the task. However, the committee cautions against assuming that altering the statute alone will solve all difficulties related to FDA's regulatory authorities. FDA needs considerable new resources to perform optimally in a fast changing, challenging environment, including resources to support its regulatory activities, such as regulatory oversight of direct-to-consumer (DTC) advertising and staff with training and expertise in drug regulation (see Chapter 7 for more discussion of resources).

This chapter briefly summarizes the history of drug regulation, describes the use of the agency's authority during the preapproval and postapproval processes, identifies needed changes, and makes recommendations to strengthen or clarify FDA's authority.

HISTORY OF FDA DRUG REGULATION

The foundation of FDA's regulatory authorities was laid in the 1906 Pure Food and Drug Act, which focused on misbranding and adulteration. In keeping with other consumer product laws, it focused on postmarketing remedies only. That is, if a drug already on the market was proven to be a hazard, it could be seized and further sales halted.

In the wake of deaths due to elixir of sulfanilamide in 1937, the 1906 law was replaced with a stronger form of regulation in the Federal Food, Drug, and Cosmetic (FD&C) Act of 1938. The new law changed the emphasis to the period of time before a drug enters the market, and required manufacturers to notify FDA before beginning testing on human subjects and to submit proof of the drug's safety (though not of its efficacy) (Hutt, 1992). The requirement was a major advance in drug regulation, but it was nonetheless still somewhat weak, as marketing could begin 60 days after submission of the information to the FDA unless the FDA affirmatively found the drug to be unsafe.

The statutory scheme for drug regulation went through yet another revision in 1962, after thousands of European children with limb defects were born to mothers who had been administered thalidomide (Kaplan, 1995; FDA, 2006). The Drug Amendments of 1962 shifted the burden of proof from FDA (which previously had to prove harm to keep a drug from being marketed) to manufacturers, who now were required to demonstrate both safety and efficacy prior to receipt of marketing approval (Hutt, 1991). The early 1960s also marked the crystallization of clinical trials into the sequence of phase 1, 2, 3 trials still in use today and described in greater detail in Chapter 2 (DHEW, 1963).

The FDA's ability to form judgments about the safety and efficacy of drugs depends upon the submission of data, usually from drug company sponsors, rather than on the use of data developed independently or on its own initiative. As a result, the statutory scheme governing drug approval in the United States has also included a series of measures to provide an incentive for third parties to develop safety and efficacy data for use by FDA. These incentives include patent extensions (the Drug Price Competition and Patent Term Extension Act of 1984), and periods of market exclusivity in exchange for developing information about new drugs, new indications for old drugs, and new information about the action of old drugs in special populations, such as children (The Orphan Drug Act of 1982; The FDA Modernization Act of 1997 [FDAMA]; the Best Pharmaceuticals for Children Act of 2002). Thus, the statutory scheme is characterized by carrots rather than sticks, in that the development of new information on drug safety and efficacy is achieved more by creating incentives than by issuing mandates.

The 1938 FD&C Act, as amended several times, defines FDA's regulatory jurisdiction and its enforcement powers. The statute empowers FDA to bring enforcement actions through administrative procedures (warning letters, adverse publicity, recalls, and withdrawals of product approvals) and judicial procedures (seizure, injunction, and prosecution) (Bass, 1997; Levine, 2002). FDA's enforcement authority is derived by delegation from the secretary of the Department of Health and Human Services (DHHS) to the commissioner of food and drugs (Bass, 1997). Regulations contained in the *Code of Federal Regulations* empower FDA to enforce the FD&C Act and other statutes, as appropriate. FDA's ability to regulate is also influenced by Congress and its "oversight jurisdiction" exercised by holding congressional hearings (Hutt, 1991). The judiciary branch also may influence FDA regulation, when FDA's interpretations of the statute and its development of regulations are successfully challenged in court.

AN AGING AND INADEQUATE STATUTORY FRAMEWORK

The statutory authority for drug regulation was constructed decades ago, and it remains largely unchanged. The existing regulatory framework is structured around the premarketing testing process; few tools are available for addressing postmarketing safety issues, short of the blunt instruments to respond to clear-cut adulteration and misbranding. As described in Chapter 1, the sciences of drug discovery and development, the practice of medicine and the extent of drug use, and the information environment in which health care providers practice and patients learn about drugs and interact with the health care delivery system have all changed. It is time to reassess and strengthen FDA's postmarketing authorities and tools in view of these changes. The carefully controlled clinical trials currently conducted premarket under the existing statutory framework consists of study populations that are commonly different in composition and health status from populations that will use the marketed drug. Study populations are chosen for a legitimate reason: to make data from the trials clearer and thus to make safety and efficacy testing more efficient. After approval, drugs are used by larger and more heterogeneous populations, and by people who have comorbidities or are taking multiple prescription and over-the-counter drugs and dietary supplements. Furthermore, the promotion of drugs has moved beyond health care providers, and substantial industry investment goes into directly targeting consumers. It also has become more important to recognize that the assessment of a drug's risk-benefit profile does not remain static after approval. Every effort must be made to monitor the performance of drugs on the market, to identify safety problems early, and to address them effectively. FDA's ability to regulate drugs effectively in a rapidly changing context requires reconsideration of the laws and a clarification and strengthening of the agency's regulatory authority.

Below, the committee describes main aspects and weaknesses of FDA's authority before and after approval.

FDA Authority Preapproval

A primary regulatory activity of the FDA Center for Drug Evaluation and Research (CDER) is shepherding products through phase 1, 2, and 3 trials. If at any point during clinical trials, the agency "does not believe, or cannot confirm, that the study can be conducted without unreasonable risk to the subjects/patients", the agency has the statutory authority to impose a clinical hold on the trial (CDER et al., 1998). This suspends further progress in the study until the underlying reasons for the hold (e.g., adverse events or other safety questions) are addressed. Center review teams can also ask sponsors to develop and submit for review, when appropriate, plans for postmarketing safety surveillance and study to monitor previously undocumented, unexpected risks, and a risk management program when there are known risks. Other risk management measures and data from epidemiologic studies may be needed if safety signals are identified and confirmed when a drug has been on the market, including label changes, communication to health care providers, restriction of marketing, and public health advisories. In recent years, CDER has developed guidance for industry on preparing and evaluating risk minimization action plans (RiskMAPs), which may include an array of educational and administrative activities to address risks that are known at the time of approval.

There appear to be several conditions FDA can impose at the time of approval, for example, requiring distribution limited to a specific medical specialty, distribution with required periodic screening to avoid contraindicated use, and distribution with mandatory enrollment in a registry. Certainly such conditions have been imposed in the past, for example with teratogenic drugs such as thalidomide and isotretinoin. However, varying interpretations by occupants of the general counsel's office of the FDA's authority has led to significant variation in the willingness of the FDA to consider using conditions on sale as a condition of approval. And in general, such conditions are even more difficult to put in place after the drug has been approved for marketing, as efforts to impose such conditions nearly always depend upon voluntary compliance by the manufacturer rather than on the threat of withdrawal of the drug from the market as an imminent health hazard.

The Prescription Drug User Fee Act of 1992 (PDUFA) complicated FDA's ability to use its authority before approval. FDA's existing statute required that drug review be completed in 180 days; in practice, that goal proved largely impossible to achieve (Kaplan, 1995). The desire of patients and the general public for more rapid access to important drugs was among the primary drivers of congressional action to speed up the drug approval process. The enactment of PDUFA secured user-fee funds dedicated to enabling FDA drug review divisions to retain the staff and other resources needed to shorten the length of the approval process. PDUFA has clearly expedited agency decision making and has probably led to efficiencies in distinguishing important from less important issues in the final stages of the review process. However, there is concern that the rapid pace of the process needed to meet PDUFA goals (see Chapters 2 and 3) creates an environment that makes it hard or close to impossible for CDER reviewers to pursue safety concerns as carefully as they would in a less frenetic setting (GAO, 2002b; DHHS and OIG, 2003; Levine, 2006; Nickas, 2006; IOM Staff Notes, 2005–2006). Some also have serious concerns that the regulator has been "captured" by industry it regulates, that the agency is less willing to use the regulatory authority at its disposal (see Chapter 3). Patient expectations and misperceptions about drugs, the ever broader array of drugs, the complexity of actual drug use in the real world, and the intense pace of preapproval activities all suggest that FDA needs stronger authority postapproval to conduct adequate surveillance and oversee and enforce safety studies.

FDA Authority After Approval

The primary expression of FDA's authority is the threat to withhold or withdraw approval; but because a drug may offer unique benefits to a population in need, the threat of postapproval withdrawal can ring hollow.

Authority to Compel Completion of Postmarketing Commitments

Many postmarketing study commitments—a key activity requested by the agency to help to narrow the remaining uncertainty about an approved drug's safety—are not met and many are never undertaken. As described in Chapter 4, postmarketing studies are often planned and designed as an afterthought late in the review process, just before approval, and sometimes the study designs may not be the most useful, necessary, or even practicable (IOM, 2005). That appears to be at least partly a result of the frenetic pace of the review process, but it may also reflect the agency's awareness of its limited authority after approval.

FDA's statutory authority to require postmarketing studies has been a subject of debate for decades. Although the agency has interpreted FD&C Act section 505(k), which grants it power to require "records and reports" from sponsors as giving it the authority to mandate postmarketing studies, this interpretation has been contested by the industry (Steenburg, 2006). Several commissioners have admitted that the agency's interpretation of the statute made it vulnerable to court challenges. In 1977, the Review Panel on New Drug Regulation also found that the statute did not give FDA that authority. Many of the Panel's recommendations were incorporated into the 1979 Drug Regulation Reform Act (S. 1075, Kennedy) which passed Senate but failed to garner support in the House (DHEW, 1977; Steenburg, 2006). The panel's final report asserted that "rather than delay approval of a drug pending additional studies, FDA should have the authority to require a sponsor to conduct additional research as a condition of approval when a drug has been shown to be safe and effective for its intended use, but questions remain, for example, with regard to its long term effects" (DHEW, 1977). The 1979 bill included a provision to allow FDA to require postapproval studies (Dorsen and Miller, 1979). The 1996 Inspector General found that the FDA "tradition" of asking for voluntary postmarketing studies was not supported by statute in most cases (DHHS and OIG, 1996).

FDAMA (which included the reauthorization of PDUFA) added a provision to the FD&C Act requiring sponsor submission of annual updates on progress in meeting postmarketing study commitments. However, PDUFA provided no resources or new authorities to enable the agency to enforce that provision. FDA was required to develop and publish a rule on the reporting format and to report annually on sponsor performance in the *Federal Register*. The 2005 *Federal Register* notice on sponsor progress in meeting postmarketing study commitments showed that 797 (65 percent) of New Drug Applications (NDAs) and abbreviated NDA-related postmarketing commitments are "pending" (they are neither "ongoing" nor "delayed") and 47 percent of annual reports on studies that were due were not submitted to FDA. FDA's limited authority after marketing and its inability to enforce implementation and fulfillment of important and necessary postmarketing commitments have been at the core of many proposals for strengthening FDA's authority (GAO, 2002b; van der Linden et al., 2003; Ganslaw, 2005; Grassley, 2005; Thaul, 2005). A recent DHHS Office of the Inspector General (OIG) report on FDA's monitoring of postmarketing commitments noted that FDA has authority to require postmarketing studies only in certain cases (such as accelerated approval) and that 91 percent of postmarketing commitments between 1990 and 2004 were requested by the agency rather than being required by statute or regulation (DHHS and OIG, 2006). The report also found that postmarketing study commitments do not have a high priority in FDA, the agency lacks a system for managing postmarketing study commitments and the existing database of commitments is not consistently populated with information from commitment letters or from annual status reports, one-third of annual status (required by FDAMA) reports on postmarketing commitments are not submitted or are incomplete, and many completed reports lack useful information. The OIG report also concluded that FDA has no recourse when sponsors do not make progress or do not report on their commitments (DHHS and OIG,

2006). It is clear that FDA authority to require postmarketing studies (in cases other than accelerated approval, etc.) is at best unclear, and statutory change is needed to enable FDA to require such studies when necessary and appropriate.

Authority to Unilaterally Impose Risk-Reducing Remedies, Such as Label Changes and Distribution Restrictions

During the drug development process and up to the point of approval, FDA has a great deal of power. Its communications with sponsors at meetings and in written exchanges (including approval and other letters issued while an NDA is under review) carry enormous weight; sponsors are highly motivated to accede to FDA's requests and demands during this time to avoid any delay in the approval of their product. After approval, however, unless a case meets the statutory definition of fraud or misbranding or the high threshold for proving imminent hazard to the health of the public, FDA's regulatory and enforcement options generally lie at the ends of the spectrum of regulatory actions: do nothing or precipitate the voluntary withdrawal of the drug.[1] FDA relies on firms to withdraw drugs from the market voluntarily when safety issues are revealed. Doing nothing implies not acting on potential threats to the health of the public, and precipitating withdrawal implies taking the drug from patients who need it, so neither is a satisfactory option. Currently, most actions involve softer remedies negotiated with a drug sponsor; FDA cannot unilaterally compel label changes, addition of boxed warnings, or fulfillment of postmarketing study commitments. Nor can it unilaterally restrict marketing, change the content of a package insert (including Medication Guides[2]), or change the content of other documents intended for the public. The process of negotiation works well in many cases, but for some products the process can be long and have potentially adverse repercussions for safety. The diminished FDA authority after approval is of concern because knowledge of a drug's risk-benefit profile is never complete at the time of approval.

FDA takes several approaches to monitoring postmarketing safety. CDER staff members review Adverse Event Reporting System (AERS) reports using data mining techniques for automated monitoring of the AERS database, conduct retrospective and observational studies using external administrative databases, and track the status of phase 4 studies. CDER

---

[1]Withdrawals are almost always voluntary rather than mandated by FDA. According to its statute, FDA can institute recalls only for devices and baby formula (Adams et al., 1997).

[2]Medication Guides, or MedGuides, are patient-specific labeling for prescription drug products determined by FDA to have "serious and significant public health concern requiring distribution of FDA-approved patient information" (21 CFR 208.1, 4-1-05 Edition, p. 114) (CDER, 2006).

staff also evaluate and oversee sponsor-designed efforts to manage known risks, such as developing and implementing RiskMAPs for specific products, and negotiate with sponsors on actions needed to confirm and address just-identified risks. Such actions may include additional study, label changes, and risk communication including Dear Health Professional letters. If safety problems are identified, FDA can ask the sponsor to propose label language but cannot require specific language to describe the newly identified risks. Often, companies argue strongly against label changes, limitation of market-ing, boxed warnings, and so on.

Regulatory Oversight of Sponsor Promotional Activities

Pharmaceutical companies engage in various activities to promote their products to the public and to health care providers. Historically, health care professionals have been the primary target of such promotional activities; even at the time of this writing, more than 80 percent of promotional bud-gets are spent on reaching prescribers through such activities as "detailing" (in-person promotion by sales representatives in the health care setting) and sponsorship of professional educational opportunities (Rosenthal et al., 2002). An increasing proportion of promotional funds goes toward DTC advertising, which is an increasingly contentious area of drug regulation (GAO, 2002a). In 2006, the United States and New Zealand were the only nations that permitted DTC advertising of prescription drugs. However, the European Medicines Agency has for some time considered allowing DTC advertising for three disease categories (HIV/AIDS, diabetes, and asthma and other respiratory conditions). (See Box 5-1 for a history of FDA DTCA regulation.)

Around the turn of the 20th century, some analysts became concerned that regulation of DTC advertising was not keeping pace with the rapid evolution in advertising, and the debate that began with the introduction of DTC advertising became multifaceted (Hunt, 1998). Consumer groups, insurers, providers, and others have identified several interrelated concerns about DTC advertising, such as its influence on drug pricing, patient behav-ior, and prescriber behavior. A 2002 report from the Government Account-ability Office concluded that DTC advertising appears to increase spending on prescription drugs and drug utilization (GAO, 2002a). One concern is that advertising may lead to more rapid uptake of a new drug, which, in cases where the drug in question is later found to present greater risks than older drugs in the same class, could potentially dramatically increase the exposure to that particular drug, even among patients who are not good candidates for it. That exemplifies the continuing tension between safety concerns and benefits that outweigh the risks for certain patients. Also, DTC advertising may distort use patterns within classes of drugs, often driving use of more costly but no more effective therapies at the expense of older, cheaper options (e.g., generics).

As a communication or educational tool, DTC advertising appears to have mixed effects. There is evidence that advertisements have raised awareness about certain health conditions and led people to visit their health care provider and in some cases, receive needed diagnosis and treatment (Ostrove, 2000; Calfee, 2002; Aikin, 2003; Almasi et al., 2006) (see Box 5-2 for a sample of public opinion of DTC advertising). Advertisements about drugs may increase consumer familiarity with products available to treat their particular condition(s), perhaps empowering them to initiate discussion about therapy with their health care provider, and in some cases, to alert a less well-informed provider to a particular therapy (Wilkes et al., 2000; Lyles, 2002; Almasi et al., 2006). On a potentially more negative note, viewers of television prescription drug advertisements may learn more about the benefits than about the risks. Also, DTC advertising has been shown to have an effect on physician prescribing patterns (Aikin, 2003; Mintzes et al., 2003; Aikin et al., 2005; Weissman et al., 2004; Spence et al., 2005).

FDA's authority to regulate prescription drug advertisements is found in Section 502(n) of the FD&C Act, and Title 21 of the *Code of Federal Regulations* (CFR) section 202.1 is the source of the implementing regulations that describe the content required in such advertisements (Behrman, 2005). Specifically, regulations require that print advertisements must disclose every risk listed in the FDA-approved label as part of a brief summary, but broadcast advertisements may either contain a brief summary of side effects and contraindications or make "adequate provision" for conveying the product's complete labeling information, that is, a toll-free telephone number or Web site. FDA can regulate advertising that is false or misleading, but its regulatory actions must harmonize with First Amendment protections of truthful commercial speech.

FDA does not have the authority to approve drug advertisements or require that advertising materials be reviewed prior to their use. The agency can require and enforce corrective action only after a drug advertisement has been broadcast (Woodcock et al., 2003). To avoid having to issue a correction after beginning a marketing activity, a majority of sponsors submit advertising materials for comment to the CDER Division of Drug Marketing and Communication (DDMAC) before airing them (Woodcock et al., 2003) (see Box 5-3).

The history of court challenges to restrictions on DTC advertising is lengthy and instructive. Attempts to ban DTC advertising have foundered due in part to uncertainty as to whether such a prohibition is constitutional. Drug advertising has been held to be commercial speech deserving First Amendment protection (Virginia State Board of Pharmacy v. Virginia Citizens Consumer Council, Inc., 425 U.S. 748, 762 [1976]). In Central

---

BOX 5-1
History of FDA's DTC Advertising Regulation

As a variety of social changes began to transform the passive patient into an empowered seeker and contributor of knowledge and information, the patient-provider relationship and other interactions and spheres of influence around it changed as well. As early as 1968, FDA developed the first patient package insert in recognition of the need to instruct patients on the use of a drug, the inhalational product isoproterenol (Pines, 1999). In the 1970s and 1980s, more health-related information was made available to the general public (such as the *Physician's Desk Reference*), cable television experimented with physician-oriented channels, and pharmaceutical companies began to advertise in print to patients. As FDA and the industry reoriented some of their communication activities to target patients, the agency worked in two different directions: furthering its own role in communicating to patients through patient package inserts (see Chapter 6) and making determinations about how to regulate and ascertain the public health implications of emerging industry promotional efforts directed at consumers (Pines, 1999; DHHS et al., 2005).

FDA's authority in that respect originates in the FD&C Act, which gave FDA authority over drug labeling and gave the Federal Trade Commission (FTC) authority over advertising (Kaplan, 1995). Current statutes give FDA and FTC overlapping and concurrent authority over the labeling of FDA-regulated products and over advertising of prescription drugs and devices. FTC is responsible for regulating false or deceptive claims about products other than prescription drugs and FDA has primary jurisdiction over false and misleading labeling of all jointly regulated products and, on the basis of the definition of advertising as an extension of labeling, over DTC advertising (Adams et al., 1997; Pines, 1999; Palumbo and Mullins, 2002).

In 1983, FDA requested a voluntary moratorium on all drug advertising to

---

Hudson Gas & Electric Corp. v. Public Service Commission (447 U.S. 557 (1980)), the Court stated that a governmental restriction upon commercial speech is lawful only if the asserted governmental interest in the restriction is substantial, that the speech restriction directly advances the governmental interest asserted, and that the speech restriction is not more extensive than is necessary to serve the asserted governmental interest. If the government cannot demonstrate that it meets all three prongs of the Central Hudson test, the speech restriction is unlawful. In Thompson v. Western States Medical Center, 535 U.S. 357 (2002), the Supreme Court applied the Central Hudson test and ruled that the statutory ban on advertising of compounded drugs allow the agency to determine where there were adequate statutory protections for consumers (Palumbo and Mullins, 2002). After its internal decision making and discussion with academic, consumer, health care, and other communities, the agency concluded in the *Federal Register* (1985-Notice 50 FR 36677) that "current regulations governing prescription drug advertising provide sufficient safeguards to protect consumers." The notice also stated that DTC advertising must meet the same requirements as advertising to physicians, including the "brief summary" of risk information required by statute (21 CFR 202.1).

In the 1990s, as DTC advertising progressed from print to television, pharmaceutical companies found they could not make product claims in advertisements, because that required presenting the statutorily "brief summary" of safety and contraindications information. The television equivalent of the page of minuscule print on the back of magazine advertisements "would take a minute or more at a barely readable scrolling rate" (Woodcock et al., 2003). For this reason, DTC advertisements did not make product claims and generally consisted of "help-seeking" and "reminder" advertisements. The former described an identifiable condition and urged viewers to "see your doctor," while the latter mentioned the name of a product without the indication. Advertisements that talked about the disease, but not the drug, or about the drug without mentioning the indication left viewers confused and led FDA to reconsider the entire subject of DTC advertising (Pines, 1999). In 1997, FDA produced the draft *Guidance for Industry: Consumer-Directed Broadcast Advertisements*. That document, issued in final form in 1999, allowed television product claim advertisements, finding that they could meet the statutory requirement and make "adequate provision" for the information contained in the brief summary by providing a toll-free number or Web site where consumers could receive the complete information contained in the drug's label.

violated commercial speech rights. How the court would react to restrictions short of outright ban on DTC advertisements is unclear, but it is worth noting that in the western states decision the court was unsympathetic to the argument that DTC advertisements of compounded drugs might affect physician prescribing practices, to the detriment of their patients. The same court cases are relevant to whether FDA can require prior approval of the advertisements. If courts were to conclude that this amounts to a "prior restraint" on First Amendment protected speech, FDA would have to show a compelling government purpose for such a policy.

FDA's regulation of promotional activities was challenged in court by

---

BOX 5-2
Public Perspectives on DTC Advertising

It has been suggested that DTC advertising is associated with the transformation in the role of patients from passive to actively contributing to the health care encounter (shared decision making). A study of 1999 Princeton Survey Research Associates data found that more than 40% of consumers have used DTC advertisement information in their decision-making process and used information learned from a DTC advertisement to discuss a prescription drug with their health care provider (Deshpande et al., 2004). The study also found that consumers believe advertisements are more effective in communicating benefits than risks of prescription drugs.

An online survey conducted for the Wall Street Journal in 2005 (Harris Interactive, 2005) found that only 35% of American adults believe FDA does a good or excellent job in its oversight of DTC advertising. When asked whether they thought banning DTC advertising for a period of time after a prescription drug is approved by FDA so "doctors have time to become familiar with the drug," 51% agreed. Only 26% of respondents agreed that banning DTC advertising is not a good idea because "it is how many patients learn about new treatments that might be right for them."

---

the Washington Legal Foundation in 1994. In its lawsuit, the Foundation claimed FDA had no statutory grounds for regulating companies' truthful statements even if they did not adhere to FDA's requirements for "fair balance" and "full disclosure." Although the lawsuit involved off-label promotion to health care providers, the decision against FDA was sweeping and many believe it limits FDA's ability to regulate DTC advertising. Washington Legal Foundation continues to scrutinize FDA's actions regarding DTC advertising on First Amendment grounds (FDA, 2002), and in June 2005, the Foundation launched its "DDMAC Watch," charging that FDA/DDMAC requirements exceed the statutory requirement of full disclosure of risks and that the division does not fully demonstrate how it determines that a given advertisement is misleading to consumers (Washington Legal Foundation, 2005).

In response to the debate about the effects of DTC advertising on prescription drug use and, ultimately, on drug safety, Senator Frist called for a 2-year moratorium on DTC advertising (Pharma Marketletter July 6, 2005). The Pharmaceutical Research and Manufacturers of America (PhRMA) issued 15 guiding principles on the advertising of prescription drugs (see Box 5-4). One of the principles called for submitting advertising material to FDA prior to broadcast, and informing the agency about the intended time of initial airing. The principles also urged companies to cooperate with FDA to alter or remove DTC advertising when safety issues about an advertised prescription drug arise. Twenty-three drug companies agreed to the new guidelines, and at least two, Bristol-Meyers Squibb and Pfizer, announced moratoria (for 1 year, and 6 months, respectively) on DTC advertising for newly approved drugs. That was an important action, and one that is consonant with the committee's views about the value of limiting marketing of

---

BOX 5-3
The Division of Drug Marketing and Communication

The CDER office responsible for reviewing DTC advertisements and other sponsor promotional materials is the Division of Drug Marketing and Communication (DDMAC). Whether or not an advertisement is reviewed in a timely manner depends on the resources available for review activities—DDMAC is small and has limited resources. A forthcoming report from the Government Accountability Office reviews DDMAC's work and resources.

In 2005 the Division's staff of 35 received 53,000 pieces of promotional material (up from 36,700 in 2002) (Winter, 2005; Woodcock et al., 2003). When a company submits material, the appropriate DDMAC staff members (including a social scientist, regulatory counsel, and others) meet to review the proposed promotional material and make a decision. "Drugs that are new products, have new indications, are first in a class to have broadcast advertisements, or are being advertised in a broadcast medium for the first time have more extensive reviews" (Woodcock et al., 2003). There are several regulatory tools CDER's DDMAC can employ against companies that engage in violative promotional practices. These include

- Untitled letters (or "notice of violation" letters), requiring sponsors to discontinue use of false or misleading advertising materials.
- Warning letters, issued to sponsors for more serious violations than those addressed by untitled letters (i.e., those posing potentially serious health risks to the public).
- Injunctions and consent decrees.
- Referrals for criminal investigation or prosecution.
- Seizures.

BOX 5-4
PhRMA's 15 Guiding Principles on DTC Advertising (2005)

- Potential public health benefit
- Accurate and not misleading
- Educational
- Identify product as prescription not OTC
- Foster responsible communication between patient and provider
- Educate providers about new medicine or new indication for an appropriate (given all facts about the drug, the condition, etc.) length of time before beginning DTC advertising
- Working with FDA, alter or discontinue DTC advertising if indicated by new risk information
- Submit all new DTC TV advertisements to FDA before releasing them
- DTC TV and print advertisements should inform about non-drug options (e.g., lifestyle and diet change) when appropriate
- DTC advertisements that identify a product by name should include indications and major risks
- Design advertisements to present benefits and risks in a balanced, clear way
- Respect seriousness of conditions and drugs
- Content and placement should be age-appropriate
- Encouraged: promote health and disease awareness as part of DTC advertising
- Encouraged: include information for uninsured and underinsured where feasible

new molecular entities in order to prevent potentially rapid uptake of a new drug about which considerable uncertainty remains.

Rationale for Strengthening Drug Regulation

The "Bully Pulpit" Is Not Enough

A response to the concern about FDA's limited postmarketing authority (see Box 5-5 for two interesting exceptions) is that FDA has and can use its "bully pulpit," its influence, to compel action on the part of a sponsor. The committee learned in conversations with and from literature about several former FDA leaders that even in cases where authority was not clear-cut, the agency was able to use its bully pulpit to powerful effect in its interactions with sponsors (IOM Staff Notes, 2005–2006). However, consumer organizations, legislators, scientists, and others who have called for strengthening and clarifying FDA regulatory authority have provided numerous examples of cases where the agency was unable to effect desired changes. The committee asserts that the bully pulpit route leaves potentially critical regulatory action vulnerable to a subjective and highly variable process of exercising individual or agency influence, and to the vicissitudes of changing attitudes toward regulation. That is why FDA's authorities must be clarified and strengthened to empower the agency to take rapid and decisive actions when necessary and appropriate.

BOX 5-5
Two Exceptions in FDA's Regulatory Authority

Pediatric drugs and accelerated approval drugs provide two important incentive mechanisms with which to circumvent the imbalance in regulatory authority pre- and postapproval, and may be instructive as models for strengthening the statutory authorities available to FDA. The FDA Modernization Act of 1997 included patent exclusivity provisions as an incentive for sponsors who conducted studies of approved drugs in pediatric populations, and the 2002 Best Pharmaceuticals for Children Act renewed those incentives. That legislation exemplifies the "carrot" approach to motivating conduct and completion of studies: no study, no extended period of exclusivity. The "stick" approach to enforcing study commitments, which has not worked so well, is illustrated by accelerated approvals on the basis of surrogate endpoints (e.g., for cancer drugs) "which allows products to be used in nonresearch clinical care settings before they have been reliably established to have a favorable benefit-to-risk profile" (Fleming, 2005). Here again, however, FDA's authority to enforce these commitments rests on withdrawing approval if the company does not complete the requisite studies and the high value of such therapeutic agents makes withdrawal undesirable. FDA's authority to enforce should be made explicit, as it is for accelerated approvals, and the agency should also be given additional tools to enforce that authority. The power to withdraw is not a realistic tool as demonstrated by an FDA study of 8 drugs granted accelerated approvals. The average length of time for completion of required validation studies was 10 years, and it is unclear what FDA is able to do if studies are inconclusive (Fleming, 2005).

*Approval Should Not Be the "Last Call" for Realistic Regulatory Action
on Safety*

In acknowledgement of the complexity of regulatory decision-making, the multiple conflicting interests involved, and the undesirability of delaying the approval of important drugs, the committee has sought to recommend tools that will allow FDA greater regulatory flexibility postapproval and throughout a drug's lifecycle. Establishing an interval for reviewing all accumulated information about new molecular entities (NMEs) will provide FDA with the authority to take necessary regulatory action when appropriate. For most drugs, the review of the drug's performance for renewal of approval will be a relatively simple process. For others, the review of postapproval data will give FDA an opportunity to reconsider the drug's risk-benefit profile and respond to safety issues.

Over the years, patient groups and industry representatives have expressed concern that regulatory actions that are too risk-averse could stifle innovation in drug development. Longer and larger preapproval trials to improve certainty about a drug's risk and benefit at the time of approval are often not possible, because the extremely broad-based testing in complex populations needed to get a better picture of postapproval use and risks would slow drug development unacceptably in many disease settings. Many scientists agree that CDER needs better resources for research and surveillance and better regulatory tools to manage risk-benefit uncertainty after approval (Deyo, 2004; Avorn, 2006; Ray and Stein, 2006). In earlier chapters, the committee described an organizational culture and a scientific milieu that encourage thinking about and preparing to address postmarketing safety issues much earlier in the development and review process. In this chapter, the committee calls for strengthening FDA's authority so that the point of approval would no longer be the "last call" for major regulatory action.

The committee finds that FDA's authority is built on an aging regulatory framework, that FDA's largely all-or-nothing regulatory tools limit its ability to regulate effectively after approval, and that strengthened agency authority would greatly mitigate the concern that fast review and approval may sacrifice safety. Current enforcement options limit FDA's ability to regulate in a manner that matches the agency's mission—protecting and advancing the health of the public. FDA's strongest tools are largely all-or-nothing, and these are unrealistic options in light of patients' needs for given drugs. The agency needs a more nuanced set of tools to respond to uncertainty, to reduce advertising that drives rapid uptake of new drugs, or to compel additional studies in the actual patient populations who take the drug after its approval.

STRENGTHENING FDA'S REGULATORY AUTHORITIES

The committee has examined five areas of regulation in which it believes that FDA's authority requires strengthening. The committee reasserts the importance of a regulatory system that is dynamic and flexible; a key aspect is that most NDAs and approvals pose few issues of concern and little or no need for unusual postapproval monitoring and risk management. For most drugs, the existing interaction between regulator and sponsor is adequate—incoming safety information does not reveal extremely serious unlabeled adverse events (AEs), and regulatory re-examination (for new indications and labeling changes) is more or less routine. The committee's recommendations for regulatory change apply mainly to what may be a smaller proportion of drugs—which cannot always be identified beforehand—that have complex risk-benefit assessments and both lingering and emergent safety concerns. Possible examples may be found among drugs that are similar to those with a poor safety record, NMEs with unique modes of action, drugs for which preclinical testing revealed a potential for clinical safety problems, and so on. First, clarification or strengthening of existing authority for use postapproval is needed to take important regulatory action out of the realm of negotiation and the bully pulpit. Second, FDA needs a new way to address DTC advertising that has provoked great interest and debate in recent years. Third, FDA needs sufficient enforcement tools to ensure that regulatory requirements imposed at or after approval are fulfilled. Fourth, FDA needs to develop a major strategy to improve public and health care provider awareness that approval is not the end of uncertainty and that as new drugs enter the market, more information about their benefits and risks is likely to become available. Fifth, regulation of drugs in the United States would be greatly strengthened by requiring a milestone in each drug's lifecycle that triggers a comprehensive review of consolidated safety and efficacy data and of the status of postmarketing conditions and commitments.

Conditions and Restrictions on Distribution Throughout the Drug Lifecycle

The committee has found that FDA has some ability to ask for and negotiate with sponsors about various risk management and other actions. For example, marketing of isotretinoin is conditioned on a four-step RiskMAP (iPLEDGE) that consists of: registration of and an educational program for patients, pharmacies, prescribers, and distributors; implementation of an education program for the four groups just listed; implementation of a reporting and data collection system for serious AEs in compliance with statutory requirements and as pertaining to the sale and dispensing of isotretinoin outside the iPLEDGE program; and implementation of a plan to monitor and minimize drug exposure during pregnancy through a pregnancy registry (Houn, 2006). It must be noted here that the iPLEDGE program has drawn criticism from providers and patients who find its requirements onerous and the administration of the program inadequate (Ritter, 2006). In another example, FDA issued a public health advisory pertaining to the multiple sclerosis drug natalizumab after an unexpected serious AE surfaced. The sponsor later withdrew natalizumab from the market and began working with CDER staff to develop a risk management program (including restricted distribution through certified infusion centers and so on). FDA convened the appropriate advisory committee to review the sponsor's proposed risk management program and CDER's evaluation of it. The advisory committee recommended that natalizumab be returned to the market with the necessary safeguards; after additional FDA consideration, Tysabri was returned to the market in July 2006. Another important example is clozapine, an antipsychotic whose use was conditioned on regular blood work showing that agranulocytosis, a potentially fatal side effect of the drug, was not emerging. Even more recently, FDA suggested 5-year followup of patients on the HIV drug class of CCR5 antagonists, which target a novel pathway and pose a serious risk of worsening the disease.

The committee believes that although FDA is able to negotiate for label changes (including warnings), and to impose restrictions or conditions on distribution at approval, it exercises those options inconsistently and lacks both the ability to require sponsor agreement with label changes and compliance with conditions imposed after approval and enforcement threats short of withdrawal. The conditions on the distribution of isotretinoin were implemented at the conclusion of an extremely long process. Label change negotiations for some drugs with emergent safety problems (such as cisapride, rofecoxib) have been unreasonably drawn out, and sponsors have made great effort to soften the language preferred by FDA (Harris and Koli, 2005). Such delays and barriers to timely action are problematic given the seriousness of the AEs which such label changes and similar measures are intended to warn about and to prevent (Kweder, 2004).

FDA's regulatory authorities do not give the agency sufficient flexibility to address safety concerns quickly during a drug's lifecycle and as consistent with the agency's public health mission. No drug is thoroughly understood at the time of approval, but most drugs perform effectively and without major safety concerns once they are on the market. FDA needs more a consistent approach and more nuanced range of enforcement measures to act when an approved drug's risk-benefit profile is in question and when safety concerns arise after marketing.

FDA needs new authority or a clarification of existing authority to apply restrictions and conditions on distribution from the regulatory "tool kit" described below. Some of the regulatory options described have already been used in some cases, but are often exercised at the point of approval. In general, even if FDA is successful in placing a condition or restriction at the time of approval, doing so after marketing is substantially more challenging. For example, FDA's authority over labels is limited to approving the contents of a label prepared by the sponsor, after a sometimes lengthy process of negotiation about the language. Although FDA may disagree with the sponsor and request certain changes, it is the committee's understanding that the agency cannot compel the sponsor to make changes.

> **5.1: The committee recommends that Congress ensure that the Food and Drug Administration has the ability to require such postmarketing risk assessment and risk management programs as are needed to monitor and ensure safe use of drug products. These conditions may be imposed both before and after approval of a new drug, new indication, or new dosage, as well as after identification of new contraindications or patterns of adverse events. The limitations imposed should match the specific safety concerns and benefits presented by the drug product. The risk assessment and risk management program may include:**

a. Distribution conditioned on compliance with agency-initiated changes in drug labels.
b. Distribution conditioned on specific warnings to be incorporated into all promotional materials (including broadcast direct to consumer [DTC] advertising).
c. Distribution conditioned on a moratorium on DTC advertising.
d. Distribution restricted to certain facilities, pharmacists, or physicians with special training or experience.
e. Distribution conditioned on the performance of specified medical procedures.
f. Distribution conditioned on the performance of specified additional clinical trials or other studies.
g. Distribution conditioned on the maintenance of an active adverse event surveillance system.

As with any grant of regulatory authority, FDA authority to revise labels, require conditions on distribution, and to impose penalties must be accompanied by administrative procedures that protect the due process rights of affected parties. These procedures, as generally used throughout federal law, include adequate notice, opportunity for response, and avenues of appeal within the agency and, typically, with the courts. In this fashion, statutory authority to impose restrictions and remedies is neither dictatorial nor unlimited. It does, however, provide the FDA with a wider range of remedies and a stronger base from which to negotiate voluntary actions, while still providing affected parties an avenue of relief from what they may perceive as unwarranted or overly burdensome actions.

The committee also finds that FDA needs enforcement tools to ensure that the regulatory requirements described above are applied and met. Specifically, FDA does not have the set of flexible regulatory actions that it needs to enforce necessary and important postmarketing commitments effectively.

5.2: The committee recommends that Congress provide oversight and enact any needed legislation to ensure compliance by both the Food and Drug Administration and drug sponsors with the provisions listed above. FDA needs increased enforcement authority and better enforcement tools directed at drug sponsors, which should include fines, injunctions, and withdrawal of drug approval.

The agency's timely performance of the required postmarketing safety reviews could be listed as one of the goals associated with PDUFA and reported on in the goals letter to Congress (see Chapter 3).

A Symbol to Denote Limited Knowledge About New Drugs

A recurring theme in this report is the committee's concern that the public and even health care providers may base their choices and behaviors related to prescription drugs on inaccurate assumptions. For example, there may be a lack of general awareness that FDA approval does not represent a lifetime guarantee of safety or the end of uncertainty, that the understanding of a drug's risk-benefit profile evolves over the drug's lifecycle, and that new drugs are approved on the basis of carefully controlled limited testing in relatively small populations and under circumstances that may differ greatly from a drug's use after marketing.

The committee believes that a symbol or icon could be added to the labels and all materials associated with new drugs, new combinations of active substances, and new delivery systems to alert patients and the general public that such products are new and that the knowledge available about their performance is often incomplete. In the United Kingdom, a black triangle marks every newly marketed drug approved by the Medicines and Health products Regulatory Agency (MHRA). The black triangle signifies that a pharmaceutical product is under intense scrutiny of regulatory authorities, and the symbol is placed next to the product name in the British National Formulary and in the British pharmaceutical industry's compendium of drugs approved for marketing (MHRA, 2006). The black triangle program has an additional purpose of alerting National Health Service providers to report all adverse reactions (rather than only serious ones) associated with drugs labeled with the symbol. Study of reporting patterns indicates that despite the request for both serious event and non-serious event reporting, providers are five times more likely to report a serious than a non-serious adverse drug reaction (Heeley et al., 2001). Therefore, it is not clear whether the black triangle program in the United Kingdom was successful in increasing provider reporting. However, the black triangle was not intended as a tool to inform or educate consumers, so evidence from the United Kingdom would not necessarily be informative in the case of a somewhat different use for such a symbol. The committee believes that marking the label and all promotional material for newly approved drugs or indications with a special symbol and communicating its meaning to patients and consumers may help to increase awareness of the nature of newly approved therapies, for example, the incompleteness of information on safety.

5.3: The committee recommends that Congress amend the FD&C Act to require that product labels carry a special symbol such as the black triangle used in the United Kingdom or an equivalent symbol for new drugs, new combinations of active substances, and new systems of delivery of existing drugs. The FDA should restrict direct-to-consumer advertising during the period of time the special symbol is in effect.

The symbol should remain on the drug label and related materials for 2 years unless FDA chooses to shorten or extend the period on a case-by-case basis. The committee believes that companies should refrain from DTC advertising during the black triangle period, and would favor imposition of a formal moratorium on such advertising. Such restraints may be necessary because DTC advertising has the ability to dramatically increase the uptake of a newly approved drug. In some cases, that may expose larger numbers of people (compared with a lower-key market introduction) to a new drug with not-yet-documented safety concerns. Recognizing the legal uncertainties surrounding such an imposition, the committee suggests that at the very least any DTC advertising during this period should include explicit notice that the data related to risks and benefits associated with the product are less extensive than those related to alternative products that have been in use for a longer period and should include a caution to speak to one's health care provider about alternatives. If a moratorium on DTC advertising for the time that the special symbol is in effect is deemed to be inconsistent with First Amendment protections of commercial speech, the committee believes that it is necessary to require placement of the symbol on all promotional materials, patient or consumer information, and all DTC advertising while the special symbol is in effect.

Products carrying the special notation also would be subject to heightened postmarketing scrutiny, with measures that include:

- Prompt review of individual 15-day reports of AEs (sponsors are required to report serious, unexpected AEs to the agency within 15 calendar days)[3] in addition to review of regular tabulations of such reports.
- Followup of these reports as needed to obtain additional information, such as that on related health factors and resolution of AEs, that may be helpful in assessing role of product and overall impact of AEs.
- Scheduling of regular meetings of postmarketing and premarket reviewers at which summaries of recent reports of AEs related to newly approved products prepared by the postmarketing reviewers would be discussed.
- Preparation of annual summaries of reports received on new products to be posted on the FDA Web site—not simply a list or tabulation, but a thoughtful interpretation of the reported experiences and what they mean for continued use of the drug.

The committee believes that a broad-based discussion of the most appropriate symbol for a US audience would be desirable before the program is launched, and an evaluation of the effect of such a program on public awareness and knowledge would be important.

Periodic Review of Data on New Molecular Entities

In 1977, the Review Panel on New Drug Regulation found that "FDA even lacks a basis for judging whether the approved drug and the approved labeling are still correct, since there is no comprehensive system for gathering and utilizing data on an approved drug's performance and effect" (Department of Health Review Panel on New Drug Regulation, 1977:91). This continues to be the case.

The committee finds that a lifecycle approach to risk and benefit would be facilitated by establishing a milestone in a drug's lifecycle for a comprehensive review of consolidated safety and efficacy data and the status of postmarketing conditions and commitments (see Chapter 4 for discussion of the assessment of risks and benefits). There is no systematic CDER review of

---

[3]Refer to the *Code of Federal Regulations*, 21 CFR 314.80.

accumulated knowledge about a drug a year or more after its approval for marketing. In 2005, the European Medicines Agency enacted a new statute requiring that prescription drug marketing authorizations in the European Union be reviewed and, if appropriate, renewed at 5 years after initial approval (EMEA, 2005).[4]

> 5.4: The committee recommends that FDA evaluate all new data on new molecular entities no later than 5 years after approval. Sponsors will submit a report of accumulated data relevant to drug safety and efficacy, including any additional data published in a peer-reviewed journal, and will report on the status of any applicable conditions imposed on the distribution of the drug called for at or after the time of approval.

As described above, such conditions on distribution may include a moratorium on DTC advertising, postmarketing studies, monitoring (such as registries, active surveillance, and so on), and restricted distribution. The 5-year report would include results of postmarketing studies, outcomes of monitoring, and, where applicable, the extent of DTC advertising (examples of all advertisements and total expenditure) during the first 5 years. For most drugs, the committee expects the 5-year "review" process to entail nothing more than a one-page FDA letter agreeing with the sponsor's summary of all accumulated (or consolidated) safety and efficacy information. On rare occasions, as a consequence of the review, regulatory action including suspension or withdrawal of approval (for example, if evidence of imminent public health hazard emerged in the course of the review) would be a possibility. This recommendation is not intended to preclude any regulatory action, and it does not constitute a request for new authority for FDA, rather, for the creation of a milestone moment in a drug's lifecycle that would allow FDA to review what has been learned during a drug's first 5 years on the market.

REFERENCES

Adams DG, Cooper RM, Kahan JS, Eds. 1997. *Fundamentals of Law and Regulation: An In-Depth Look at Therapeutic Products.* Vol. 2. Washington, DC: FDLI.

---

[4]Product safety specialists from the Center for Biologics Evaluation and Research routinely develop reviews of the postmarket safety experience with a new vaccine within 2–3 years of the time the vaccine is licensed. These reviews are published in journals and are available on the FDA Web site's Vaccine Adverse Event System page.

Aikin KJ. 2003 (September 22). *The Impact of Direct-to-Consumer Prescription Drug Advertising on the Physician-Patient Relationship.* PowerPoint presentated at the Food and Drug Administration Direct-to-Consumer Promotion Public Meeting. Washington, DC: FDA.

Aikin KJ, Swasy JL, Braman AC. 2005. *Patient and Physician Attitudes and Behaviors Associated with DTC Promotion of Prescription Drugs—Summary of FDA Survey Research Results.* Final report: DHHS.

Almasi EA, Stafford RS, Kravitz RL, Mansfield PR. 2006. What are the public health effects of direct-to-consumer drug advertising? *PLoS Med* 3(3):e145.

Avorn J. 2006. Evaluating drug effects in the post-Vioxx world: there must be a better way. *Circulation* 113(18):2173-2176.

Bass IS. 1997. Enforcement powers of the Food and Drug Administration: drug and devices. In: Adams DG, Cooper RM, Kahan JS, Eds. *Fundamentals of Law and Regulation.* Vol. II. Washington, DC: FDLI. Pp. 55-92.

Behrman R. 2005 (November 4). *Adverse Reactions: Information In, Information Out.* PowerPoint presented at the Institute of Medicine Forum for Drug Discovery, Development, and Translation Workshop on the Role of Consumers and Healthcare Professionals in Adverse Drug Event Reporting: Key Challenges and Opportunities. Washington, DC: IOM.

Calfee JE. 2002. Public policy issues in direct-to-consumer advertising of prescription drugs. *J Pub Pol Marketing* 21(2):174-193.

CDER (Center for Drug Evaluation and Research). 2006. *Medication Guides.* [Online]. Available: http://www.fda.gov/cder/Offices/ODS/medication_guides.htm [accessed September 18, 2006].

CDER, FDA (Food and Drug Administration), DHHS (Department of Health and Human Services). 1998. *The CDER Handbook.* [Online]. Available: http://www.fda.gov/cder/handbook/handbook.pdf [accessed November 14, 2005].

Department of Health Review Panel on New Drug Regulation. 1977. *Final Report.* Dorsen N, Weiner N, Astin AV, Cohen MN, Cornelius CE, Hamilton RW, Rall DP, Eds. Washington, DC.

Deshpande A, Menon A, Perri M, Zinkhan G. 2004. Direct-to-consumer advertising and its utility in health care decision making: a consumer perspective. *J Heal Comm* 9:499-513.

Deyo RA. 2004. Gaps, tensions, and conflicts in the FDA approval process: implications for clinical practice. *J Am Board Fam Pract* 17(2):142-149.

DHEW. 1963. Final rule on investigational drugs. *Fed Reg* 28(179):179-180.

DHEW (Department of Health Review Panel on New Drug Regulation), Dorsen N, Weiner N, Astin AV, Cohen MN, Cornelius CE, Hamilton RW, Rall DP. 1977. *Final Report.* Washington, DC: DHEW.

DHHS (Department of Health and Human Services), OIG (Office of Inspector General). 1996. *Postmarketing Studies of Prescription Drugs.* OEI-03-94-00760. Washington, DC: OIG.

DHHS, OIG. 2003. *FDA's Review Process for New Drug Applications: A Management Review.* OEI-01-01-00590. Washington, DC: OIG.

DHHS, OIG. 2006. *FDA's Monitoring of Postmarketing Study Committements.* OEI-01-04-00390. Washington, DC: OIG.

DHHS, FDA (Food and Drug Administration), Berhman RE. 2005. *The Impact of Direct-to-Consumer Drug Advertising on Seniors' Health and Health Care Costs.* Statement of Rachel E. Berhman, September 29, 2005, before the Special Committee on Aging, United States Senate.

Dorsen N, Miller JM. 1979. The drug regulation process and the challenge of regulatory reform. *Ann Intern Med* 91(6):908-913.

EMEA (European Medicines Agency). 2005. *Guideline on the Processing of Renewals in the Centralized Procedure.* ENTR/F2/KK D. Brussels, Belgium: EMEA.

FDA. 1999. *Milestones in US Food and Drug Law.* [Online]. Available: http://www.fda.gov/opacom/backgrounders/miles.html [accessed July 7, 2006].

FDA (Dockets Management Branch). 2002. *Comments on Submissions Concerning First Amendment Issues Docket No. 02N-0209.* [Online]. Available: http://www.wlf.org/upload/FDA10-28-02.pdf [accessed September 18, 2006].

FDA. 2006. *Thalidomide Information.* [Online]. Available: http://www.fda.gov/cder/news/thalinfo/default.htm [accessed July 1, 2005].

Fleming TR. 2005. Surrogate endpoints and FDA's accelerated approval process. *Health Aff (Millwood)* 24(1):67-78.

Ganslaw LS. 2005. Drug Safety: New Legal/Regulatory Approaches. *FDLI* July/August (4)7-10.

GAO. 2002a. *Prescription Drugs: FDA Oversight of Direct-to-Consumer Advertising Has Limitations.* GAO-03-177. Washington, DC: GAO.

GAO. 2002b. *Food and Drug Administration: Effect of User Fees on Drug Approval Times, Withdrawals, and Other Agency Activities.* GAO-02-958. Washington, DC: GAO.

Grassley C. 2005. A bill to amend the Federal Food, Drug, and Cosmetic Act with respect to drug safety, and for other purposes. S.930. 109th Cong., 1st Sess. April 27, 2005.

Harris G, Koli E. 2005. *Lucrative Drug, Danger Signals and the FDA.* [Online]. Available: http://www.nytimes.com/2005/06/10/business/10drug.html? [accessed October 4, 2005].

Harris Interactive. 2005. Majority of US adults think it is a good idea to forbid direct-to-consumer advertising for new prescription drugs when they first come to market. *Wall Street Journal Online Health-Care Poll* 4(14).

Heeley E, Riley J, Layton D, Wilton LV, Shakir SA. 2001. Prescription-event monitoring and reporting of adverse drug reactions. *Lancet* 358(9296):1872-1873.

Houn, F. 2006. *Letter to Hoffman La-Roche, Attention: Ellen Carey.* [Online]. Available: http://www.fda.gov/cder/foi/appletter/2005/018662s056ltr.pdf [accessed July 1, 2005].

Hunt M. 1998. *Direct-to-Consumer Advertising of Prescription Drugs.* National Health Policy Forum. Washington, DC: The George Washington University.

Hutt PB. 1991. Appendix A: the impact of regulation and reimbursement on pharmaceutical innovation. In: Insitute of Medicine. *The Changing Economics of Medical Technology.* Washington, DC: National Academy Press.

Hutt PB. 1992. Chapter 17: the regulation of drug products by the United States Food and Drug Administration. In: Griffin JP, O'Grady J. *The Textbook of Pharmaceutical Medicine.* London, UK: Blackwell BMJ Books.

IOM (Institute of Medicine). 2005 (January 17). *Transcript: Meeting Three of the IOM Committee on the Assessment of the US Drug Safety System, Workshop, Advancing the Methods and Application of Risk-Benefit Assessment of Medicines.* Janury 17, 2005, Washington, DC: IOM.

Kaplan AH. 1995. Fifty years of drug amendments revisited: in easy-to-swallow capsule form. *Food Drug Law J* 50 Spec:179-196.

Kweder S. 2004. *Statement of Sandra Kweder, M.D. Deputy Director, Office of New Drugs Center for Drug Evaluation and Research, US Food and Drug Administration,* before the Committee on Finance, United States Senate.

Levine A. 2002. FDA enforcement: how it works. In: Pina KR, Pines WL, Eds. *A Practical Guide to Food and Drug Law and Regulation.* 2nd Ed. Washington, DC: Food and Drug Law Institute. Pp. 271-298.

Levine A. 2006 (January 19). *Presentation to the Institute of Medicine Committee on the Assessment of the US Drug Safety System,* Meeting Four. Washington, DC: IOM.

Lyles A. 2002. Direct marketing of pharmaceuticals to consumers. *Annu Rev Public Health* 23:73-91.

MHRA. 2006. *Black Triangle Scheme*. [Online]. Available: http://www.mhra.gov.uk/home/ idcplg?IdcService=SS_GET_PAGE&useSecondary=true&ssDocName=CON024119 [accessed July 13, 2006].

Mintzes B, Barer ML, Kravitz RL, Bassett K, Lexchin J, Kazanjian A, Evans RG, Pan R, Marion SA. 2003. How does direct-to-consumer advertising (DTCA) affect prescribing? A survey in primary care environments with and without legal DTCA. *Can Med Assoc J* 169(5):405-412.

Nickas J. 2006 (January 19). *A Biotechnology Industry Perspective*. PowerPoint presentation to the Institute of Medicine Committee on the Assessment of the US Drug Safety System, Meeting Four. Washington, DC: IOM.

Ostrove NM. 2000 (August 8-9). *FDA's Research About Consumer-Directed Prescription Drug Promotion*. PowerPoint presentation at Pharmaceutical Pricing Practices, Utilization and Costs.

Palumbo FB, Mullins CD. 2002. The development of direct-to-consumer prescription drug advertising regulation. *Food Drug Law J* 57(3):423-443.

Pines WL. 1999. A history and perspective on direct-to-consumer promotion. *Food Drug Law J* 54(4):489-518.

Ray WA, Stein CM. 2006. Reform of drug regulation—beyond an independent drug-safety board. *N Engl J Med* 354(2):194-201.

Ritter J. 2006. *Acne Drug Registry Irritates Patients: Rules for Avoiding Pregnancy*. [Online]. Available: http://www.findarticles.com/p/articles/mi_qn4155/is_20060821/ai_n16674372 [accessed August 21, 2006].

Rosenthal MB, Berndt ER, Donohue JM, Frank RG, Epstein AM. 2002. Promotion of prescription drugs to consumers. *N Engl J Med* 346(7):498-505.

Spence M, Cheetham C, Millares M, Teleki S, Schweitzer S. 2005 (November 1-2). *Direct-to-Consumer Advertising of Cox-2 Inhibitors: Effect on Appropriateness of Treatment*. Presented at the FDA Public Hearing on Comsumer-Directed Promotion of Medical Products. Washington, DC: FDA.

Steenburg C. 2006. The Food and Drug Administration's use of postmarketing (phase IV) study requirements: exception to the rule? *Food Drug Law J* 61(2):1-91.

Thaul S. 2005. *Drug Safety and Effectiveness: Issues and Action Options After FDA Approval*. [Online]. Available: http://www.law.umaryland.edu/marshall/crsreports/crsdocuments/ RL3279703082005.pdf [accessed June 27, 2005].

van der Linden PD, Sturkenboom MC, Herings RM, Leufkens HM, Rowlands S, Stricker BH. 2003. Increased risk of achilles tendon rupture with quinolone antibacterial use, especially in elderly patients taking oral corticosteroids. *Arch Intern Med* 163(15):1801-1807.

Washington Legal Foundation. 2005. *WLF Launches "FDA/DDMAC Watch"*. [Online]. Available: http://www.wlf.org/upload/062105RS.pdf [accessed October 10, 2005].

Weissman JS, Blumenthal D, Silk AJ, Newman M, Zapert K, Leitman R, Feibelmann S. 2004. Physicians report on patient encounters involving direct-to-consumer advertising. *Health Aff* Web Exclusive:W4-W219.

Wilkes MS, Bell RA, Kravitz RL. 2000. Direct-to-consumer prescription drug advertising: trends, impact, and implications. *Health Aff (Millwood)* 19(2):110-128.

Winter G. 2005. *Inside DDMAC: A Conversation with Thomas Abrams*. [Online]. Available: http://www.pharmexec.com/pharmexec/content/printContentPopup.jsp?id=256550 [accessed December 1, 2005].

Woodcock J, DHHS, FDA. 2003. *Statement by Janet Woodcock, MD Director, Center for Drug Evaluation and Research US Drug Administration, Department of Health and Human Services*, July 22, 2003, before the Senate Special Committee on Aging.

6

Communicating About Safety

"Information is ultimately what permits people to make meaningful choices about whether or not to take new drugs" (Greenberg, 2003).

"1962—Consumer Bill of Rights is proclaimed by President John F. Kennedy in a message to Congress. Included are the right to safety, the right to be informed, the right to choose, and the right to be heard" (FDA Milestones).[1]

Patients use the medications approved by the Food and Drug Administration (FDA) and prescribed by health care providers. Despite that, patients historically have been left out of the loop in much of the communication that has occurred among the biomedical research, health care, and pharmaceutical enterprises and government regulators. As described in Chapter 1, social and technological changes have transformed the practice of medicine, the role of patients, and the information environment that surrounds patients and physicians and influences their interactions (Henwood et al., 2003). Public interest in and knowledge about drugs have also evolved greatly due to direct-to-consumer (DTC) prescription drug advertising, ever wider Internet and e-mail access and breadth of information, a shift in the formerly passive role of patient, and the emergence of a powerful patient advocacy movement (Atkin and Wallack, 1990; Dupuits, 2002; Pew Internet and American Life Project, 2003, 2004, 2005). Finally, the recent safety concerns about widely used, well-known drugs and drug classes, from antidepressants to anti-inflammatory drugs, have further mobilized public interest in drug safety issues. As noted earlier, FDA, the pharmaceutical industry, the health care delivery system, and other stakeholders have begun to grapple with serious questions about when to inform patients and consumers about risk, how to communicate effectively, and what information is needed for personal health, health care system, and regulatory decision making.

This chapter is intended not to provide a comprehensive assessment of communication issues in the drug system but rather to describe briefly major

---

[1]http://www.fda.gov/opacom/backgrounders/miles.html.

177

communication efforts at FDA, discuss some of the challenges that have complicated those activities, and to suggest two specific areas for improvement and makes appropriate recommendations.

Pharmaceutical products constitute 11 percent of the health care dollar (Smith et al., 2005). They are characterized by complex risk-benefit profiles, long and complicated research processes, and high visibility. They have the potential to provide important health benefits, from reducing risk of death to improving quality of life, and they are subject to extensive regulatory oversight. Those are some of the reasons why effective and timely risk communication about drugs is essential.

Roles and Needs of Providers and Patients

Despite the greater role patients play in their own health care, and the health care delivery system's recognition of that role, most of the communication "transactions" in the drug safety system occur among regulators, sponsors, providers, and payors. There are two types of information that may be communicated: information directed outward from stakeholders in the drug safety system (such as education, risk communication, promotional information), and information directed toward the drug safety system from those who experience drug safety problems directly or indirectly (including drug event reporting by patients or providers).

Communication Between the Public and the Drug Safety System

The Committee on the Assessment of the Drug Safety System did not endeavor to conduct a comprehensive examination of the communication needs of patients and the general public. Another IOM committee addressed these issues extensively in their report, *Preventing Medication Errors* (2007). That report recommended specific steps the health care delivery system, FDA, and other federal agencies could take to improve the availability, accessibility, quality, and quantity of patient and consumer information about drugs and their risks and benefits (see Box 6-1 and Appendix A). The present chapter focuses only on two areas where the committee believes FDA could strengthen its programs targeting patients' and consumers' communication needs.

Consumers and patients seek to access the information they need about the drugs they use through an incomplete and imperfect patchwork of sources (Brann and Anderson, 2002). These sources are of varying reliability and usefulness, and they include health care providers and pharmacists, DTC advertising, printed information made available by pharmacies, FDA-required patient package inserts for a limited number of drugs, information from a wide variety of sources made available on the Internet, and so on. Providers develop their knowledge about prescription drugs through a variety of means, including journal articles, interactions with company sales representatives, continuing education, professional associations, communication or education provided by their practice, hospital, or health system, and communiqués from FDA (either direct for those who request FDA electronic communications, or through professional associations that subscribe to or relay FDA's public health advisories).

FDA communicates to the public and to providers about drug safety concerns through public health advisories and warning. Some components of FDA's risk communication are under development, as described in Appendix A. For example, the agency has established a Drug Watch Web site intended for timely communication of safety issues to the public, but concerns arose about communicating complex issues of scientific uncertainty, explaining complex data clearly and in a way that is useful to patients (FDA, 2005). At the time of this writing, the committee had not yet learned of a resolution of these issues.

FDA has historically focused most of its communication activities on health care providers who prescribe FDA-approved drugs and serve as the "learned intermediary" between drug production and regulation and patients. That is evident in the dense, technical language of prescription drug labeling rules. In recent years, FDA has acknowledged the importance of communicating with and to patients and the general public by including them in its mission, which calls for "advancing the public health by . . . helping the public get the accurate, science-based information they need to use medicines and foods to improve their health." FDA has also reoriented some of its information and communication toward patients and the public, and has held several public hearings on issues related to communication and DTC advertising.

At least three types of the Center for Drug Evaluation and Research (CDER) regulatory activities involve communication-related activities pertinent to patients and the public. First, FDA has authority over prescription drug advertising developed and published or broadcast by sponsors, and CDER's Division of Drug Marketing and Communication sends untitled letters[2] and warning letters to sponsors whose advertisements do not convey a fair balance of risk and benefit information. Second, all of FDA's advisory committees include consumer representatives. Those committees' meetings are open to the public and routinely include opportunity for public comment on the issues under discussion. Some committee meetings may address risk communication issues. Third, FDA provides information about prescription drugs and other FDA-approved therapies on its Web site, and in print information about prescription drugs in general on a very small scale.

---

[2]See Chapter 5 for explanation.

BOX 6-1
Recommendations Pertaining to Consumers from
Preventing Medication Errors

Recommendation 1: To improve the quality and safety of the medication-use process, specific measures should be instituted to strengthen patients' capacities for sound medication self-management. Specifically:

- Patients' rights regarding safety and quality in health care and medication use should be formalized at the state and/or federal levels and ensured at every point of care.
- Patients (or their surrogates) should maintain an active list of all prescription drugs, over-the-counter (OTC) drugs, and dietary supplements they are taking; the reasons for taking them; and any known drug allergies. Every provider involved in the medication-use process for a patient should have access to this list.
- Providers should take definitive action to educate patients (or their surrogates) about the safe and effective use of medications. They should provide information about side effects, contraindications, and how to handle adverse reactions, as well as where to obtain additional objective, high-quality information.
- Consultation on their medications should be available to patients at key points along the medication-use process (during clinical decision making in ambulatory and inpatient care, at hospital discharge, and at the pharmacy).

Recommendation 2: Government agencies (i.e., the Agency for Healthcare Research and Quality [AHRQ], the Centers for Medicare and Medicaid Services [CMS], FDA, and the National Library of Medicine [NLM]) should enhance the resource base for consumer-oriented drug information and

The Role of Other Government Agencies

Other agencies in the Department of Health and Human Services (DHHS), such as the Agency for Healthcare Research and Quality (AHRQ), the National Institutes of Health (NIH), and the Centers for Medicare and Medicaid Services play a role in public communication about drug risk and benefit. For example, AHRQ's Effective Health Care Program develops consumer summaries of reports prepared by its DEcIDE (Developing Evidence to Inform Decisions about Effectiveness) network—prescription drug outcomes are one focus of the network—and other material on evidence-based practice. NIH conducts or sponsors clinical trials and does make medication self-management support. Such efforts require standardization of pharmacy medication information leaflets, improvement of online medication resources, establishment of a national drug information telephone helpline, the development of personal health records, and the development of a national medication safety dissemination plan.

- Pharmacy medication information leaflets should be standardized to a format designed for readability, comprehensibility, and usefulness to consumers. The leaflets should be made available to consumers in a manner that accommodates their individual needs, such as those associated with variations in literacy, language, age, and visual acuity.
- NLM should be designated as the chief agency responsible for Internet health information resources for consumers. Drug information should be provided through a consumers' version of the DailyMed program, with links to NLM's Medline Plus program for general health and additional drug information.
- FDA, CMS, and NLM working together should undertake a full evaluation of various methods for building and funding a national network of drug information helplines.
- CMS, FDA, and NLM should collaborate to confirm a minimum data set for personal health records and develop requirements for vendor self-certification of compliance. Vendors should take the initiative to improve the use and functionality of personal health records by incorporating basic tools to support consumers' medication self-management.
- A national plan should be developed for widespread distribution and promotion of medication safety information. Health care provider, community-based, consumer, and government organizations should serve as the foundation for such efforts.

SOURCE: IOM (2007).

public announcements about major health findings from them, good and bad. Recent studies from the Women's Health Initiative have generated such communications (e.g., about the benefits and risks of Hormone Replacement Therapy) in postmenopausal women. Through NLM, NIH also operates the clinicaltrials.gov trial registration Web site (discussed in Chapter 4).

Communicating Between Providers and the Drug Safety System

Although the present report acknowledges general areas of opportunity and challenges, it does not discuss the communication roles and needs of providers in great detail. The IOM report *Preventing Medication Errors* (2007) describes challenges in this area, including barriers to implementing and perfecting the use of information technology. That report also recommends several measures to improve communication to providers by government agencies and health systems (see Box 6-2 and Appendix C).

In the health care delivery system, information about drug safety, and particularly risk management, is integrated into drug prescribing and distribution systems (e.g., claims databases that issue alerts when two drugs with potential interactions are prescribed for the same patient). In its work,

---

BOX 6-2
Recommendations Pertaining to Providers (and Patients) from
Preventing Medication Errors

Recommendation 3: All health care organizations should immediately make complete patient-information and decision-support tools available to clinicians and patients. Health care systems should capture information on medication safety and use this information to improve the safety of their care delivery systems. Health care organizations should implement the appropriate systems to enable providers to:

- Have *access to comprehensive reference information* concerning medications and related health data.
- Communicate patient-specific medication-related information in an interoperable format.
- Assess the safety of medication use through active monitoring and use these monitoring data to inform the implementation of prevention strategies.
- Write prescriptions electronically by 2010 and all pharmacies to be able to receive them electronically, also by 2010. All prescribers should have plans in place by 2008 to implement electronic prescribing.
- *Subject prescriptions to evidence-based, current clinical decision support.*
- Have the appropriate competencies for each step of the medication use process.
- Make effective use of well-designed technologies, which will vary by setting.

Recommendation 5: Industry and government should collaborate to establish standards affecting drug-related health information technologies, specifically:

the committee learned about a wide variety of communication opportunities and challenges related to involving the general public and disease groups (such as online support groups) in reporting drug-related adverse events, about a movement to counteract commercial pharmaceutical company "detailing" with neutral "academic detailing" (Avorn, 2005), about First Amendment-based opposition to calls for increased FDA regulation (including banning) of DTC advertising, etc.

Providers, including physicians and pharmacists, are encouraged to report adverse drug reactions experienced by their patients to the manufac-

- The NLM should take the lead in developing a common drug nomenclature for use in all clinical information technology systems based on the standards for the national health information infrastructure.
- *AHRQ should take the lead in organizing safety alert mechanisms by severity, frequency, and clinical importance to improve clinical value and acceptance.*
- AHRQ should take the lead in developing intelligent prompting mechanisms specific to a patient's unique characteristics and needs; provider prescribing, ordering, and error patterns; and *evidence-based best-practice guidelines.*
- AHRQ should take the lead in developing user interface designs based on the principles of cognitive and human factors and the context of the clinical environment.
- AHRQ should support additional research to determine specifications for alert mechanisms and intelligent prompting, and optimum designs for user interfaces.

Recommendation 7: Oversight and regulatory organizations and payers should use legislation, regulation, accreditation, and payment mechanisms and the media to motivate the adoption of practices and technologies that can reduce medication errors, and to ensure that professionals have the competencies required to deliver medications safely.

- Medication error reporting should be promoted more aggressively by all stakeholders (with a single national taxonomy used for data storage and analysis).
- Accreditation bodies responsible for the oversight of professional education should require more training in improving medication management practices and clinical pharmacology.

turer or to FDA's Adverse Event Reporting System (providers may report through the MedWatch portal). Although proposals have been made in the United States and Europe to mandate provider reporting, there is little evidence that such attempts would be successful. Furthermore, spontaneous reporting is only one component of an effective drug safety surveillance program, and should not be relied on as the sole or primary source of information. Finally, the quality of spontaneous reports is an important concern; a large quantity of incomplete and poorly executed reports would be unhelpful.

How Industry Communicates to the Public and Patients

The frequently dangerous patent medicines that led to the Pure Food and Drugs Act of 1906 and the Food, Drug, and Cosmetic Act of 1938 were advertised directly to consumers with their colorful labels and claims, but modern prescription drugs, as products of biomedical science are promoted largely to health care providers, mostly to physicians. About 86 percent of industry promotional budgets still pay for "sampling" (providing free samples to providers), detailing (drug promotion to individual providers), and advertising in professional journals (Kaiser Family Foundation, 2004). However, the 1980s were a period of increased advertising directed at patients, known in some contexts as consumers—the term intended to reflect the changing role of patients to more active engagement with the health care system and involvement in their own health care.[3] In 2005, pharmaceutical manufacturers spent an estimated $4.2 billion on DTC advertising (and $7.2 billion on professional promotion through journal advertising and sales representative contacts) (IMS Health, 2006). A more recent development in pharmaceutical promotion is relationship marketing, in which companies customize their promotional and informational efforts to target patients who have specific diseases, such as diabetics who use a specific product (Ahearne et al., 2005).

FDA's Challenges in Communicating to the Public and Patients

FDA faces a number of challenges in improving its internal and external communication. As noted in Chapters 1 and 3, CDER has recognized that its credibility can be compromised by adverse publicity with respect to drug

---

[3]The mention of the term consumer is not intended to reflect the committee's views on its validity. The committee is aware of the favorable sides of health consumerism—such as empowerment and self-management—and of the more unfavorable aspects, including the commodification of health. It is also aware of the reality that access to health care and the level of health literacy (IOM, 2005) determine whether a patient has the opportunity to make health care choices and to form productive relationships with health care providers.

BOX 6-3
FDA Response to the December 2005 Public Meeting Input

In December 2005, FDA held a public hearing on communication of drug safety information. The hearing was intended to facilitate discussion on FDA's risk communication with health care providers and patients/ consumers. The following topics presented to FDA at the meeting were noted as needing improvement and attention:

- Engaging health care professionals.
- Improving Internet access for patient information.
- Maintaining benefit-risk balance in communications.
- Standardizing one-way communications.
- Addressing needs of those with low health literacy and poor English-language skills.

---

safety, and it has made efforts to improve transparency and communication, including establishing the Drug Watch Web site (currently under discussion by the agency), charging its recently constituted Drug Safety Oversight Board (DSB, discussed in Chapter 3) with (among other things) oversight of external communication, and creating a new Office of Safety Policy and Communication. However, the guidance document on the purpose and functioning of the Drug Watch Web site is being reconsidered because of concerns about needlessly alarming the public and about releasing safety data without proper context and analysis (DHHS et al., 2005a,b; personal communication, S. Cummins, FDA, 2006). Representatives of consumer organizations that participated in the December 2005 hearing on drug safety communication told the agency about their concerns and criticisms of the FDA Web site and offered specific suggestions for improving it and making it more user-friendly and broadly accessible (see Box 6-3).

Consumer Medication Information

It may surprise many Americans to know that most prescription drugs have only a physician package insert and lack patient package inserts (also known as patient information leaflets), which provide information about a drug's use, risks, and benefits in clearer, more accessible language appropriate for a lay reader (IOM, 2007). The types of patient package information required by FDA to accompany dispensed drugs include information on oral contraceptives and estrogens (required since 1968 by regulation, 21 CFR

310.501 and 310.515, respectively) and medication guides (MedGuides), which are developed by sponsors (and approved by FDA) from the label text for several hundred drugs that "pose serious and significant public health concern" (CDER, 2006). When patients receive what FDA calls consumer medication information it is in the form of a leaflet developed by health care organizations, or more likely, content included by pharmaceutical software providers with the software that they sell to pharmacies. Sponsors may also choose to prepare patient package inserts, which requires FDA approval. Until 1996, there were no standards and no requirements for the minimal useful information to be provided in patient leaflets.

In 1979 and 1980, FDA published in the *Federal Register* the draft, and then the final rule requiring written patient information for prescription drugs (CDER and CBER, 2006). The draft rule addressed all prescription drugs, but the final focused only on a limited number of prescription drugs. In 1982, FDA revoked those regulations, partly in response to assurances by the pharmaceutical industry, by health care professional organizations, and private-sector developers of medication information that the objectives of the final rule would be better achieved without regulation.

The absence of FDA-approved literature on some drugs that are on the market has been criticized by consumer advocates and other parties, and it seems to be a result of legislative obstacles due to private-sector resistance, long-standing claims that regulation in this regard might interfere with the practice of medicine and pharmacy, and finally, FDA's lack of resources. According to the current deputy commissioner for operations, "the Agency [in 1980] published a rule requiring FDA approved patient labeling[4] for ten drugs/drug classes," with the expectation that this would be extended to all prescription drugs. In 1982, "the rule was revoked in favor of private sector efforts to provide patient information that FDA would monitor" (Woodcock, 2002). In 1996, Congress opted to leave consumer medication information in the hands of private-sector content providers and instead tasked FDA with oversight to ensure that 95 percent of consumer medication information meets quality standards by 2006. The quality standards were defined by a broad consortium, the Steering Committee for the Collaborative Development of a Long-Range Action Plan for the Provision of Useful Prescription Medicine Information, which was established to develop an action plan for the secretary of DHHS in 1996.[5] FDA expects to complete its review of the quality of consumer medication information in 2007 (see Box 6-4).

---

[4]FDA uses the term labeling to refer to any FDA-approved materials based on the formal label on which FDA and the sponsor agree at the time on approval or to change in the label after marketing.

[5]The action plan is available online at http://www.fda.gov/cder/offices/ods/keystone.pdf.

BOX 6-4
Criteria for Useful Consumer Medication Information

Written prescription medicine information should be
  (1) scientifically accurate
  (2) unbiased in content and tone
  (3) sufficiently specific and comprehensive
  (4) presented in an understandable and legible format that is readily
       comprehensible to consumers
  (5) timely and up-to-date
  (6) useful

SOURCE: Steering Committee for the Collaborative Development of a Long-Range Action Plan for the Provision of Useful Prescription Medicine Information (1996).

One function of the DSB (described in more detail in Chapter 3), now located in the Office of Safety Policy and Communication, is to produce patient information sheets for every drug, to be posted on the FDA/CDER Web site. The sheets are intended to provide safety alerts and other emerging information to consumers about specific drugs. However, a footnote to the Drug Watch guidance developed by CDER seems to suggest that the center's long-term goal is to develop patient information sheets (and provider sheets) for every drug on the market (FDA, 2005; Galson, 2005; confirmed by S. Galson, personal communication, February 22, 2006).

Improving Communication with the Public

CDER uses the expertise of 17 advisory committees (and the Drug Safety and Risk Management advisory committee) charged with advising FDA and the center on issues related to broad classes of drugs (such as oncologic, cardiovascular, and renal). Although communication issues related to specific drugs may emerge in the committees' work, the existing committees are chartered to review and evaluate safety and efficacy data (on marketed or investigational human drug products) and to make recommendations to the agency.[6] The committee has found a 1996 reference to an FDA Committee on Patient Education (1996). To our knowledge, there is no advisory

---

[6]http://www.fda.gov/cder/audiences/acspage/index.htm.

committee devoted to advising the agency (and CDER specifically) on public communication issues that arise during the lifecycle of drugs.

The committee remains perplexed about the tasks of the new DSB, and how they relate to the center's other plans for improving communication. The DSB, discussed in Chapter 3, has the dual purpose of addressing disagreements among CDER offices or divisions and assisting the center in communicating about drug safety issues to patients (Meadows, 2006; Throckmorton, 2006). As the committee noted in Chapter 3, assigning the two functions to the same internal body may not be effective. Both sets of activities require substantial expertise and resources, and from a management point of view, it seemed unusual that the two functions would be assigned to the same group. Although the committee realizes that the appearance of internal CDER conflict over how drug safety issues are identified, defined, and addressed became associated in the press with poor and delayed communication to the public about those drug safety issues, the committee believes that these two areas should be managed separately. Also, the DSB does not possess substantial expertise in the area of risk communication and consumer or patient behavior. For these reasons, the committee believes that a separate, external entity is needed to advise the agency on the diverse communication needs of the public and patients and on the best evidence on risk communication tools and strategies.

Several FDA centers, including CDER, the Center for Biologics Evaluation and Research (CBER), and the Center for Devices and Radiological Health (CDRH), share similar communication challenges. An advisory committee on consumer and patient communication issues could have a dual function, serving as a conduit for public input into FDA's decision making (for example, through surveys), and an advisor to the agency on a range of communication issues. Other government agencies have advisory committees that involve consumers and patients (see Box 6-5).

The presence of consumer representatives in FDA's advisory committee process is limited to one member per committee, and communication issues understandably constitute just a small component of advisory committees' work. We believe that the agency, and especially CDER, would benefit from having a new advisory committee focused entirely on communication with the public, including risk communication. Public communication issues cut across CDER, CBER, and CDRH such as when and how to warn, how and what to communicate, so the proposed committee should serve all relevant centers.

6.1: The committee recommends that Congress enact legislation establishing a new FDA advisory committee on communication with patients and consumers. The committee would be composed of members who represent consumer and patient perspectives and

organizations. The advisory committee would advise CDER and other centers on communication issues related to efficacy, safety, and use during the lifecycle of drugs and other medical products, and it would support the centers in their mission to "help the public get the accurate, science-based information they need to use medicines and foods to improve their health."

The proposed advisory committee should also have the role of developing and implementing a comprehensive consumer information program at FDA. The expertise needed on the advisory committee may include consumer and patient perspectives (adult, children, chronic conditions, new reader, consumer organizations, disease specific advocacy groups, and patient safety advocacy groups), risk communication, health literacy, social marketing expertise, public relations expertise, social sciences expertise with an emphasis on qualitative research and survey science, journalism, and ethics. The advisory committee could develop standards for effective communication of risk and benefit information, patient-provider communication, and patient participation in the generation of drug safety information and data, and apply available expertise and evidence to refine the structure and content of public health advisories, develop more robust standards for FDA's assessment of DTC advertising. It would, like all other advisory committees, be based in the Office of the Commissioner, but it would work closely with the new CDER Office of Safety Policy and Communication.[7]

The scope of work for the new CDER Office of Safety Policy and Communication is still under development. Given the reactive, fragmentary, and short-lived nature of previous CDER initiatives and organizational changes, the committee believes that special attention and commitment will be required to allow the new office to succeed. It will be essential to have its scope and goals clearly defined, and for its work to be given a high priority in CDER.

> **6.2: The committee recommends that the new Office of Drug Safety Policy and Communication should develop a cohesive risk communication plan that includes, at a minimum, a review of all center risk communication activities, evaluation and revision of communication tools for clarity and consistency, and priority-setting to ensure efficient use of resources.** The work of the office should be evaluated after one year.

---

[7]The Advisory Committee Oversight and Management Staff in the Office of the Commissioner works in collaboration with FDA centers to ensure consistent development, implementation, and operations of the FDA advisory committees (FDA, 2003).

BOX 6-5
Examples of Federal Advisory Committees
on Consumer Issues

Two DHHS agencies have successfully used consumer advisory committees to obtain input from consumers. The NIH Director's Council of Public Representatives (COPR) advises the NIH director on "matters related to medical research, NIH policies and programs, and public participation in agency activities." The COPR has held workshops and issued reports on enhancing public input in research priority-setting, on strengthening public trust in the research enterprise, and on the organizational structure and management of NIH. The COPR Web site also provides information about the cost of running the council: $222,351 for operations and member expenses and $124,118 for 1.30 full-time equivalents of staff. NIH sponsors a public lecture series at which NIH scientists discuss their work in a manner appropriate for a lay audience (NIH, 2006); this series is another example of reaching out to understand consumer concerns.

The National Cancer Institute (NCI) Office of Liaison Activities launched the Director's Consumer Liaison Group (DCLG) in 1997; it is NCI's first and only consumer advisory group. The DCLG makes recommendations to the director of NCI from the consumer advocate perspective on a wide variety of issues, programs, and research priorities. The 15 members include advocates, survivors, family members, and health care professionals and are chosen by the NCI director from a pool of applicants. The DCLG complies with the provisions of the Federal Advisory Committee Act. (NCI, 2006a,b). It also provides a forum for the cancer advocacy community. At the time of this writing, plans were being made for a summit titled "Listening and Learning Together: Building a Bridge of Trust" to bring together many segments of the cancer community to give them a voice in shaping the interaction and collaboration between NCI and consumers (NCI, 2006c). In 2003, NCI contracted with a consulting firm to conduct a survey of the cancer advocacy community and, among other things, to measure and track advocacy organizations' perceptions of the DCLG. The survey found that DCLG was known in the cancer advocacy community, and 69% percent of respondents thought that the group would be more effective if it worked strategically with NCI rather than monitoring or participating in the implementation of NCI's strategic plan. Respondents also wanted to see the DCLG more involved in research, clinical trials, survivorship, health disparities, and communication.

REFERENCES

Ahearne M, Bhattacharya CB, Gruen T. 2005. Antecedents and consequences of customer-company identification: expanding the role of relationship marketing. *J Appl Psychol* 90(3):574-585.

Atkin C, Wallack L. 1990. *Mass Communication and Public Health: Complexities and Conflicts.* London: Sage.

Avorn J. 2005 (October 24). *Professional Interactions.* PowerPoint presentation at the Institute of Medicine 2005 Annual Meeting. Washington, DC: IOM.

Brann M, Anderson JG. 2002. E-medicine and health care consumers: recognizing current problems and possible resolutions for a safer environment. *Health Care Anal* 10(4):403-415.

CBER (Center for Biologics Evaluation and Research), CDER (Center for Drug Evaluation and Research). 2006. *Guidance Useful Written Consumer Medication Information (CMI).* Rockville, MD: FDA.

CDER (Center for Drug Evaluation and Research). 2006. *Medication Guides.* [Online]. Available: http://www.fda.gov/cder/Offices/ODS/medication_guides.htm [accessed September 18, 2006].

DHHS, FDA, CDER. 2005a. *FDA's Communication of Drug Safety Information: Transcript.* [Online]. Available: http://www.fda.gov/cder/meeting/RiskComm2005/1207fda.pdf [accessed March, 2006].

DHHS, FDA, CDER. 2005b. *FDA's Communication of Drug Safety Information: Transcript.* [Online]. Available: http://www.fda.gov/cder/meeting/RiskComm2005/1208fda.pdf [accessed March, 2006].

Dupuits FMHM. 2002. The effects of the internet on pharmaceutical consumers and providers. *Dis Manage Outcomes* 10(11):679-691.

FDA (Food and Drug Administration). 2003. *Advisory Committee Oversight and Management Staff.* [Online]. Available: http://www.fda.gov/oc/advisory/missionandstaff.html [accessed April 18, 2006].

FDA. 2005. *FDA's "Drug Watch" for Emerging Drug Safety Information Draft Guidance.* Rockville, MD: FDA.

Galson S. 2005. *Statement of Steven Galson, M.D., M.P.H, Acting Director Center for Drug Evaluation and Research, US Food and Drug Administration, Department of Health and Human Services,* at the May 5, 2005, Committee on Government Reform, United States House of Representatives.

Greenberg MD. 2003. Information, paternalism, and rational decision-making: the balance of FDA new drug approval. *Alb L J Sci & Tech* Summer/Fall:1-16.

Henwood F, Wyatt S, Hart A, Smith J. 2003. "Ignorance is bliss sometimes": constraints on the emergence of the "informed patient" in the changing landscapes of health information. *Sociol Health Illn* 25(6):589-607.

IMS Health. 2006. *IMS Health Reports Global Pharmaceutical Market Grew 7 Percent in 2005, to $602 Billion.* [Online]. Available: http://www.imshealth.com/ims/portal/front/articleC/0,2777,6599_3665_77491316,00.html [accessed August 28, 2006].

IOM (Institute of Medicine). 2005. *Health Literacy: A Prescription to End Confusion.* Washington, DC: The National Academies Press.

IOM. 2007. *Preventing Medication Errors: Quality Chasm Series.* Washington, DC: The National Academies Press.

Kaiser Family Foundation. 2004. *Trends and Indicators in the Changing Health Care Marketplace.* [Online]. Available: http://www.kff.org/insurance/7031/print-sec1.cfm [accessed October 10, 2005].

Meadows M. 2006. Keeping up with drug safety information. *FDA Consumer Magazine* May/June.

NCI (National Cancer Institute). 2006a. *Director's Consumer Liaison Group: Charter Summary*. [Online]. Available: http://deainfo.nci.nih.gov/advisory/dclg/dclgchr.htm [accessed April 20, 2006].

NCI. 2006b. *Director's Consumer Liaison Group: Fact Sheet*. [Online]. Available: http://la.cancer.gov/DCLGFactSheet2006.pdf [accessed April 20, 2006].

NCI, Office of Liaison Activities. 2006c. *Listening and Learning Together: Building a Bridge of Trust*. [Online]. Available: http://www.palladianpartners.com/NCISummit2006/welcome.htm [accessed June 8, 2006].

NIH (National Institutes of Health). 2006. *About COPR*. [Online]. Available: http://copr.nih.gov/mission.asp [accessed July 13, 2006].

Pew Internet & American Life Project. 2003. *Internet Health Resources: Health Searches and Email Have Become More Commonplace, but There Is Room for Improvement in Searches and Overall Internet Access*. [Online]. Available: http://www.pewinternet.org/pdfs/PIP_Health_Report_July_2003.pdf [accessed October 14, 2005].

Pew Internet & American Life Project. 2004. *Prescription Drugs Online: One in Four Americans Have Looked Online for Drug Information, But Few Have Ventured into the Online Drug Marketplace*. [Online]. Available: http://www.pewinternet.org/pdfs/PIP_Prescription_Drugs_Online.pdf [accessed Octpber 17, 2005].

Pew Internet & American Life Project. 2005. *Health Information Online: Eight in Ten Internet Users Have Looked for Health Information Online, With Increased Interest in Diet, Fitness, Drugs, Health Insurance, Experimental Treatments, and Particular Doctors and Hospitals*. [Online]. Available: http://www.pewinternet.org/pdfs/PIP_Healthtopics_May05.pdf [accessed October 17, 2005].

Smith C, Cowan C, Sensenig A, Catlin A, the Health Accounts Team. 2005. Health spending growth slows in 2003. *Health Aff (Millwood)* 24(1):185-194.

Steering Committee for the Collaborative Development of a Long-Range Action Plan for the Provision of Useful Prescription Medicine Information.1996. *Action Plan for the Provision of Useful Prescription Medicine Information*. [Online]. Available: http://www.fda.gov/cder/offices/ods/keystone.pdf [accessed July 18, 2006].

Throckmorton DC. 2006 (March 31). *Drug Safety Oversight Board: Recent Activities*. PowerPoint presentation to the FDA Science Advisory Board. Bethesda, MD: FDA.

Woodcock J. 2002. *Statement by Janet Woodcock, MD, Director, Center for Drug Administration Before the Subcommittee on Oversight and Investigations* before the Committee on Energy and Commerce, US House of Representatives.

7

Resources for the Drug Safety System

The Food and Drug Administration (FDA) lacks the resources needed to accomplish its large and complex mission today, let alone to position itself for an increasingly challenging future. Despite the fact that so much has changed in drug discovery and development, in the number and complexity of FDA's congressionally mandated responsibilities, in the practice of medicine, the structuring and delivery of health care, the way drugs are used, the role of patients and consumers, and the information environment, FDA appropriations for new drug review have remained roughly flat (in constant dollars) since the passing of the Prescription Drug User Fee Act (PDUFA) (Thompson, 2000; GAO, 2002).[1] User fees have led to an overall increase in resources for new drug review, but activities not funded by user fees have received a smaller portion of FDA's total budget. There is little dispute that FDA in general is, and the Center for Drug Evaluation and Research (CDER) specifically remains, severely underfunded (Goldhammer, 2005; Wolfe, 2006). There is widespread agreement that resources for postmarketing drug safety work are especially inadequate and that resource limitations have hobbled the agency's ability to improve and expand this essential

---

[1]Also of note: "Total FDA appropriations each year (exclusive of user fees and rent payments to GSA) must total at least as much as FDA received in FY 1997, adjusted for inflation at the rate of change in the Consumer Price index since FY 1997. . . . FDA meets this trigger consistently, even though for most years since FY 1997 FDA did not receive increases to cover the cost of pay increases and inflation for its core programs—which was the original intent of this trigger. FDA meets this trigger primarily because FDA has received appropriation increases earmarked for specific initiatives since FY 1997 (e.g., food safety, tobacco, counter-terrorism)" (FDA, 2003).

component of its mission. Continued resource shortages will impede the agency's ability to use new and future scientific and technological advances in drug research across the lifecycle. In particular, the limited resources could impede the agency's ability to detect risks of new drugs in a timely fashion, analyze emerging drug safety data, and effectively communicate that information to the public in the ways envisioned in the committee's report. For fiscal year 2006, CDER's enacted budget was $517,557,000, with $297,716,000 from congressional appropriations and $219,841,000 (or 42.5 percent of the total budget) from user fees (see Figures 7-1 and 7-2 for more information on trends in CDER funding and staffing).

Although PDUFA has facilitated substantial expansion of CDER staff, especially in the Office of New Drugs (OND), growth has been largely to shorten review times and improve related processes, including interactions with industry representatives and the development of guidances, rather than strategic with respect to the full breadth of functions and disciplines needed to operate the largest center of a world-class regulatory agency. PDUFA I and II did not allow for the use of PDUFA funds to support postmarketing drug safety work. PDUFA III allowed for a very restricted amount of funds to be used for very specific and narrow postmarketing safety work (postmarketing surveillance of drugs for 2–3 years after approval) (FDA,

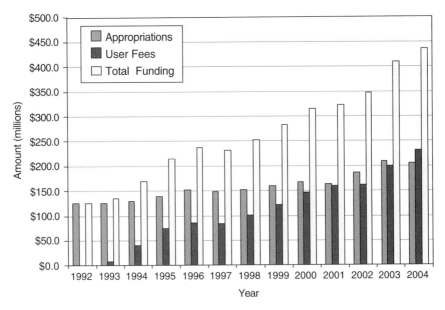

FIGURE 7-1 History of CDER funding.
SOURCE: PDUFA White Paper (FDA, 2005b).

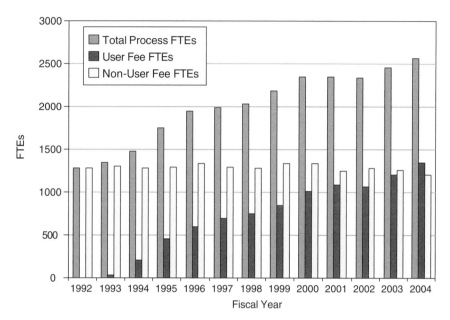

FIGURE 7-2 History of CDER staffing.
SOURCE: PDUFA White Paper (FDA, 2005b).

2003). These restrictions have contributed to a troubling resource imbalance between OND and other CDER units (e.g., postmarketing safety activities, compliance). Some effects or correlates of the resource imbalance between OND and the Office of Drug Safety (ODS)/ Office of Surveillance and Epidemiology (OSE) are discussed in Chapter 3.

The committee recognizes that the recommendations in this report come with a price tag, one that is most likely large and believes it would be ill-advised to expect CDER to take on the many new responsibilities called for in this report without new funds for strengthening the number and expertise of staff, for intramural and extramural research, and for information technology. On the other hand, the committee believes that full implementation of the recommendations it offers is essential. Although some of the recommendations are more far-reaching than others, the committee believes each of its recommendations will serve to improve the drug safety system.

For the past 15 years, user fees have supported a steadily increasing share of CDER's work. Many have argued that relying so heavily on industry funds is inherently inappropriate and damaging to the reputation and functioning of CDER, indeed, of any regulatory entity. Some CDER staff, as well as some public advocates (Wolfe, 2006) have expressed discomfort with this funding (DHHS and OIG, 2003; GAO, 2006; IOM Staff Notes,

2005–2006; Union of Concerned Scientists, 2006) based on real or perceived "capture" of the agency, that is, that the center's increasing dependence on industry funding in itself creates a sense of obligation "to please" on the part of the agency. The Pharmaceutical Research and Manufacturers of America (PhRMA) itself has expressed a concern about this perception.

> "We share a concern with FDA about the current balance between the user fee portion and the appropriated portion of the review process," PhRMA's Goldhammer says. As industry funding approaches half of the review budget, "it has led to a perceptual issue that industry is paying for the review process and that the American public, through its tax moneys, is not. We would hope that can be dealt with in some way because we don't want there to be the perception that this is an industry-driven program" (Thompson, 2000).

The effects of user-fee funding are experienced differently by different staff at CDER (IOM Staff Notes, 2005–2006). Some staff recognize no impact on their day-to-day work of the source of their salary and support the principle and practice of the user-fee system, while others expressed concerns about the workload and time pressures that they feel have accompanied the PDUFA funding,[2] cognizant that if industry were displeased with CDER performance and worked to eliminate user fees (and appropriations did not increase to close the shortfall), staff would have to be eliminated. Yet other CDER staff, particularly CDER leadership and managers, describe PDUFA as setting necessary performance goals that any responsible agency should employ regardless of links to funding source, and deny that the goals are used as anything more than targets. Indeed, the goals allow for review times longer than the 6- and 10-month approval targets in up to 10 percent of the cases for standard-rated and priority-rated new drug applications. However, if CDER were to consistently miss the goals for time-to-approval, the pharmaceutical industry would push for changes in PDUFA fees or other arrangements in the following round of negotiations. This reality would undoubtedly put pressure on CDER management to meet these targets.

For some staff and policy analysts, user-fee funding, combined with industry's considerable role in shaping PDUFA-associated goals and expectations, further reinforces the perception that the industry has become a primary driver of the agency's priorities and performance.[3] The notion

---

[2]As described in Chapter 2, some CDER new drug review staff assert that the workload pressures to meet PDUFA goals are compounded by industry submissions that are not well organized, submissions that come in on paper or with data that are not easily reanalyzed, or on suboptimal management by their direct supervisors or team leaders. Some of these CDER staff also reported that the biggest pressures come from 6-month priority approvals and not from standard applications, the goal for which is 10 months for approval.

[3]Zelenay has proposed eliminating the PDUFA sunset clause as a means to reduce the industry's bargaining power (Zelenay, 2005).

of "regulatory capture"[4] has been employed to describe the state of affairs created or, more likely, exacerbated by the user-fee system,[5] namely, that powerful industry interests control or strongly influence the regulatory agency's decision making.

Some have argued that eliminating industry funding for regulatory review is in the best interest of the credibility of the drug safety system. Others have argued that industry receives a valuable service (timely approval of their products) and should be expected to pay for this,[6] as long as agency independence and the credibility of its scientific review remain intact. Others argue that without extra funding from user-fee revenue, the delays in new drug review observed prior to user fees will return since FDA budgets will then be subject to fluctuations in the policitical climate and increased pressures to reduce government spending. This too may compromise the effectiveness of our drug approval system.

As described elsewhere in the report, PDUFA has included an extensive number of performance goals (see Appendix C for a complete listing). CDER reports yearly to Congress on how well it has met those goals (in the performance goals letter[7] submitted by the Secretary of the Department of Health and Human Services (DHHS), see, for example, http://www.fda.gov/cder/pdufa/default.htm). Along with performance goals, PDUFA includes restrictions on how CDER can use its funds. Each round of PDUFA negotiations has led to more demands on CDER and continued restrictions on CDER's flexibility. The committee is not concerned about the existence of performance goals in principle,[8] but finds the limitations or "strings" that direct how CDER can use PDUFA funds the most troubling aspect of the arrangement.[9]

7.1: To support improvements in drug safety and efficacy activities over a product's lifecycle, the committee recommends that the Administration should request and Congress should approve sub-

---

[4]Adapted from the capture theory of regulation advanced by Stigler (1971) and critiqued by Laffont and Tirole (1991) and by Carpenter and Ting (2004).

[5]The industry has a powerful influence on the political process and on the regulatory environment whether or not it funds the agency.

[6]Similar arguments have been made regarding user-fee programs for other regulatory agencies.

[7]http://energycommerce.house.gov/107/hearings/03062002Hearing502/print.htm.

[8]See Chapter 3 for a recommendation regarding institution of safety goals.

[9]The committee is aware that other regulatory agencies, for example the Environmental Protection Agency and the Federal Communications Commission, are supported in part by specific user-fee programs. Some user fees go directly into the Treasury; other user fees go to the agency and offset congressional appropriations. The committee has not done an exhaustive analysis of other user-fee programs but is of the understanding that they are not associated with significant requirements on how the agency uses the fees to achieve programmatic goals.

stantially increased resources in both funds and personnel for the Food and Drug Administration.

The committee favors appropriations from general revenues, rather than user fees, to support the full spectrum of new drug safety responsibilities proposed in this report. This preference is based on the expectation that CDER will continue to review and approve drugs in a timely manner and that increasing attention to drug safety will not occur at the expense of efficacy reviews but rather it will complement efficacy review for a life-cycle approach to drugs. Congressional appropriations from general tax revenues are a mechanism by which the public can directly, fairly, and effectively invest in the FDA's postmarket drug safety activities. However, if appropriations are not sufficient to fund these activities and user fees are required, Congress should greatly reduce current restrictions on how CDER uses PDUFA funds. Should the sources described above be insufficient, alternatives that could be considered and evaluated by Congress include but are likely not limited to a user fee associated with the consumption of prescription medications and a sales tax on purchase of marketing services by pharmaceutical companies.

By some estimates, more than a billion prescriptions are written each year in the United States. A small tax on prescriptions could generate significant funding to implement the recommendations made in this report. A tax of ten cents on every prescription, for example, would generate more than $100 million for the FDA budget. The administrative costs of collecting such a tax would need to be considered as well as the ultimate incidence of the tax. For example, collecting the tax from retailers or consumers at the point of sale might have higher administrative costs than collecting it from manufacturers. On the other hand, manufacturers might not know how many prescriptions were filled out of a given amount of product sold to a wholesales or retailer. An alternative approach might be to tax manufacturers based on the value of sales (perhaps net of rebates). This would have the advantage of more heavily taxing more expensive drugs, which would tend to be the newest ones and the ones around which there is greatest uncertainty about safety. Regardless of the taxation method used, it must be considered that the ultimate incidence of the tax will be on consumers and will be regressive. This tax would likely also have an effect on the costs of and access to pharmaceuticals.

Another tax-based proposal would seek to accomplish two goals—revenue enhancement and deterrence of excessive DTC advertising. A direct tax on DTC advertising for newer drugs would have the advantage of linking the decision to impose a tax with the finding that newer drugs necessarily suffer from greater uncertainty with respect to safety and efficacy in the general population, which is more heterogeneous than that studied in the preapproval clinical trials. On the other hand, taxation of protected speech can raise constitutional objections that have yet to be fully litigated before the courts. An alternative is to deny the tax deductibility of pharmaceutical advertising. Just such a proposal was made in H.R. 1655: America Rx Act, although in that case the resulting revenues were to be used to offer discounts on prescription drugs to those in need.

Regardless of the source of the funds, the committee reiterates that the functioning of a drug safety system that assesses a drug's risks and benefits throughout its lifecycle is too important a public health need to continue to be underfunded.

The committee was charged with reviewing CDER's resources but concluded that it was not feasible to do a financial audit of CDER or a detailed calculation of the costs for CDER or other stakeholders, including the pharmaceutical industry, of implementing the recommendations in this report. Convention dictates that federal agencies do not publicly articulate resource needs that differ from those offered in the President's budget, so the committee was unable to understand fully what CDER and FDA leadership estimate is needed to meet current objectives, let alone the expanded responsibilities the committee envisions for the future. Thus, the committee can only offer general guidance and estimates of resources that will be required to implement its recommendations; it does so with the caveat that this list is most likely incomplete and is but a starting point for discussions between FDA and congressional appropriations committees. CDER will need carefully to assess their resource needs in light of the recommendations in this report.

Staff: The first three 5-year cycles of PDUFA funding and accompanying process improvements have led to dramatic shortening of the time required for new drug approval, in great part due to the significant staff increases, primarily in OND. The committee asserts that the next phase of improvements, including staff increases, should focus on the postmarket activities recommended in this report.

The committee notes certain facts about current staffing. CDER estimated that in 2004 it devoted 700 full-time equivalents (FTEs) for premarket safety work and 393 FTEs (or 36 percent of total safety-related FTEs) for postmarket safety work (FDA, 2005a,b). PDUFA funding supported 1320 FTEs for new drug review in 2004 and appropriations supported 1287 FTEs (FDA, 2005a,b). CDER staff devoted to new drug review has approximately doubled in the PDUFA era. Between 1996 and 2004, new drug review FTEs supported by PDUFA increased by 125 percent (from 600 to 1320) whereas ODS staff increased by 75 percent (from 52 to 90)[10] (FDA, 2005a,b).

The committee recognizes that CDER will require a significant increase

---

[10]In 2004 eight of the ODS staff were funded by PDUFA.

in staff to meet the new responsibilities described in this report. CDER will require new staff, for example, to participate more actively in efforts to generate more and better safety analyses, such as through an expanded epidemiology contracts program; participate in new drug review teams; develop more consistent approaches to risk-benefit assessment both premarket and postmarket; evaluate risk minimization action plans; work with other federal agencies and departments in their efforts to improve their drug safety-related activities; evaluate industry-submitted 5-year reviews; routinely assess and make public emerging safety and effectiveness information, and consider appropriate imposition of the newly clarified conditions on distribution. The committee's recommendations will require additional staff throughout CDER and with varied expertise, for example, epidemiology, statistics, public health, medicine, pharmacy, informatics, programming, law, regulatory policy, communication, as well as project management and administration.

The committee recognizes that increases in postmarket safety staff must be phased in over time. As CDER begins to implement the recommendations in this report and gradually increase their staff, the size of the needed increase will become apparent to CDER and the Congress. Congress can ensure this by requesting that CDER perform and make publicly available a formal evaluation of staff needs, perhaps in the form of a work audit. The FDA commissioner can serve an important role as a champion within the government and in discussions with Congress for needed resources. The committee also recognizes that other federal partners in drug safety will require additional staff to achieve a fully functioning postmarket drug safety system, as described in Chapter 4.

Research funds: ODS/OSE is the CDER component most likely to have primary responsibility for implementing the extramural and intramural research activities called for in the report. The committee was concerned by the very small and inadequate amount of funds for the epidemiology contracts programs in particular. CDER will also require funds for extramural contracts to improve their passive and active surveillance activities, in addition to increased intramural use of drug utilization databases and other datasets such as the General Practice Research Database.

The committee provides several estimates of needed funds for intramural and extramural research. The committee's lower bound estimate is that an expanded epidemiology contracts program would cost $10 million.[11] The committee estimates that other agencies/departments also require similar resources for epidemiology research contracts. The committee offers as a

---

[11]The current epidemiology contract program, funded at approximately $1 million, is insufficient to complete one major study. The committee asserts that at least 10 drug safety hypotheses could be explored through this or a similar program per year.

more ambitious estimate that the epidemiology contracts program at CDER should be expanded to $60 million.[12] This upper bound estimate does not include the costs for research to be conducted by other DHHS agencies or other departments, such as the Centers for Medicare and Medicaid Services or the Department of Veterans Affairs.

The committee acknowledges that a financial investment will be required for the success of the public-private partnership (PPP) it recommends for the prioritization and planning of confirmatory drug safety and efficacy studies. The federal partners will require dedicated staff to make this partnership successful, in addition to research funds for studies. The committee anticipates that pharmaceutical companies and other health care industries will also fund some of this research.

The committee offers a lower bound estimate of $20 million per year for start-up and administrative costs of the PPP. This is based on an estimate for a research institute recently proposed to advance the Critical Path Initiative.[13] As Chapter 4 describes, the PPP will have responsibility for prioritizing and planning postmarket studies to address public health concerns, will help advise on the design of such studies (including the postmarket study commitments agreed upon by CDER and industry), and will facilitate necessary collaborations between government agencies and departments, and the pharmaceutical industry. Some studies conducted under the aegis of the PPP will require new resources. Other studies will be ones likely done absent the PPP. In these cases the PPP brings added value to the research by advising on study design, but the conduct of the research itself will not require incremental funds.

An upper bound estimate for the PPP should include the cost of a large clinical trial. Although not all studies to be conducted under the aegis of the PPP are large, complicated, and expensive, some necessary studies will require significant new resources. The committee asserts that at least one major drug safety question that is best answered with prospective research of some magnitude could be addressed each year under the aegis of the PPP. Some of these studies would be epidemiology studies using existing data, such as those also conducted under the epidemiology contracts program. Other studies would address narrowly defined safety concerns in specific populations. As described in Chapter 4, some, if not most, of these studies would not be incremental costs to the system, because they would have occurred absent the PPP. However, it is not unreasonable to anticipate, and

---

[12]This is based on testimony to Congress in 2000 that an expanded epidemiology contracts program would cost $50 million (Federal News Service, 2000). Using the Consumer Price Index, this would cost $60 million in 2006.

[13]The Enhancing Drug Safety and Innovation Act of 2006 (S. 3807) authorizes appropriations for the Reagan-Udall Institute.

it would be naïve to suggest otherwise, that on occasion significant new resources will be required to fund a large, prospective, randomized clinical trial to answer drug safety questions of pressing public health concern. Thus, an upper bound estimate of the resources needed for the PPP on such occasions is on the order of $150 million[14] to be spread out over the period of time the study is conducted.

Information technology (IT): The committee concluded from its conversations with individual CDER staff that CDER's IT systems are antiquated. Upgrades of staff workstations are clearly part of CDER and FDA plans, but there will be additional IT needs (e.g., servers, programmers, and training) to implement several of the recommendations in Chapter 4 that should be included in budget projections.

Other resource needs: The committee was tasked to assess only one aspect, drug safety, of CDER responsibilities. There are many important areas of CDER work that the committee did not assess, for example compliance, inspections, and the prevention of medication errors. The committee also realizes that the already-initiated PDUFA IV negotiations will likely result in additional requirements on CDER. The committee notes that both of these factors could very well require additional funds for staff and research.

It is critical that CDER assess the center's resource needs with particular attention to ensuring that funding for premarketing product review and postmarketing risk-benefit assessments is commensurate with:

1. The breadth of both sets of programs and activities, and
2. Their importance in achieving a lifecycle approach to drug safety and efficacy that translates into how FDA regulates, studies, and communicates about drugs with stakeholders in industry, health care, academic research, and the public.

This process must be conducted with a keen awareness of the expectations, needs, and perspectives of all stakeholders in the system and in a transparent manner. It is incumbent on the leadership of the agency and the center, as well as the Administration, to present to Congress a full review and analysis of the levels of funding needed to fulfill the mission of the center and the vision the committee has set forth. While resources might not be immediately available, a public statement acknowledging the resource needs is essential.

FDA's centennial offers an occasion to celebrate the past and to give serious consideration to what is needed to strengthen the agency's central

---

[14]For example, the Clinical Antipsychotic Trials of Intervention Effectiveness cost $42.6 million; the Antihypertensive and Lipid-Lowering Treatment to Prevent Heart Attacks trial cost $125 million; the Study of Tamoxifen and Raloxifene trial cost $118 million.

role in assuring the safety and efficacy of prescription drugs now and in the future. Also, PDUFA reauthorization is just months away, and major legislation addressing drug regulation has been prepared and considered.[15] These circumstances make this a golden moment of opportunity to improve fundamentally the way FDA regulation considers and responds to the evolving understanding of risks and benefits of drugs, and the way all stakeholders in the drug safety system perceive, study, and communicate about those risks and benefits. As described in Chapter 1, there have been many commissions and reports addressing issues similar to those contained in this report. It is the committee's fervent hope that Congress, FDA, and the other stakeholders will seize the gathering momentum to invigorate the drug safety system. The agency's credibility and its ability to protect and promote optimally the health of the American people cannot wait another year or another decade.

REFERENCES

Carpenter D, Ting MM. 2004. *A Theory of Approval Regulation.* [Online]. Available: http://people.hmdc.harvard.edu/~dcarpent/endosub-20040214.pdf [accessed October 10, 2005].

DHHS (Department of Health and Human Services), OIG (Office of Inspector General). 2003. *FDA's Review Process for New Drug Applications: a Management Review.* OEI-01-01-00590. Washington, DC: OIG, FDA.

FDA (Food and Drug Administration). 2003. *PDUFA III Five Year Plan.* [Online]. Available: http://www.fda.gov/oc/pdufa3/2003plan/default.htm [accessed October 10, 2005].

FDA. 2005a. *Center for Drug Evaluation and Research—Activities and Level of Effort Devoted to Drug Safety.* Submitted to the Institute of Medicine Committee on the Assessment of the US Drug Safety System by FDA.

FDA. 2005b. *White Paper, Prescription Drug User Fee Act (PDUFA): Adding Resources and Improving Performance in FDA Review of New Drug Applications.* [Online]. Available: http://www.fda.gov/oc/pdufa/PDUFAWhitePaper.pdf [accessed December 5, 2005].

Federal News Service. 2000. *Prepared Testimony of Richard Platt, MD, MSC, Professor of Ambulatory Care and Prevention Harvard Medical School Director of Research Harvard Pilgrim Health Care.*

GAO. 2002. *Food and Drug Administration: Effect of User Fees on Drug Approval Times, Withdrawals, and Other Agency Activities.* GAO-02-958. Washington, DC: GAO.

GAO. 2006. *Drug Safety: Improvement Needed in FDA's Postmarket Decision-Making and Oversight Process.* GAO-06-402. Washington, DC: GAO.

Goldhammer A. 2005 (June 8). *Statement of the Pharmaceutical Research and Manufacturers of America to Institute of Medicine.* Presentation to the Institute of Medicine Committee on the Assessment of the US Drug Safety System. Washington, DC: IOM.

Laffont J, Tirole J. 1991. The politics of government decision-making: a theory of regulatory capture. *Quart J Econ* 106(4):1089-1127.

Stigler G. 1971. The theory of economic regulation. *Bell J Econ Manage Sci* 2:2-21.

Thompson L. 2000. User fees for faster drug reviews. Are they helping or hurting the public health? *FDA Consum* 34(5):25-29.

---

[15]The Enhancing Drug Safety and Innovation Act of 2006, http://help.senate.gov/S___.pdf.

Union of Concerned Scientists (UCS). 2006. *FDA Scientists Pressured to Exclude, Alter Findings; Scientists Fear Retaliation for Voicing Safety Concerns.* [Online]. Available: http://www.ucsusa.org/news/press_release/fda-scientists-pressured.html [accessed July 24, 2006].

Wolfe S. 2006. *Public Citizen: The 100th Anniversary of the FDA: The Sleeping Watchdog Whose Master Is Increasingly the Regulated Industries.* [Online]. Available: http://www.pharmalive.com/News/index.cfm?articleid=353196&categoryid=54 [accessed July 11, 2006].

Zelenay JL. 2005. The Prescription Drug User Fee Act: is a faster Food and Drug Administration always a better Food and Drug Administration? *Food Drug Law J* 60(2):261-338.

Appendix A

Moving Target: Changes at FDA During the Course of the Study[1]

DRUG SAFETY INITIATIVES

Many of the recent changes stem from the 2004 Food and Drug Administration (FDA) Drug Safety Initiative. The purpose of the initiative is to create a culture of openness and to enhance oversight in FDA. To achieve that FDA has established the Drug Safety Oversight Board (DSB), proposed a Drug Watch Web page, and is soliciting public input on how to expand and establish communication channels with the public to increase transparency (FDA, 2005d).

DRUG SAFETY OVERSIGHT BOARD

The DSB was established in February 2005 (FDA, 2005d) to help FDA realize its vision of culture of openness, enhanced oversight, and transparency in decision making. The DSB is charged with identifying, tracking, and overseeing the management of important drug safety issues in the Center for Drug Evaluation and Research (CDER) (CDER, 2005). A separate board task is to facilitate timely external communication of drug safety issues. Board members—all appointed by the FDA commissioner—include FDA staff, medical experts in other Department of Health and Human Services agencies, and other government departments, and medical experts and representatives of patient and consumer groups. The DSB has 31 members. It

---

[1]This section was compiled by Institute of Medicine staff with guidance from the Committee on the Assessment of the US Drug Safety System.

met nine times from its inception through June 2006, and it has generally discussed Patient Information Sheets, Public Health Advisories distributed by CDER, and ways to strengthen CDER's risk communication efforts.

DRUG WATCH

A Drug Watch Web page was proposed as part of FDA's drug safety initiative in February 2005 to improve communication with the public on drug safety issues by putting information out as quickly as possible in an easily accessible format. The goal of the proposed Drug Watch program is to help patients and health care professionals make informed decisions on the use of prescription drugs. Drug Watch will include emerging data and risk information in a consumer-friendly form (information sheets) for healthcare professionals and patients regarding drugs for which FDA is actively assessing incoming safety information (FDA, 2005b,d).

A draft guidance on Drug Watch released in May 2005 (FDA, 2005f) discussed how the inclusion of a drug on Drug Watch would not signify that the drug is dangerous or should not be used; it only means that FDA is investigating emerging safety signals. The information on each drug would vary but could include "factual information about newly observed, serious adverse events associated with the use of a drug that have been reported to FDA"; "information about significant emerging risks that FDA believes may be associated with a drug, but that might be avoided by appropriate patient selection, monitoring, or use of concomitant therapy"; and notice of an important risk minimization procedure that has been put into place by the sponsor to alert healthcare providers and patients that there has been a change in how a drug should be prescribed, dispensed, or used (FDA, 2005f). The DSB role in overseeing the Drug Watch program was described above.

STRUCTURAL CHANGES AND LEADERSHIP CHANGES IN THE CENTER FOR DRUG EVALUATION AND RESEARCH

In September 2004, CDER announced that it would be restructuring the Office of New Drugs (OND) and has implemented this in phases throughout 2005–2006 (FDA and CDER, 2005). Phase I of the reorganization involved the elimination of the Office of Drug Evaluation V (ODE V), which began in May 2005 and is now complete. Phase II began in July 2005 with the operation of the new Office of Oncology Drug Products. It also involved the split of the Division of Neuropharmacological Drug Products in ODE I into two new divisions: Neurology and Psychiatry. Phase III began in September 2005 with reassignment of staff in the Division of Therapeutic Biological Internal Medicine Products and the Division of Review Management Policy in ODE VI to other ODEs and divisions in OND, so that ODE VI could be eliminated (FDA and CDER, 2005).

In October 2005, in his "State of CDER" address to center employees, Steven Galson outlined a proposed center reorganization to "better align staff functions with CDER's goals and FDA's public health mission" (FDA, 2005j). According to Dr. Galson, the three goals of the reorganization are to position CDER to be able to participate fully in the Critical Path Initiative (CPI), to increase visibility and a cross-center approach to drug safety, and to centralize risk communication efforts (FDA, 2006a).

As of May 15, 2006, the changes that Dr. Galson outlined in 2005 were put into effect (FDA and CDER, 2005). The reorganization resulted in the lifting of the status (to be at the same level as OND) of the Office of Drug Safety (ODS) whose name was changed to Office of Surveillance and Epidemiology (OSE) and which now reports to the office of the center director. That was done in part to address the perception that drug safety is solely the responsibility of ODS. A new office that reports to the center director and serves as a catalyst for CPI activities was created, with clinical pharmacology and the office of biostatistics reporting to that office. Another change was elevating the Office of Policy and Communication to the office of the center director.

LEADERSHIP CHANGES IN THE
FOOD AND DRUG ADMINISTRATION

Over the course of this study, several changes in leadership have taken place in FDA. When the study began, Lester M. Crawford was the acting commissioner; he was confirmed in July 2005 (FDA, 2005i). Soon after his permanent appointment, Dr. Crawford made several changes in FDA leadership, including appointing a new deputy commissioner for medical and scientific affairs, deputy commissioner for operations and chief operating officer, deputy commissioner for international and special programs, and associate commissioner for legislation (FDA, 2005h).

In September 2005, Dr. Crawford abruptly resigned as FDA commissioner (two months after confirmation). Shortly thereafter, President Bush appointed Andrew C. von Eschenbach as the new acting commissioner, and he is still serving in this capacity. In March 2006, President Bush nominated Dr. von Eschenbach to be the permanent head of the agency; as of June 2006, confirmation hearings have not yet taken place.

In June 2005, FDA announced its search for a new director of drug safety in CDER (FDA, 2005g). In late July 2005, the agency announced that CDER Acting Director Steven Galson would be director. In September 2005, FDA announced that it had selected Douglas Throckmorton as the deputy director of CDER. In October 2005, Gerald Dal Pan was named director of ODS. In April 2006, FDA announced the appointment of Paul Seligman as the CDER associate director for safety policy and communication; this was a newly created position to provide oversight of drug safety issues and policies in CDER (FDA, 2006c).

During the study process, the committee referred to newly released FDA and CDER guidance documents and reports. FDA made additional important changes and undertook reviews of some of its programs. Those are described below.

RECENT MATERIALS FROM THE
FOOD AND DRUG ADMINISTRATION

Guidance Documents

In March 2005, FDA released three final guidance documents to help develop new ways to improve methods of assessing and monitoring risks associated with drugs in clinical development:

- *Guidance for Industry: Premarketing Risk Assessment* (FDA et al., 2005). This guidance focuses on what pharmaceutical companies should consider throughout the clinical trial process to improve the assessment and reporting of safety, to assess important safety issues during trial registration and best practices for the use of data from preapproval safety evaluations, and to build on FDA and International Conference on Harmonisation guidances related to preapproval safety assessments.
- *Guidance for Industry: Development and Use of Risk Minimization Action Plans* (FDA, 2005a). This guidance outlines steps that pharmaceutical companies can take to address goals and objectives related to risk and suggests tools to minimize known risks posed by drugs. These include the consistent use and definition of terms; a framework for ensuring that benefits exceed risks; obtaining input from the public, patients, and health care professionals when deciding to initiate, revise, or end risk minimization plans; and making certain that risk minimization efforts are successful by evaluating risk minimization action plans.
- *Guidance for Industry: Good Pharmacovigilance Practices and Pharmacoepidemiologic Assessment* (FDA, 2005e). This guidance discusses how to increase postmarketing vigilance to identify safety signals, investigation of the signals, interpreting the signals in terms of risk, and using pharmacovigilance plans to speed the acquisition of safety information with unusual safety signals.

Those guidance documents were issued as part of FDA's effort to minimize risks while preserving the benefits of medical products. FDA stated that the guidance documents are part of the drug safety initiative announced in 2004 (FDA, 2005d) to improve drug safety and the commitment to transparency (FDA News, 2005a).

FDA released a final guidance in January 2006 titled "Guidance for Industry, Investigators, and Reviewers Exploratory IND Studies" (CDER, 2006). It was one FDA step to "advance the earliest phases of clinical research in the development of innovative medical treatments" (FDA News, 2006a). The guidance discusses specific steps to be taken when exploratory clinical studies on humans are done under an investigational new drug to make the process more efficient and safe.

Reports

In November 2005, FDA announced the availability of a white paper titled *Prescription Drug User Fee Act (PDUFA): Adding Resources and Improving Performance in FDA Review of New Drug Applications* (FDA, 2005c). It was released shortly after FDA requested public input on PDUFA provisions for FDA to consider during the renewal process for 2007 (FDA, 2005k). The white paper describes PDUFA goals, how they were implemented or achieved by CDER, and the changes that have resulted from PDUFA (that is, hiring of more medical reviewers, shorter approval times, greater consistency, and increased workload) (FDA, 2005c).

In February 2006, a report commissioned by FDA, *Evaluation of FDA's First Cycle Review Performance—Retrospective Analysis* was released[2] (FDA News, 2006c). It showed a positive correlation between receiving approval on the first review cycle and pharmaceutical company consultation with FDA before the beginning of the final phase of human testing (the end of phase 2). The commissioner of FDA stated that "these meetings have become one of the most valuable aspects of the drug development process" (FDA News, 2006c). Deficiencies in safety assessment during the Investigational New Drug process were cited in the report as a main cause of multiple review cycles, which potentially could have been avoided if a "milestone meeting" had taken place where CDER staff could have made suggestions for improving the quality of the initial applications (FDA News, 2006c).

---

[2]The report was written by Booz Allen Hamilton in relation to the Prescription Drug User Fee Amendments of 2002 (PDUFA III).

OTHER RELEVANT CHANGES AT
THE FOOD AND DRUG ADMINISTRATION AND
THE CENTER FOR DRUG EVALUATION AND RESEARCH

Labeling

On November 2, 2005, FDA started requiring that drug manufacturers submit prescription drug label information to FDA in a new electronic format. That was intended to allow patients and healthcare providers to obtain information in FDA-approved package inserts ("labels") with greater ease (FDA News, 2006c). Drug manufacturers are now required to provide FDA with accurate and up-to-date product and prescribing information in a structured product labeling that can be electronically managed. These labels will be the main source of information for a new interagency Web site, "DailyMed," a health information clearinghouse, which will provide up-to-date information to consumers and healthcare providers free (National Library of Medicine, 2006).

In January 2006, FDA announced a change in the prescription drug format for the package insert to provide clear and concise information so that healthcare providers can make better use of the drug label to minimize risk and medical errors in their patients (FDA News, 2006c). The final rule was the first revision in 25 years and now requires that prescription information for new and recently approved products meet new criteria. The change was aimed at increasing the readability and accessibility of label information and drawing health professionals and consumers' attention to the most important pieces of drug information before a product is prescribed. The changes include the insertion of a "highlights" section that includes concise information on the risks and benefits related to the drug, a table of contents in the label, the date of initial approval of the drug, a toll-free number, and Internet reporting information.

The labeling rule also established an important change in statutory interpretation: preempting state product liability laws on the basis of FDA's approved label. The preamble to the labeling rule states that state laws and judicial decisions that would have the effect of finding FDA-approved labels inadequate or misleading are preempted by the federal rule (21 CFR Parts 201, 314, and 601). That position has partial support in existing case law, and FDA's assertion of federal preemption under the new labeling rule has not yet been tested in court (National Conference of State Legislatures, 2006).

PROGRAM REVIEWS OR EVALUATIONS

Advisory Committees

In May 2006, CDER announced that it was launching an internal assessment of its Advisory Committee meeting system to establish best practices surrounding that process. The assessment will be led by senior management in CDER and will take a comprehensive look at current practices for nominating committee members, screening for conflicts of interest, choosing expertise for specific meeting topics, and utilizing Special Government Employees.

Postmarketing Study Commitments

In April 2006, FDA contracted with Booz Allen Hamilton for an evaluation of FDA's postmarket study process (phase IV commitments) for collecting medical information (FDA Press Release, 2006). The evaluation will comment on how FDA can increase consistency in requesting, facilitating, and reviewing postmarketing commitments among centers. Ultimately, this will help FDA to request focused studies that result in the information needed to assess safety postmarket.

Partnerships

In August 2005, FDA and the Association of American Medical Colleges (AAMC) released the joint report *Drug Development Science Obstacles and Opportunities for Collaborations*, which describes an array of opportunities for scientific breakthroughs to be undertaken through collaboration to reach the goals of CPI (AAMC, 2006; AAMC et al., 2005; DeClaire, 2005). The report states that those partnerships should focus on greater sharing of knowledge, regulatory and legislative relief, earlier evaluation of drugs in humans, and improved education and training for health professionals. Some of the kinds of collaboration outlined in the report are to develop mechanisms to learn from failed drug targets, establish joint models for biomarker validation, set up a consortium to analyze and learn from failed clinical trials, and develop agreements for sharing of information restricted as intellectual property.

In November 2005, FDA, the European Commission, and the European Medicines Agency extended by 5 years a confidentiality agreement that began in September 2003 (FDA and EMEA, 2004; DeClaire, 2005; FDA et al., 2005). The types of information covered by the agreement are legal and regulatory issues, scientific advice, orphan drug designation, inspection reports, marketing authorization procedures, and postmarketing surveillance. The implementation of the confidentiality agreement was planned to take place in several stages and is described in the implementation plan finalized in September 2004 (FDA and EMEA, 2004).

FDA announced that the agency would partner with the Agency for Healthcare Research and Quality (AHRQ) to launch an effort aimed at increasing research collaboration and to foster communication between the two agencies in December 2005 (FDA News, 2006b). FDA leaders stated that the collaboration will increase their understanding of health outcomes of prescription drugs, which will lead to better information to provide to the public. One component of the collaboration was assignment of a member of senior CDER leadership to a 12-month detail at AHRQ's Center for Outcomes and Evidence as senior adviser in pharmaceutical outcomes research (FDA News, 2006b).

CRITICAL PATH INITIATIVE AND PARTNERSHIPS

In March 2004, FDA released the report entitled *Innovation or Stagnation?—Challenge and Opportunity on the Critical Path to New Medical Products* (the Critical Path Initiative) (FDA, 2004). The report discussed the lack of innovative technologies and science in recent years to help to make drug development less expensive and more efficient. The goal of the CPI is to make safe and effective treatments available to the public quicker by using scientific innovations. The three dimensions outlined in the CPI report are safety assessment, evaluation of medical utility, and product industrialization.

FDA called for assistance from the public, academic researchers, funding agencies, and industry to help to reach that goal because it does not believe that it can get there alone. A major objective of the CPI is to encourage new and increased collaborations among a broad array of experts to develop innovative tools.

To reach its goal, FDA has partnered with the World Health Organization, the Bill and Melinda Gates Foundation, biotechnology research firms, AAMC, and others. After receiving feedback from those and other stakeholders, FDA released the *Critical Path Opportunities Report* in March 2006 to identify the initiative's six kinds of priority-targeted research. One related to safety is the use of biomarkers to predict the performance of a product during development and thus reduce uncertainties about safety or effectiveness. If the biomarkers can be identified, validated, and shown to improve health outcomes, FDA believes that these priorities "will increase efficiency, predictability, and productivity of new medical products" (FDA, 2004, 2006b).

The main element related to drug safety in the CPI is improving tools for assessing safety to detect drug safety issues as early as possible. Today, safety issues are usually found during clinical trials or when drugs are on the market. Tests for finding safety problems earlier are few and not reliable. The CPI highlights that there are great efforts to be made and that a new safety toolkit would include the ability to predict failures due to safety before human testing in clinical trials and to demonstrate safety before a drug is on the market. The safety toolkit would lead to better safety standards by helping to predict safety performance efficiently and quickly and will decrease uncertainty.

FDA announced its partnership with the Critical Path Institute (C-Path) in December 2005 to help it to reach the goals of the CPI (FDA, 2006d). C-Path is an independent, publicly funded, nonprofit organization founded by FDA, the University of Arizona, and SRI International. It was created to fulfill the mission of the CPI, which is to "create innovative collaborations in education and research that enable the safe acceleration of the process for developing new medical products" (The Critical Path Institute, 2006). FDA leaders stated that some of the projects developed by C-Path will help to achieve many of the objectives outlined in the opportunities list discussed above.

In March 2006, shortly after the release of the *Opportunities Report*, FDA announced that it will be taking on an advisory role in the new Predictive Safety Testing Consortium of C-Path and five pharmaceutical companies. The partnership will "share internally developed laboratory methods to predict the safety of new treatments before they are tested in humans" (FDA, 2006b). The collaboration is in line with the public-private partnerships stressed as a major need to improve drug development in the CPI. CDER's J. Woodcock commented that this is a "concrete example of the power of the collaborative nature of the Critical Path Initiative."

REFERENCES

AAMC (Association of American Medical Colleges), FDA, Center for Drug Development Science at the University of California, San Francisco. 2005. *Drug Development Science Obstacles and Opportunities for Collaboration Among Academia, Industry and Government.* [Online]. Available: https://services.aamc.org/Publications/showfile.cfm?file=version45. pdf [accessed October 10, 2005].

AAMC. 2006. *Collaboration Key to Overcoming Obstacles to Drug Development.* [Online]. Available: http://www.aamc.org/newsroom/pressrel/2005/050815.htm [accessed June 14, 2006].

CDER (Center for Drug Evaluation and Research). 2005. *Drug Safety Oversight Board (DSB), MAPP 4151-3.* [Online]. Available: http://www.fda.gov/cder/mapp/4151-3.pdf [accessed June 20, 2005].

CDER. 2006. *Guidance for Industry, Investigators, and Reviewers Exploratory IND Studies.* Rockville, MD: CDER.

The Critical Path Institute. 2006. *Welcome to C-Path.* [Online]. Available: http://www.c-path. org/ [accessed June 14, 2006].

DeClaire J. 2005. *Which Drugs Should Health Plans Cover?* [Online]. Available: http://

www.eurekalert.org/pub_releases/2005-10/ghcc-wds102805.php [accessed December 14, 2004].

FDA (Food and Drug Administration). 2004. *Innovation Stagnation: Challenge and Opportunity on the Critical Path to New Medical Products.* [Online]. Available:http://www.fda. gov/oc/initiatives/criticalpath/whitepaper.pdf [accessed October 10, 2005].

FDA. 2005a. *Guidance for Industry: Development and Use of Risk Minimization Action Plans.* March 2005. Rockville, MD: FDA.

FDA. 2005b. *Questions and Answers (Qs & As) Proposed Drug Watch Program.* [Online]. Available: http://www.fda.gov/cder/guidance/6657qs&asext5-2.pdf [accessed May 6, 2005].

FDA. 2005c. *White Paper, Prescription Drug User Fee Act (PDUFA): Adding Resources and Improving Performance in FDA Review of New Drug Applications.* [Online]. Available: http://www.fda.gov/oc/pdufa/PDUFAWhitePaper.pdf [accessed December 5, 2005].

FDA. 2005d. *FDA Fact Sheet: FDA Improvement in Drug Safety Monitoring.* [Online]. Available: http://www.fda.gov/oc/factsheets/drugsafety.html [accessed February 23, 2005].

FDA. 2005e. *Guidance for Industry Good Pharmacovigilance Practices and Pharmacoepidemiologic Assessment.* Rockville, MD: FDA.

FDA. 2005f. *Guidance FDA's "Drug Watch" for Emerging Drug Safety Information Draft Guidance.* Rockville, MD: FDA.

FDA. 2005g. *New Leadership for Safer Drugs.* [Online]. Available: http://www.fda.gov/bbs/ topics/NEWS/2005/NEW01195.html [accessed July 11, 2005].

FDA. 2005h. *FDA Commissioner Announces Important Personnel Changes.* [Online]. Available: http://www.fda.gov/bbs/topics/news/2005/new01215.html [July 29, 2005].

FDA. 2005i. *FDA's Center for Drug Evaluation and Research Gets Permanent Leadership.* [Online]. Available: http://www.fda.gov/bbs/topics/news/2005/new01214.html [accessed July 29, 2005].

FDA. 2005j. *FDA Names New Director of Drug Safety, Goals for Center for Drug Reorganization Announced.* [Online]. Available: http://www.fda.gov/bbs/topics/news/2005/ new01245.html [accessed October 20, 2005].

FDA. 2005k. *FDA Seeks Public Input on Renewal process for Prescription Drug User Fee Act (PDUFA).* [Online]. Available: http://www.fda.gov/bbs/topics/news/2005/NEW01259. html [accessed June 15, 2006].

FDA. 2006a. *CDER Reorganization Chart and Description.* [Online]. Available: http://www. fda.gov/cder/cderorg/ond_reorg.htm [accessed June 21, 2006].

FDA. 2006b. *Critical Path Opportunities Report.* [Online]. Available: http://www.fda.gov/oc/ initiatives/criticalpath/reports/opp_report.pdf [accessed June 2, 2006].

FDA. 2006c. *FDA Names First Associate Center Director for Safety Policy and Communication in the Center for Drug Evaluation and Research FDA Centralizes Drug Safety Policy and Communication.* [Online]. Available: http://www.fda.gov/bbs/topics/NEWS/2006/ NEW01359.html [accessed May 25, 2006].

FDA. 2006d. *FDA Announces Partnership with Critical Path Institute to Conduct Essential Research to Spur Medical Innovation.* [Online]. Available: http://www.fda.gov/bbs/topics/NEWS/2005/NEW01276.html [accessed June 14, 2006].

FDA, CDER. 2005. *Office of New Drugs Reorganization.* [Online]. Available: http://www.fda. gov/cder/cderorg/ond_reorg.htm [accessed June 21, 2005].

FDA, CDER, CBER (Center for Biologics Evaluation and Research). 2005. *Guidance for Industry: Premarketing Risk Assessment.* Rockville, MD: FDA.

FDA, EMEA (European Medicines Agency). 2004. [Online]. Available: http://www.emea. eu.int/pdfs/general/direct/internationalcoop/EMEA-FDAconfidentialityimplement%20. pdf [accessed June 6, 2005].

FDA, EU (European Union), EMEA. 2005. *FDA and EU (European Commission and EMEA) Extend Confidentiality Arrangements for Five More Years.* [Online]. Available: http://www.fda.gov/bbs/topics/news/2005/NEW01257.html [accessed June 6, 2005].

FDA News. 2005. *FDA Issues Final Risk Management Guidance's.* [Online]. Available: http://www.fda.gov/bbs/topics/news/2005/NEW01169.html [accessed March 24, 2005].

FDA News. 2006a. *FDA Issues Advice to Make Earliest Stages of Clinical Drug Development More Efficient.* [Online]. Available: http://www.fda.gov/bbs/topics/news/2006/NEW01296.html [accessed March 9, 2006].

FDA News. 2006b. *FDA to Strengthen Research and Communication with AHRQ.* [Online]. Available: http://www.fda.gov/bbs/topics/news/2005/NEW01286.html [accessed January 3, 2006].

FDA News. 2006c. *FDA Announces New Prescription Drug Information Format to Improve Patient Safety.* [Online]. Available: http://www.fda.gov/bbs/topics/news/2005/NEW01272.html [accessed March 9, 2006].

FDA News. 2006d. *Report Demonstrates Benefits of Earlier Meetings with FDA to Make Drug Review Process More Efficient.* [Online]. Available: http://www.fda.gov/bbs/topics/news/2006/NEW01312.html [accessed June 15, 2006].

FDA Press Release. 2006 (April 5). *FDA Awards Contract to Assess Postmarketing Study Commitment Decision-Making Process Analysis Will Lead to a More Standardized Approach.* [Online]. Available: http://www.boozallen.com/home/industries_article/2323260?1pid=386491 [accessed May 26, 2006].

National Conference of State Legislatures. 2006. *FDA Final Rule on Prescription Drug Labeling.* [Online]. Available: http://www.ncsl.org/statefed/health/FDArule.htm [accessed July 3, 2006].

National Library of Medicine. 2006. *About DailyMed.* [Online]. Available: http://dailymed.nlm.nih.gov/dailymed/about.cfm [August 28, 2006].

Appendix B

Acronyms

ADR	adverse drug report
AE	adverse event
AER	adverse event review
AERS	Adverse Event Reporting System
AHRQ	Agency for Healthcare Research and Quality
BLA	biologics license application
CBER	Center for Biologics Evaluation and Research
CDC	Centers for Disease Control and Prevention
CDER	Center for Drug Evaluation and Research
CDRH	Center for Devices and Radiological Health
CERTS	Center for Education and Research Therapeutics
CFR	Code of Federal Regulations
CFSAN	Center for Food Safety and Applied Nutrition
CGMPs	Current Good Manufacturing Practices
CMS	Centers for Medicare and Medicaid Services
COPR	Council of Public Representatives
CVM	Center for Veterinary Medicine
DDMAC	Division of Drug Marketing, Advertising and Communication
DDRE	Division of Drug Risk Evaluation
DHHS	Department of Health and Human Services
DSaRM	Drug Safety and Risk Management Advisory Committee

DSB   Drug Safety Oversight Board
DTCA   direct-to-consumer advertising

ELA   established license application
EMEA   European Medicines Agency
EU   European Union

FAA   Federal Aviation Administration
FDA   Food and Drug Administration
FDAMA   Food and Drug Administration Modernization Act of 1997
FD&C Act   Federal Food, Drug, and Cosmetic Act
FOIA   Freedom of Information Act
FTC   Federal Trade Commission
FTE   full-time equivalent
FY   fiscal year

GAO   Government Accountability Office
GGP   good guidance practice
GLP   good laboratory practice
GMP   good manufacturing practice
GPRD   General Practice Research Database
GRMP   good review manufacturing practice

HIPAA   Health Insurance Portability and Accountability Act

IND   Investigational New Drug
IOM   Institute of Medicine
IRB   institutional review board
IT   information technology

MaPP   Manual of Policies and Procedures
MHRA   Medicines and Healthcare Products Regulatory Agency

NAS   National Academy of Sciences
NASA   National Aeronautics and Space Administration
NCTR   National Center for Toxicological Research
NDA   New Drug Application
NIH   National Institutes of Health
NME   new molecular entity
NSAID   non-steroidal anti-inflammatory drug

ODE   Office of Drug Evaluation
ODS   Office of Drug Safety

OIG	Office of Inspector General
OMB	Office of Management and Budget
OMP	Office of Medical Policy
OND	Office of New Drugs
OP	Office of Planning
OPaSS	Office of Pharmacoepidemiology and Statistical Science
OSE	Office of Surveillance and Epidemiology
PDUFA	Prescription Drug User Fee Act
PLA	product license application
RiskMAP	risk minimization action plan
SRS	Spontaneous Reporting System
UK	United Kingdom
USDA	US Department of Agriculture
VSD	Vaccine Safety Datalink
WHO	World Health Organization

Appendix C

PDUFA Performance Goals—All Years

The following list presents by fiscal year the performance measures set forth in the letters referenced in Section 102(3) of the PDUFA. In those letters, the timing of a number of the goals was conditional either (1) on the date (July 2, 1993) upon which a supplemental appropriation was enacted to permit FDA to collect PDUFA user fees, or (2) a specific performance interval (e.g., 6 or 12 months after submission). Table C-1 lists the 29 goals by fiscal year with appropriate goal measurement dates:

TABLE C-1 PDUFA Performance Goals, FY 1993–FY 1997

Interim Goals by Fiscal Year	Timing of Measurement	Measurement Date[a]
Interim Goals of FY 93		
1. Establish an industry/FDA working group upon initiation of the user fee program.	Supplemental appropriation date	July 2, 1993
2. Initiate a pilot computer-assisted PLA review (CAPLAR) program during FY 93.	End of FY 93	Sept. 30, 1993
Interim Goal of FY 94		
1. Review and act upon 55 percent of complete NDA and PLA/ELA submissions received during FY 94 within 12 months after submission date.	12 months after end of FY 94	Sept. 30, 1995
2. Review and act upon 55 percent of efficacy supplements[b] received during FY 94 within 12 months after submission date.	12 months after end of FY 94	Sept. 30, 1995

221

TABLE C-1 Continued

Interim Goals by Fiscal Year	Timing of Measurement	Measurement Date[a]
3. Review and act upon 55 percent of manufacturing supplements[b] received during FY 94 within 6 months after submission date.	6 months after end of FY 94	Mar. 31, 1995
4. Review and act upon 55 percent of manufacturing applications received during FY 94 within 6 months after the resubmission date.	6 months after end of FY 94	Mar. 31, 1995
5. Implement performance tracking and monthly monitoring of CBER performance within 6 months of initial user fee payments.	6 months after 7/2/93	July 2, 1994
6. Implement project management methodology for all NDA reviews within 12 months of the initiation of user fee payments.	12 months after 7/2/93	July 2, 1994

Interim Goals of FY 95

1. Review and act upon 70 percent of complete NDA and PLA/ELA submissions received during FY 95 within 12 months after submission date.	12 months after end of FY 95	Sept. 30, 1996
2. Review and act upon 70 percent of efficacy supplements received during FY 95 within 12 months after submission date.	12 months after end of FY 95	Sept. 30, 1996
3. Review and act upon 70 percent of manufacturing supplements received during FY 95 within 6 months after submission date.	6 months after end of FY 95	Mar. 31, 1996
4. Review and act upon 70 percent of resubmitted applications received during FY 95 within 6 months after the resubmission date.	6 months after end of FY 95	Mar. 31, 1996
5. Recruit and bring on board 50 percent of FDA incremental review staff by first quarter of FY 95.	3 months after end of FY 94	Dec. 31, 1994
6. Implement project management methodology for all PLA/ELA reviews within 18 months of user fee payments.	18 months after 7/2/93	Jan. 2, 1995
7. Eliminate overdue backlogs of efficacy and manufacturing supplements to NDAs within 18 months of initiation of user fee payments.	18 months after 7/2/93	Jan. 2, 1995
8. Eliminate overdue of NDAs within 24 months of initiation of user fees.	24 months after 7/2/93	Jan. 2, 1995
9. Eliminate overdue backlogs of PLAs, ELAs and PLA/ELA supplements within 24 months of initiation of user fees.	24 months after 7/2/93	Jan. 2, 1995
10. Adopt uniform computer-assisted NDA standards during FY 95.	End of FY 95	Sept. 30, 1995

Interim Goals of FY 96

1. Review and act upon 80 percent of complete NDA and PLA/ELA submissions receive during FY 96 within 12 months after submission date.	12 months after end of FY 96	Sept. 30, 1997

TABLE C-1 Continued

Interim Goals by Fiscal Year	Timing of Measurement	Measurement Date[a]
2. Review and act upon 80 percent of efficacy supplements received during FY 96 within 12 months after submission date.	12 months after end of FY 96	Sept. 30, 1997
3. Review and act upon 80 percent of manufacturing supplements received during FY 96 within 6 months after submission date.	6 months after end of FY 96	Mar. 31, 1997
4. Review and act upon 80 percent of resubmitted applications received during FY 96 within 6 months after the resubmission date.	6 months after end of FY 96	Mar. 31, 1997
Five-Year Goals of FY 97		
1. Review 90 percent of complete PLAs, ELAs, and NDAs for priority applications within 6 months after submission date.	6 months after end of FY 97	Mar. 31, 1998
2. Review 90 percent of complete PLAs, ELAs, and NDAs for standard applications within 12 months after submission date.	12 months after end of FY 97	Sept. 30, 1998
3. Review 90 percent of priority supplements to PLAs, ELAs, and NDAs within 6 months after submission date.	6 months after end of FY 97	Mar. 31, 1998
4. Review 90 percent of standard supplements to PLAs, ELAs, and NDAs that require review of clinical data (efficacy supplements) within 12 months after submission.	12 months after end of FY 97	Sept. 30, 1998
5. Review 90 percent of supplements to PLAs, ELAs, and NDAs that do not require review of clinical data (manufacturing supplements) within 6 months after submission date.	6 months after end of FY 97	Mar. 31, 1998
6. Review 90 percent of complete applications resubmitted following receipt of a non-approval letter within 6 months after the resubmission date.	6 months after end of FY 97	Mar. 31, 1998
7. Total review staff increment recruited and on board by end of FY 97.	End of FY 97	Sept. 30, 1997

[a]The statute allows three additional months for review of original NDA, PLA, or ELA submissions that involve major amendments within the last three months of their usual 6- or 12-month review intervals. In these cases, the measurement dates shown in this Appendix move forward by 3 months.

[b]The term "supplement" applies to both drug and biologic submissions. It includes "amendments" to biologic submissions.

SOURCE: FDA (Food and Drug Administration). 1995. *Appendix A: PDUFA Performance Goals, FY 199–FY 1997.* [Online]. Available: http://www.fda.gov/ope/pdufa/report95/appenda.html [accessed June 21, 2006].

ENCLOSURE
PDUFA REAUTHORIZATION PERFORMANCE
GOALS AND PROCEDURES

The performance goals and procedures of the FDA Center for Drug Evaluation and Research (CDER) and the Center for Biologics Evaluation and Research (CBER), as agreed to under the reauthorization of the prescription drug user fee program in the "Food and Drug Administration Modernization Act of 1997," are summarized as follows:

I. FIVE-YEAR REVIEW PERFORMANCE GOALS

Fiscal year 1998
1. Review and act on 90 percent of standard original New Drug Application (NDAs) and Product License Applications (PLAs)/Biologic License Applications (BLAs) filed during fiscal year 1998 within 12 months of receipt.
2. Review and act on 90 percent of priority original NDA and PLA/BLA submissions filed during fiscal year 1998 within 6 months of receipt.
3. Review and act on 90 percent of standard efficacy supplements filed during fiscal year 1992 within 12 months of receipt.
4. Review and act on 90 percent of priority efficacy supplements filed during fiscal year 1998 within 6 months of receipt.
5. Review and act on 90 percent of manufacturing supplements filed during fiscal year 1998 within 6 months of receipt.
6. Review and act on 90 percent of all resubmitted original applications filed during fiscal year 1998 within 6 months of receipt, and review and act on 30 percent of Class 1 resubmitted original applications within 2 months of receipt.

Fiscal year 1999
1. Review and act on 90 percent of standard original NDA and PLA/BLA submission filed during fiscal year 1999 within 12 months of receipt and review and act on 30 percent within 10 months of receipt.
2. Review and act on 90 percent of priority original NDA and PLA/BLA submission filed during fiscal year 1999 within 6 months of receipt.
3. Review and act on 90 percent of standard efficacy supplements filed during fiscal year 1999 within 12 months of receipt and review and act on 30 percent with in 10 months of receipt.

4. Review and act on 90 percent of priority efficacy supplements filed during fiscal year 1999 within 6 months of receipt.
5. Review and act on 90 percent of manufacturing supplements filed during fiscal year 1999 within 6 months of receipt and review and act on 30 percent of manufacturing supplements requiring prior approval within 4 months of receipt.
6. Review and act on 90 percent of Class 1 resubmitted original applications filed during fiscal year 1999 within 4 months of receipt and review and act on 50 percent within 2 months of receipt.
7. Review and act on 90 percent of Class 2 resubmitted original applications filed during fiscal year 1999 within 6 months of receipt.

Fiscal year 2000
1. Review and act on 90 percent of standard original NDA and PLA/BLA submissions filed during fiscal year 2000 within 12 months of receipt and review and act on 50 percent within 10 months of receipt.
2. Review and act on 90 percent of priority original NDA and PLA/BLA submissions filed during fiscal year 2000 within 6 months of receipt.
3. Review and act on 90 percent of standard efficacy supplements filed during fiscal year 2000 within 12 months of receipts and review and act on 50 percent within 10 months of receipt.
4. Review and act on 90 percent of priority efficacy supplements filed during fiscal year 2000 within 6 months of receipt.
5. Review and act on 90 percent of manufacturing supplements filed during fiscal year 2000 within 6 months of receipt and review and act on 50 percent of manufacturing supplements requiring prior approval within 4 months of receipt.
6. Review and act on 90 percent of Class 1 resubmitted original applications filed during fiscal year 2000 within 4 months and review and act on 50 percent within 2 months of receipt.
7. Review and act on 90 percent of Class 2 resubmitted original applications filed during fiscal year 2000 within 6 months of receipt.

Fiscal year 2001
1. Review and act on 90 percent of standard original NDA and PLA/BLA submissions filed during fiscal year 2001 within 12 months and review and act on 70 percent within 10 months of receipt.
2. Review and act on 90 percent of priority original NDA and PLA/BLA submissions filed during fiscal year 2001 within 6 months of receipt.
3. Review and act on 90 percent of standard efficacy supplements filed during fiscal year 2001 within 12 months and review and act on 70 percent within 10 months of receipt.

4. Review and act on 90 percent of priority efficacy supplements filed during fiscal year 2001 within 6 months of receipt.
5. Review and act on 90 percent of manufacturing supplements filed during fiscal year 2001 within 6 months of receipt and review and act on 70 percent within 2 months of receipt.
6. Review and act on 90 percent of Class 1 resubmitted original applications filed during the fiscal year 2001 within 4 months of receipt and review and act on 70 percent within 2 months of receipt.
7. Review and act on 90 percent of Class 2 resubmitted original applications within 6 months of receipt.

Fiscal year 2002
1. Review and act on 90 percent of standard original NDA and PLA/BLA submissions filed during fiscal year 2002 within 10 months of receipt.
2. Review and act on 90 percent of priority original NDA and PLA/BLA submissions filed during fiscal year 2002 within 6 months of receipt.
3. Review and act on 90 percent of standard efficacy supplements filed during fiscal year 2002 within 10 months of receipt.
4. Review and act on 90 percent of priority efficacy supplements filed during fiscal year 2002 within 6 months of receipt.
5. Review and act on 90 percent of manufacturing supplements filed during fiscal year 2002 within 6 months of receipt and review and act on 90 percent of manufacturing supplements requiring prior approval within 4 months of receipt.
6. Review and act on 90 percent of Class 1 resubmitted original applications filed during fiscal year 2002 within 2 months of receipt.
7. Review and act on 90 percent of Class 2 resubmitted original applications within 6 months of receipt.

These review goals are summarized in Tables C-2, C-3, and C-4:

TABLE C-2 Original NDAs/BLAs/PLAs and Efficacy Supplements

SUBMISSION COHORT	STANDARD	PRIORITY
FY 98	90% IN 12 MO	90% IN 6 MO
FY 99	30% IN 10 MO 90% IN 12 MO	90% IN 6 MO
FY 00	50% IN 10 MO 90% IN 12 MO	90% IN 6 MO
FY 01	70% IN 10 MO 90% IN 12 MO	90% IN 6 MO
FY 02	90% IN 10 MO	90% IN 6 MO

TABLE C-3 Manufacturing Supplements

SUBMISSION COHORT	MANUFACTURING SUPPLEMENTS THAT DO NOT REQUIRE PRIOR APPROVAL ("CHANGES BEING EFFECTED" OR "30-DAY SUPPLEMENTS	MANUFACTURING SUPPLEMENTS THAT DO REQUIRE PRIOR APPROVAL
FY 98	90% IN 6 MO	90% IN 6 MO
FY 99	90% IN 6 MO	30% IN 4 MO 90% IN 6 MO
FY 00	90% IN 6 MO	50% IN 4 MO 90% IN 6 MO
FY 01	90% IN 6 MO	70% IN 4 MO 90% IN 6 MO
FY 02	90% IN 6 MO	90% IN 4 MO

TABLE C-4 Resubmission of Original NDAs/BLAs/PLAs

SUBMISSION COHORT	CLASS 1	CLASS 2
FY 98	30% IN 2 MO 90% IN 6 MO	90% IN 6 MO
FY 99	50% IN 2 MO 90% IN 4 MO	90% IN 6 MO
FY 00	70% IN 2 MO 90% IN 4 MO	90% IN 6 MO
FY 01	90% IN 2 MO	90% IN 6 MO
FY 02	90% IN 2 MO	90% IN 6 MO

II. NEW MOLECULAR ENTITY (NME) PERFORMANCE GOALS

The performance goals for standard and priority original NMEs in each submission cohort will be the same as for all of the original NDAs (including NMEs) in each submission cohort but shall be reported separately.

For biological products, for purposes of this performance goal, all original BLAs/PLAs will be considered to be NMEs.

III. MEETING MANAGEMENT GOALS

A. Responses to Meeting Requests:

1. **Procedure:** Within 14 calendar days of the Agency's receipt of a request from industry for a formal meeting (i.e., a scheduled face-to-

face, teleconference, or videoconference) CBER and CDER should notify the requester in writing (letter or fax) of the date, time and the place for the meeting, as well as expected Center participants.

2. **Performance Goal:** FDA will provide this notification within 14 days for 70 percent of requests (based on request receipt cohort year) starting in FY99; 80 percent in FY00; and 90 percent in subsequent fiscal years.

B. Scheduling Meetings:

1. **Procedure:** The meeting date should reflect the next available date on which all applicable Center personnel are available to attend, consistent with the component's other business; however, the meeting should be scheduled consistent with the type of meeting requested. If the requested date for any of these types of meetings is greater than 30, 60, or 75 calendar days (as appropriate) from the date the request is received by the Agency, the meeting date should be within 14 calendar days of the date requested.

   Type A Meetings should occur within 30 calendar days of the Agency receipt of the meeting request.

   Type B Meetings should occur within 60 calendar days of the Agency receipt of the meeting request.

   Type C Meetings should occur within 75 calendar days of the Agency receipt of the meeting request.

2. **Performance Goal:** 70 percent of meetings are held within the timeframe (based on cohort year of request) starting in FY99; 80 percent in FY00; and 90 percent in subsequent fiscal years.

C. Meeting Minutes:

1. **Procedure:** The Agency will prepare minutes which will be available to the sponsor 30 calendar days after the meeting. The minutes will clearly outline the important agreements, disagreements, issues for further discussion, and action items from the meeting in bulleted form and need not be in great detail.

2. **Performance Goal:** 70 percent of minutes are issued within 30 calendar days of date of meeting (based on cohort year of meeting) starting in FY99; 80 percent in FY00; and 90 percent in subsequent fiscal years.

D. Conditions:

For a meeting to qualify for these performance goals:

1. A written request (letter or fax) should be submitted to the review division; and
2. The letter should provide:
   a. A brief statement of the purpose of the meeting;
   b. A listing of the specific objectives/outcomes the requester expects from the meeting;
   c. A proposed agenda, including estimated times needed for each agenda item;
   d. A listing of planned external attendees;
   e. A listing of requested participants/disciplines representative(s) from the Center;
   f. The appropriate time that supporting documentation (i.e., the "backgrounder") for the meeting will be sent to the Center (i.e., "x" weeks prior to the meeting, but should be received by the Center at least 2 weeks in advance of the scheduled meeting for Type A or C meetings and at least 1 month in advance of the scheduled meeting for Type B meetings); and
3. The Agency concurs that the meeting will serve a useful purpose (i.e., it is not premature or clearly unnecessary). However, requests for a "Type B" meeting will be honored except in the most unusual circumstances.

IV. CLINICAL HOLDS

A. **Procedure:** The Center should respond to a sponsor's complete response to a clinical hold within 30 days of the Agency's receipt of the submission of such sponsor response.
B. **Performance Goal:** 75 percent of such responses are provided within 30 calendar days of the Agency's receipt of the sponsor's response starting FY98 (cohort of date of receipt) and 90 percent in subsequent fiscal years.

V. MAJOR DISPUTE RESOLUTION

A. **Procedure:** For procedural or scientific matters involving the review of human drug applications and supplements (as defined in PDUFA) that cannot be resolved at the divisional level (including a request for reconsideration by the Division after reviewing any materials that are planned to be forwarded with an appeal to the next level), the response to appeals of decisions will occur within 30 calendar days of the Center's receipt of the written appeal.
B. **Performance Goal:** 70 percent of such answers are provided within 30

calendar days of the Center's receipt of the written appeal starting in FY99; 80 percent in FY00; and 90 percent in subsequent fiscal years.

C. **Conditions:**

1. Sponsors should first try to resolve the procedural or scientific issue at the Divisional level. If it cannot be resolved at that level, it should be appealed to the Office Director level (with a copy to the Division Director) and then, if necessary, to the Deputy Center Director (with a copy to the Office Director).

2. Responses should be either verbal (followed by a written confirmation within 14 calendar days of the verbal notification) or written and should ordinarily be to either deny or grant the appeal.

3. If the decision is to deny the appeal, the response should include reasons for the denial and any actions the sponsor might take in order to persuade the Agency to reverse its decision.

4. In some cases, further data or further input from others might be needed to reach a decision on the appeal. In these cases, the "response" should be the plan for obtaining that information (e.g., requesting further information from the sponsor, scheduling a meeting with the sponsor, scheduling the issue for discussion at the next scheduled available advisory committee).

5. In these cases, once the required information is received by the Agency (including any advice from an advisory committee), the person to whom the appeal was made, again has 30 calendar days from the receipt of the required information in which to either deny or grant the appeal.

6. Again, if the decision is to deny the appeal, the response should include the reasons for the denial and any actions the sponsor might take in order to persuade the Agency to reverse its decision.

7. N.B. If the Agency decides to present the issue to an advisory committee and there are not 30 days before the next scheduled advisory committee, the issue will be presented at the following scheduled committee meeting in order to allow conformance with advisory committee administrative procedures.

VI. SPECIAL PROTOCOL QUESTION ASSESSMENT AND AGREEMENT

A. **Procedure:** Upon specific request by a sponsor (including specific questions that the sponsor desires to be answered), the agency will evaluate certain protocols and issues to assess whether the design is adequate to meet scientific and regulatory requirements identified by the sponsor.

1. The sponsor should submit a limited number of specific questions about the protocol design and the scientific and regulatory requirements for which the sponsor seeks agreement (e.g., is the dose range in the carcinogenicity study adequate, considering the intended clinical dosage; are the clinical endpoints adequate to support a specific efficacy claim).

2. Within 45 days of Agency receipt of the protocol and specific questions, the Agency will provide a written response to the sponsor that includes a succinct assessment of the protocol and answers to the questions posed by the sponsor. If the agency does not agree that the protocol design, execution plans, and data analyses are adequate to achieve the goals of the sponsor, the reasons for the disagreement will be explained in the response.

3. Protocols that qualify for this program include: carcinogenicity protocols, stability protocols, and Phase 3 protocols for clinical trials that will form the primary basis of an efficacy claim. (For such Phase 3 protocols to qualify for this comprehensive protocol assessment, the sponsor must have had an end of Phase 2/pre-Phase 3 meeting with the review division so that the division is aware of the developmental context in which the protocol is being reviewed and the questions being answered).

4. N.B. For products that will be using Subpart E or Subpart H development schemes, the Phase 3 protocols mentioned in this paragraph should be construed to mean those protocols for trials that will form the primary basis of an efficacy claim no matter what phase of drug development in which they happen to be conducted.

5. If a protocol is reviewed under the process outlined above and agreement with the Agency is reached on design, execution, and analyses and if the results of the trial conducted under the protocol substantiate the hypothesis of the protocol, the Agency agrees that the data from the protocol can be used as part of the primary basis for approval of the product. The fundamental agreement here is that having agreed to the design, execution, and analyses proposed in protocols reviewed under this process, the Agency will not later alter its perspective on the issues of design, execution or analyses unless public health concerns unrecognized at the time of protocol assessment under this process are evident.

B. **Performance Goal:** 60 percent of special protocols assessments and agreement requests completed and returned to sponsor within timeframes (based on cohort year of request) starting in FY99; 70 percent in FY00; 80 percent in FY01; and 90 percent in FY02.

VII. ELECTRONIC APPLICATIONS AND SUBMISSIONS

The Agency shall develop and update its information management infrastructure to allow, by fiscal year 2002, the paperless receipt and processing of INDs and human drug applications as defined in PDUFA, and related submissions.

VIII. ADDITIONAL PROCEDURES

A. Simplification of Action Letters:
To simplify regulatory procedures, the CBER and the CDER intend to amend their regulations and processes to provide for the issuance of either an "approval" (AP) or a "complete response" (CR) action letter at the completion of a review cycle for a marketing application.

B. Timing of Sponsor Notification of Deficiencies in Applications:
To help expedite the development of drug and biologic products, CBER and CDER intend to submit deficiencies to sponsors in the form of an "information request" (IR) letter when each discipline has finished its initial review of its section of the pending application.

IX. DEFINITIONS AND EXPLANATION OF TERMS

A. The term "review and act on" is understood to mean the issuance of a complete action letter after the complete review of a filed complete application. The action letter, if it is not an approval, will set forth in detail the specific deficiencies and, where appropriate, the actions necessary to place the application in condition for approval.
B. A major amendment to an original application submitted within three months of the goal date extends the goal date by three months.
C. A resubmitted original application is a complete response to an action letter addressing all identified deficiencies.
D. Class 1 resubmitted applications are applications resubmitted after a complete response letter (or a not approvable or approvable letter) that include the following items only (or combination of these items):

1. Final printed labeling
2. Draft labeling
3. Safety updates submitted in the same format, including tabulations, as the original safety submission with new data and changes highlighted (except when large amounts of new information including important new adverse experiences not previously reported with the product are presented in the resubmission)
4. Stability updates to support provisional or final dating periods

5. Commitments to perform Phase 4 studies, including proposals for such studies
6. Assay validation data
7. Final release testing on the last 1–2 lots used to support approval
8. A minor reanalysis of data previously submitted to the application (determined by the agency as fitting the Class 1 category)
9. Other minor clarifying information (determined by the Agency as fitting the Class 1 category)
10. Other specific items may be added later as the Agency gains experience with the scheme and will be communicated via guidance documents to industry.

E. Class 2 resubmissions that include any other items, including any item that would require presentation to an advisory committee.

F. A Type A Meeting is a meeting which is necessary for an otherwise stalled drug development program to proceed (a "critical path" meeting).

G. A Type B Meeting is a 1) pre-IND, 2) end of Phase 1(for Subpart E or Subpart H or similar products) or end of Phase 2/pre-Phase 3, or 3) a pre-NDA/PLA/BLA meeting. Each requestor should usually only request 1 each of these Type B meetings for each potential application (NDA/PLA/BLA) (or combination of closely related products, i.e., same active ingredient but different dosage forms being developed concurrently).

H. A Type C Meeting is any other type of meeting.

I. The performance goals and procedures also apply to original applications and supplements for human drugs initially marketed on an over-the-counter (OTC) basis through an NDA or switched from prescription to OTC status through an NDA or supplement.

SOURCE: FDA. 2002. *Enclosure: PDUFA Reauthorization Performance Goals and Procedures*. [Online]. Available: http://www.fda.gov/oc/pdufaIIIGoals.html [accessed June 21, 2006].

ENCLOSURE
PDUFA REAUTHORIZATION PERFORMANCE
GOALS AND PROCEDURES

The performance goals and procedures of the FDA Center for Drug Evaluation and Research (CDER) and the Center for Biologics Evaluation and Research (CDER), as agreed to under the reauthorization of the prescription drug user fee program are summarized as follows:

I. REVIEW PERFORMANCE GOALS—FISCAL YEAR 2003 THROUGH 2007

A. NDA/BLA Submissions and Resubmissions:
Review and act on 90 percent of standard original NDA and BLA submissions filed during fiscal year within 10 months of receipt.

1. Review and act on 90 percent of priority original NDA and BLA submissions filed during fiscal year within 6 months of receipt.
2. Review and act on 90 percent of Class 1 resubmitted original applications filed during fiscal year within 2 months of receipt.
3. Review and act on 90 percent of Class 2 resubmitted original applications filed during fiscal year within 6 months of receipt.

Original Efficacy Supplements:

1. Review and act on 90 percent of standard efficacy supplements filed during fiscal year within 10 months of receipt.
2. Review and act on 90 percent of priority efficacy supplements filed during fiscal year within 6 months of receipt.

Resubmitted Efficacy Supplements:

Fiscal Year 2003:
1. Review and act on 90 percent of Class 1 resubmitted efficacy supplements filed during fiscal year 2003 within 6 months of receipt and review and act on 30 percent within 2 months of receipt.
2. Review and act on 90 percent of Class 2 resubmitted efficacy supplements filed during fiscal year 2003 within 6 months of receipt.

Fiscal Year 2004:

1. Review and act on 90 percent of Class 1 resubmitted efficacy supplements filed during fiscal year 2004 within 4 months of receipt and review and act on 50 percent within 2 months of receipt.
2. Review and act on 90 percent of Class 2 resubmitted original applications filed during fiscal year 2004 within 6 months of receipt.

Fiscal Year 2005:

1. Review and act on 90 percent of Class 1 resubmitted efficacy supplements filed during fiscal year 2005 within 4 months of receipt and review and act on 50 percent within 2 months of receipt.
2. Review and act on 90 percent of Class 2 resubmitted efficacy supplements within 6 months of receipt.

Fiscal Year 2006:

1. Review and act on 90 percent of Class 1 resubmitted efficacy supplements filed during fiscal year 2006 within 4 months of receipt and review and act on 80 percent within 2 months of receipt.
2. Review and act on 90 percent of Class 2 resubmitted efficacy supplements within 6 months of receipt.

Fiscal Year 2007:

1. Review and act on 90 percent of Class 1 resubmitted efficacy supplements filed during fiscal year 2007 within 2 months of receipt.
2. Review and act on 90 percent of Class 2 resubmitted efficacy supplements within 6 months of receipt.

Original Manufacturing Supplements:

1. Review and act on 90 percent of manufacturing supplements filed during fiscal year within 6 months of receipt and review and act on 90 percent of manufacturing supplements requiring prior approval within 4 months of receipt.

These review goals are summarized in Tables C-5, C-6, C-7, and C-8:

TABLE C-5 Original and Resubmitted NDAs/BLAs

SUBMISSION COHORT	STANDARD	PRIORITY
Original Applications	90% IN 10 MO	90% IN 6 MO
Class 1 Resubmissions	90% IN 2 MO	90% IN 2 MO
Class 2 Resubmissions	90% IN 6 MO	90% IN 6 MO

TABLE C-6 Original and Resubmitted Efficacy Supplements

SUBMISSION COHORT	STANDARD	PRIORITY
Original Efficacy Supplements	90% IN 10 MO	90% IN 6 MO

TABLE C-7 Resubmitted Efficacy Supplements

SUBMISSION COHORT	CLASS 1	CLASS 2
FY 2003	90% IN 6 MO 30% IN 2 MO	90% IN 6 MO
FY 2004	90% IN 4 MO 50% IN 2 MO	90% IN 6 MO
FY 2005	90% IN 4 MO 70% IN 2 MO	90% IN 6 MO
FY 2006	90% IN 4 MO 80% IN 2 MO	90% IN 6 MO
FY 2007	90% IN 2 MO	90% IN 6 MO

TABLE C-8 Manufacturing Supplements

SUBMISSION COHORT	MANUFACTURING SUPPLEMENTS NO PRIOR APPROVAL ("CHANGES BEING EFFECTED" OR "30-DAY SUPPLEMENTS")	MANUFACTURING SUPPLEMENTS THAT DO REQUIRE PRIOR APPROVAL
FY 2003–2007	90% IN 6 MO	90% IN 4 MO

II. NEW MOLECULAR ENTITY (NME) PERFORMANCE GOALS

A. The performance goals for standard and priority original NMEs in each submission cohort will be the same as for all of the original NDAs (including NMEs) in each submission cohort but shall be reported separately.

B. For biological products, for purposes of this performance goal, all original BLAs will be considered to be NMEs.

III. MEETING MANAGEMENT GOALS

A. Responses to Meeting Requests

  1. **Procedure:** Within 14 calendar days of the Agency's receipt of a request from industry for a formal meeting (i.e., a scheduled face-to-face, teleconference, or videoconference) CBER and CDER should notify the requester in writing (letter or fax) of the date, time, and place for the meeting, as well as expected Center participants.

  2. **Performance Goal:** FDA will provide notification within 14 days for 90 percent in FY 2003–2007.

B. Scheduling Meetings

1. **Procedure:** The meeting date should reflect the next available date on which all applicable Center personnel are available to attend, consistent with the component's other business; however, the meeting should be scheduled consistent with the type of meeting requested. If the requested date for any of these types of meetings is greater than 30, 60, or 75 calendar days (as appropriate) from the date the request is received by the Agency, the meeting date should be within 14 calendar days of the date requested.

    Type A Meetings should occur within 30 calendar days of the Agency receipt of the meeting request.

    Type B Meetings should occur within 60 calendar days of the Agency receipt of the meeting request.

    Type C Meetings should occur within 75 calendar days of the Agency receipt of the meeting request.

2. Performance goal: 90 percent of meetings are held within the timeframe (based on cohort year of request) from FY 03 to FY 07.

C. Meeting Minutes

1. **Procedure:** The Agency will prepare minutes which will be available to the sponsor 30 calendar days after the meeting. The minutes will clearly outline the important agreements, disagreements, issues for further discussion, and action items from the meeting in bulleted form and need not be in great detail.

2. **Performance Goal:** 90 percent of minutes are issued within 30 calendar days of date of meeting (based on cohort year of meeting) in FY03 to FY07.

D. Conditions

For a meeting to qualify for these performance goals:

1. A written request (letter or fax) should be submitted to the review division; and
2. The letter should provide:

    a. A brief statement of the purpose of the meeting;
    b. A listing of the specific objectives/outcomes the requester expects from the meeting;
    c. A proposed agenda, including estimated times needed for each agenda item;
    d. A listing of planned external attendees;

    e. A listing of requested participants/disciplines representative(s) from the Center;

    f. The approximate time that supporting documentation (i.e., the "backgrounder") for the meeting will be sent to the Center (i.e., "x" weeks prior to the meeting, but should be received by the Center at least 2 weeks in advance of the scheduled meeting for Type A meetings and at least 1 month in advance of the scheduled meeting for Type B and Type C meetings); and

    g. The Agency concurs that the meeting will serve a useful purpose (i.e., it is not premature or clearly unnecessary). However, requests for a "Type B" meeting will be honored except in the most unusual circumstances.

IV. CLINICAL HOLDS

A. **Procedure:** The Center should respond to a sponsor's complete response to a clinical hold within 30 days of the Agency's receipt of the submission of such sponsor response.

B. **Performance Goal:** 90 percent of such responses are provided within 30 calendar days of the Agency's receipt of the sponsor's response in FY03 to FY07 (cohort of date of receipt).

V. MAJOR DISPUTE RESOLUTION

A. **Procedure:** The Center should respond to a sponsor's complete response to a clinical hold within 30 days of the Agency's receipt of the submission of such sponsor response.

B. **Performance Goal:** 90 percent of such answers are provided within 30 calendar days of the Center's receipt of the written appeal in FY03 to FY07.

C. **Conditions:**

    1. Sponsors should first try to resolve the procedural or scientific issue at the Division level. If it cannot be resolved at that level, it should be appealed to the Office Director level (with a copy to the Division Director) and then, if necessary, to the Deputy Center Director.

    2. Responses should be either verbal (followed by a written confirmation within 14 calendar days of the verbal notification) or written.

    3. If the decision is to deny the appeal, the response should include reasons for the denial and any actions the sponsor might take.

    4. In some cases, further data or further input from others might be needed to reach a decision on the appeal. In these cases, the "response" should be the plan for obtaining that information (e.g.,

requesting further information from the sponsor, scheduling a meeting with the sponsor, scheduling the issue for discussion at the next scheduled available advisory committee).

5. In these cases, once the required information is received by the Agency (including any advice from an advisory committee), the person to whom the appeal was made, again has 30 calendar days from the receipt of the required information in which to either deny or grant the appeal.

6. Again, if the decision is to deny the appeal, the response should include the reasons for the denial and any actions the sponsor might take in order to persuade the Agency to reverse its decision.

7. N.B. If the Agency decides to present the issue to an advisory committee and there are not 30 days before the next scheduled advisory committee, the issue will be presented at the following scheduled committee meeting in order to allow conformance with advisory committee administrative procedures.

VI. SPECIAL PROTOCOL QUESTION ASSESSMENT AND AGREEMENT

A. **Procedure:** Upon specific request by a sponsor (including specific questions that the sponsor desires to be answered), the agency will evaluate certain protocols and issues to assess whether the design is adequate to meet scientific and regulatory requirements identified by the sponsor.

1. The sponsor should submit a limited number of specific questions about the protocol design and scientific and regulatory requirements for which the sponsor seeks agreement (e.g., is the dose range in the carcinogenicity study adequate, considering the intended clinical dosage; are the clinical endpoints adequate to support a specific efficacy claim).

2. Within 45 days of Agency receipt of the protocol and specific questions, the Agency will provide a written response to the sponsor that includes a succinct assessment of the protocol and answers to the questions posed by the sponsor. If the agency does not agree that the protocol design, execution plans, and data analyses are adequate to achieve the goals of the sponsor, the reasons for the disagreement will be explained in the response.

3. Protocols that qualify for this program include: carcinogenicity protocols, stability protocols, and Phase 3 protocols for clinical trials that will form the primary basis of an efficacy claim. (For such Phase 3 protocols to qualify for this comprehensive protocol assessment, the sponsor must have had an end of Phase 2/pre-Phase 3 meeting with the review division so that the division is aware of

the developmental context in which the protocol is being reviewed and the questions being answered.)

4. N.B. For products that will be using Subpart E or Subpart H development schemes, the Phase 3 protocols mentioned in this paragraph should be construed to mean those protocols for trials that will form the primary basis of an efficacy claim no matter what phase of drug development in which they happen to be conducted.

5. If a protocol is reviewed under the process outlined above and agreement with the Agency is reached on design, execution, and analyses and if the results of the trial conducted under the protocol substantiate the hypothesis of the protocol, the Agency agrees that the data from the protocol can be used as part of the primary basis for approval of the product. The fundamental agreement here is that having agreed to the design, execution, and analyses proposed in protocols reviewed under this process, the Agency will not later alter its perspective on the issues of design, execution, or analyses unless public health concerns unrecognized at the time of protocol assessment under this process are evident.

B. **Performance goal:** 90 percent of special protocols assessments and agreement requests completed and returned to sponsor within timeframes (based on cohort year of request) from FY 03 to FY 07.

VII. CONTINOUS MARKETING APPLICATION

To test whether providing early review of selected applications and additional feedback and advice to sponsors during drug development for selected products can further shorten drug development and review times, FDA agrees to conduct the following two pilot programs:

A. **Pilot 1—Discipline Review Letters for Pre-Submitted "Reviewable Units" of NDAs/BLAs**

1. This pilot applies to drugs and biologics that have been designated to be Fast Track drugs or biologics, pursuant to section 112 of the FDA Modernization Act (21 U.S.C. 506), have been the subject of an End-of-Phase 2 and/or a Pre-NDA/BLA meeting, and have demonstrated significant promise as a therapeutic advance in clinical trials.

2. For drugs and biologics that meet these criteria, FDA may enter into an agreement with the sponsor to accept pre-submission of one or more "reviewable units" of the application in advance of the submission of the complete NDA/BLA.

3. If following an initial review FDA finds a "reviewable unit" to be substantially complete for review (i.e., after a "filing review" similar to that performed on an NDA/BLA), FDA will initiate a review clock for the complete review of the "reviewable unit" of the NDA/BLA. The review clock would start from the date of receipt of the "reviewable unit."

4. To be considered fileable for review under paragraph 3, a "reviewable unit" must be substantially complete when submitted to FDA. Once a "reviewable unit" is "filed" by FDA, except as provided in paragraph 5 below, only minor information amendments submitted in response to FDA inquiries or requests and routine stability and safety updates will be considered during the review cycle.

5. Major amendments to the "reviewable unit" are strongly discouraged. However, in rare cases, and with prior agreement, FDA may accept and consider for review a major amendment to a "reviewable unit." To accommodate these rare cases, a major amendment to a "reviewable unit" submitted within the last three months of a 6-month review cycle may, at FDA's discretion, trigger a 3-month extension of the review clock for the "reviewable unit" in question. In no case, however, would a major amendment be accepted for review and the review clock for the "reviewable unit" extended if the extended review clock for the "reviewable unit" exceeded the review clock for the complete NDA/BLA. (See paragraph 10 below.)

6. After completion of review of the "reviewable unit" of the NDA/BLA by the appropriate discipline review team, FDA will provide written feedback to the sponsor of the review findings in the form of a discipline review letter (DRL).

7. The DRL will provide feedback on the individual "reviewable unit" from the discipline review team, and not final, definitive decisions relevant to the NDA/BLA.

8. If an application is to be presented to an advisory committee, the final DRL on the "reviewable unit" may be deferred pending completion of the advisory committee meeting and internal review and consideration of the advice received.

9. The following performance goals will apply to review of "reviewable units" of an NDA/BLA for Fast Track drugs and biologics that are submitted in advance of the complete NDA/BLA under this pilot program: a. Discipline review team review of a "reviewable unit" for a Fast Track drug or biologic will be completed and a DRL issued within 6 months of the date of the submission for 30 percent of "reviewable units" submitted in FY04; b. Discipline review team review of a "reviewable unit" for a Fast Track drug or biologic will be completed and a DRL issued within 6 months of the date of the

submission for 50 percent of "reviewable units" submitted in FY05; c. Discipline review team review of a "reviewable unit" for a Fast Track drug or biologic will be completed and a DRL issued within 6 months of the date of the submission for 70 percent "reviewable units" submitted in FY06, and d. Discipline review team review of a "reviewable unit" for a Fast Track drug or biologic will be completed and a DRL letter issued within 6 months of the date of the submission for 90 percent of "reviewable units" submitted in FY07.

10. If the complete NDA/BLA is submitted to FDA while a 6-month review clock for a "reviewable unit" is still open, FDA will adhere to the timelines and performance goals for both the "reviewable unit" and the complete NDA/BLA. For example, if a "reviewable unit" is submitted in January and the complete NDA/BLA is submitted in April, the review goal for the "reviewable unit" will be July and the review goal for the complete NDA/BLA will be October.

11. Any resubmission or amendment of a "reviewable unit" submitted by the sponsor in response to an FDA discipline review letter will not be subject to the review timelines and performance goals proposed above. FDA review of such resubmissions and amendments in advance of submission of the complete NDA/BLA will occur only as resources allow.

12. This pilot program is limited to the initial submission of an NDA/BLA and is not applicable to a resubmission in response to an FDA complete response letter following the complete review of an NDA/BLA.

13. Guidance: FDA will develop and issue a joint CDER/CBER guidance on how it intends to implement this pilot program by September 30, 2003. The guidance will describe the principles, processes, and procedures that will be followed during the pilot program. The guidance also will define what subsections of a complete technical section would be considered an acceptable "reviewable unit" for pre-submission and review and how many individual "reviewable units" from one or more technical sections of an NDA/BLA can be pre-submitted and reviewed subject to separate review clocks under this program at any given time. The pilot program will be implemented in FY 2004, after the final guidance is issued and will continue through FY 2007.

B. **Pilot 2—Frequent Scientific Feedback and Interactions During Drug Development**

1. This pilot applies to drugs and biologics that have been designated to be Fast Track drugs or biologics pursuant to section 112 of the

FDA Modernization Act (21 U.S.C. 508), that are intended to treat serious and/or life-threatening diseases, and that have been the subject of an end-of-phase 1 meeting. The pilot program is limited to one Fast Track product in each CDER and CBER review division over the course of the pilot program.

2. For drugs and biologics that meet these criteria, FDA may enter into an agreement with the sponsor to initiate a formal program of frequent scientific feedback and interactions regarding the drug development program. The feedback and interactions may take the form of regular meetings between the division and the sponsor at appropriate points during the development process, written feedback from the division following review of the sponsor's drug development plan, written feedback from the division following review of important new protocols, and written feedback from the division following review of study summaries or complete study reports submitted by the sponsor.

3. Decisions regarding what study reports would be reviewed as summaries and what study reports would be reviewed as complete study reports under this pilot program would be made in advance, following discussions between the division and the sponsor of the proposed drug development program. In making these decisions, the review division will consider the importance of the study to the drug development program, the nature of the study, and the potential value of limited (i.e., based on summaries) versus more thorough division review (i.e., based on complete study reports).

4. Guidance: FDA will develop and issue a joint CDER/CBER guidance on how it intends to implement this pilot program by September 30, 2003. The guidance will describe the principles, processes, and procedures that will be followed during the pilot program. The pilot program will be implemented in FY 2004, after the final guidance is issued and will continue through FY 2007. The full (unredacted) study report will be provided to the FDA Commissioner and a version of the study report redacted to remove confidential commercial information or other information exempt from disclosure, will be made available to the public.

C. Evaluation of the Pilot Programs

1. In FY 2004, FDA will contract with an outside expert consultant(s) to evaluate both pilot programs.

2. The consultant(s) will develop an evaluation study design that identifies key questions, data requirements, and a data collection plan, and conduct a comprehensive study of the pilot programs to help assess the value, costs, and impact of these programs to the

drug development and review process. A preliminary report will be generated by the consultant by the end of FY06.

VIII. PRE- AND PERI-NDA/BLA
RISK MANAGEMENT PLAN ACTIVITIES

A. **Submission and Review of pre-NDA/BLA meeting packages:** A pre-NDA/BLA meeting package may include a summary of relevant safety information and industry questions/discussion points regarding proposed risk management plans and discussion of the need for any post-approval risk management studies. The elements of the proposal may include:

1. assessment of clinical trial limitations and disease epidemiology
2. assessment of risk management tools to be used to address known and potential risks
3. suggestions for phase 4 epidemiology studies, if such studies are warranted
4. proposals for targeted post-approval surveillance (this would include attempts to quantify background rates of risks of concern and thresholds for actions). The pre-NDA/BLA meeting package will be reviewed and discussed by the review divisions as well as the appropriate safety group in CDER or CBER.

B. **Pre-NDA/BLA meeting with industry:** This meeting may include a discussion of the preliminary risk management plans and proposed observational studies, if warranted, as outlined above. Participants in this meeting will include product safety experts from the respective Center. The intent of these discussions will be for FDA to get a better understanding of the safety issues associated with the particular drug/biologic and the proposed risk management plans, and to provide industry with feedback on these proposals so that they can be included in the NDA/BLA submission. It is the intent of this proposal that such risk management plans and the discussions around them would focus on specific issues of concern, either based on already identified safety issues or reasonable potential focused issues of concern.

C. **Review of NDA/BLA:** The NDA/BLA submitted by industry may include the proposed risk management tools and plans, and protocols for observational studies, based on the discussions that began with the pre-NDA/BLA meeting, as described above, and may be amended as appropriate to further refine the proposal. These amendments would not normally be considered major amendments. Both the review division and the appropriate safety group will be involved in the review of the application and will try to communicate comments regarding the risk management plan as early in the review process as practicable, in the form of a discipline review letter. Items to be included in the risk management plan to assure FDA of the safety and efficacy of the drug or biologic are to be addressed prior to approval of an application. The risk management plan may contain additional items that can be used to help refine the risks and actions (e.g., background rates and observational studies) and these items may be further defined and completed after approval in accordance with time frames agreed upon at the time of product approval.

D. **Peri-Approval Submission of Observational Study Reports and Periodic Safety Update Reports (PSURs):** For NDA/BLA applications, and supplements containing clinical data, submitted on or after October 1, 2002, FDA may use user fees to review an applicant's implementation of the risk management plan for a period of up to two years post-approval for most products and for a period of up to three years for products that require risk management beyond standard labeling (e.g., a black box or bolded warning, medication guide, restricted distribution). This period is defined for purposes of the user fee goals as the peri-approval period. Issues that arise during implementation of the risk management plan (e.g., whether the plan is effective) will be reported to FDA either in the form of a PSUR or in a periodic or annual report (21 CFR 314.80 and 314.81) (ICH Guidance E2C, Clinical Safety Data Management: Periodic Safety Update Reports for Marketed Drugs) and addressed during the peri-approval period through discussions between the applicant and FDA. PSURs may be submitted and reviewed semi-annually for the first two or three years post approval to allow adequate time for implementation of risk management plans. For drugs approved under PDUFA III, FDA may use user fees to independently evaluate product utilization for drugs with important safety concerns, using drug utilization databases, for the first three years post approval. The purpose of such utilization evaluations is to evaluate whether these products are being used in a safe manner and to work pro-actively with companies during the peri-approval period to accomplish this. FDA will allocate $70,900,000 in user fees over 5 years to the activities covered in this section. FDA will track the specific amounts of user fees spent on these activities and will include in its annual report to Congress an accounting of this spending.

E. **Guidance Document Development:** By the end of Fiscal Year 04, CDER and CBER will jointly develop final guidance documents that address good risk assessment, risk management, and pharmacovigilance practices.

IX. INDEPENDENT CONSULTANTS FOR BIOTECHNOLOGY
CLINICAL TRIAL PROTOCOLS

A. **Engagement of Expert Consultant:** During the development period for a biotechnology product, a sponsor may request that FDA engage an independent expert consultant, selected by FDA, to participate in the Agency's review of the protocol for the clinical studies that are expected to serve as the primary basis for a claim.

B. **Conditions**

1. The product must be a biotechnology product (for example, DNA plasmid products, synthetic peptides of fewer than 40 amino acids, monoclonal antibodies for in vivo use, and recombinant DNA-derived products) that represents a significant advance in the treatment, diagnosis or prevention of a disease or condition, or have the potential to address an unmet medical need;

2. The product may not have been the subject of a previously granted request under this program;

3. The sponsor must submit a written request for the use of an independent consultant, describing the reasons why the consultant should be engaged (e.g., as a result of preliminary discussions with the Agency the sponsor expects substantial disagreement over the proposed protocol); and

4. The request must be designated as a "Request for Appointment of Expert Consultant" and submitted in conjunction with a formal meeting request (for example, during the end-of-Phase II meeting or a Type A, meeting).

C. **Recommendations for Consultants:** The sponsor may submit a list of recommended consultants for consideration by the Agency. The selected consultant will either be a special government employee, or will be retained by FDA under contract. The consultant's role will be advisory to FDA and FDA will remain responsible for making scientific and regulatory decisions regarding the clinical protocol in question.

D. **Denial of Requests:** FDA will grant the request unless the Agency determines that engagement of an expert consultant would not serve a useful purpose (for example it is clearly premature). FDA will engage the services of an independent consultant, of FDA's choosing, as soon as practicable. If the Agency denies the request, it will provide a written rationale to the requester within 14 days of receipt.

E. **Performance Goal Change:** Due to the time required to select and screen the consultant for potential conflicts of interest and to allow the consultant sufficient time to review the scientific issues involved, the performance goals for scheduling the formal meeting (see section III) may be extended for an additional sixty (60) days.

F. **Evaluation:** During FY 2006, FDA will conduct a study to evaluate the costs and benefits of this program for both sponsors and the Agency.

X. FIRST CYCLE REVIEW PERFORMANCE PROPOSAL

A. **Notification of Issues Identified During the Filing Review**

1. Performance Goal: For original NDA/BLA applications and efficacy supplements, FDA will report substantive deficiencies identified in the initial filing review to the sponsor by letter, telephone conference, facsimile, secure e-mail, or other expedient means.
2. The timeline for such communication will be within 14 calendar days after the 60 day filing date.
3. If no deficiencies were noted, FDA will so notify the sponsor.
4. FDA's filing review represents a preliminary review of the application and is not indicative of deficiencies that may be identified later in the review cycle.
5. FDA will provide the sponsor a notification of deficiencies prior to the goal date for 50 percent of applications in FY 2003, 70 percent in FY 2004, and 90 percent in FY 2005, FY2006, and FY 2007.

B. **Good Review Management Principles Guidance:** FDA will develop a joint CDER-CBER guidance on Good Review Management Principles (GRMPs), and publish final guidance by the end of FY 2003. The Good Review Management Principles will address, among other elements, the following:

1. The filing review process, including communication of issues identified during the filing review that may affect approval of the application.
2. Ongoing communication with the sponsor during the review process (in accordance with 21 CFR 314.102(a)), including emphasis on early communication of easily correctable deficiencies (21 CFR 314.102(b)).
3. Appropriate use of Information Request and Discipline Review letters, as well as other informal methods of communication (phone, fax, e-mail).
4. Anticipating/planning for a potential Advisory Committee meeting.
5. Completing the primary reviews—allowing time for secondary and tertiary reviews prior to the action goal date.
6. Labeling feedback—planning to provide labeling comments and scheduling time for teleconferences with the sponsor in advance of the action goal date.

C. **Training:** FDA will develop and implement a program for training all review personnel, including current employees as well as future new hires, on the good review management principles.

D. **Evaluation:** FDA will retain an independent expert consultant to undertake a study to evaluate issues associated with the conduct of first cycle reviews.

1. The study will be designed to assess current performance and changes that occur after the guidance on GRMPs is published. The study will include collection of various types of tracking data regarding actions that occur during the first cycle review, both from an FDA and industry perspective (e.g., IR letters, DR letters, draft labeling comments from FDA to the sponsor, sponsor response to FDA requests for information).

2. The study will also include an assessment of the first cycle review history of all NDAs for NMEs and all BLAs during PDUFA 3. This assessment will include a more detailed evaluation of the events that occurred during the review process with a focus on identifying best practices by FDA and industry that facilitated the review process.

3. The study will also include an assessment of the effectiveness of the training program implemented by FDA.

4. FDA will develop a statement of work for the study and will provide the public an opportunity to review and comment on the statement of work before the study is implemented. The consultant will prepare annual reports of the findings of the study and a final study report at the end of the 5-year study period. The full (un-redacted) study reports will be provided to the FDA Commissioner and a version of the study reports redacted to remove confidential commercial information or other information exempt from disclosure, will be made available to the public.

5. Development and implementation of the study of first cycle review performance will be a component of the Performance Management Plan conducted out of the Office of the Commissioner (see section X).

6. Administrative oversight of the study will rest in the Office of the Commissioner. The Office of the Commissioner will convene a joint CDER/CBER review panel on a quarterly basis as a mechanism for ongoing assessment of the application of Good Review Management Principles to actions taken on original NDA/BLA applications.

XI. IMPROVING FDA PERFORMANCE MANAGEMENT

A. **Performance Fund:** The Commissioner will use at least $7 million over five years of PDUFA III funds for initiatives targeted to improve the drug review process.

1. Funds would be made available by the Commissioner to the Centers based both on identified areas of greatest need for process improvements as well as on achievement of previously identified objectives.
2. Funds also could be used by the FDA Commissioner to diagnose why objectives are not being met, or to examine areas of concern.
3. The studies conducted under this initiative would be intended to foster:

   a. Development of programs to improve access to internal and external expertise
   b. Reviewer development programs, particularly as they relate to drug review processes,
   c. Advancing science and use of information management tools
   d. Improving both inter- and intra-Center consistency, efficiency, and effectiveness
   e. Improved reporting of management objectives
   f. Increased accountability for use of user fee revenues
   g. Focused investments on improvements in the process of drug review
   h. Improved communication between the FDA and industry

4. In deciding how to spend these funds, the Commissioner would take into consideration how to achieve greater harmonization of capabilities between CDER and CBER.

B. **First Two Initiatives:** Two specific initiatives will begin early in PDUFA III and supported from performance management initiative funds 1) evaluation of first cycle review performance, and 2) process review and analysis within the two centers.

1. First Cycle Review Performance (See section X for details on this proposed study.)
2. Process Review and Analysis

   a. In FY 2003, FDA will contract with an outside consultant to conduct a comprehensive process review and analysis within CDER and CBER. This review will involve a thorough analysis of information utilization, review management, and activity cost.
   b. The review is expected to take from 18–24 months, although its duration will depend on the type and amount of complexity of the issues uncovered during the review.
   c. The outcome of this review will be a thorough documentation

of the process, a re-map of the process indicating where efficiencies can be gained, activity-based project accounting, optimal use of review tools, and a suggested path for implementing the recommendations.

d. FDA would anticipate delivery of a report of the consultant's findings and recommendations in FY 2004–2005. The agency would consider these recommendations in planning any redesign or process reengineering to enhance performance.

3. Further Studies

In subsequent years of PDUFA III, FDA may develop other study plans that will focus on further analysis of program design, performance features and costs, to identify potential avenues for further enhancement. Future studies would be likely to include a comprehensive re-analysis of program costs following the implementation of new PDUFA III review initiatives and the adoption of any process changes following the recommendations of the year 1 and 2 studies.

XII. ELECTRONIC APPLICATIONS AND SUBMISSIONS—GOALS

A. The Agency will centralize the accountability and funding for all PDUFA Information Technology initiatives/activities for CBER, CDER, ORA and OC under the leadership of the FDA CIO. The July 2001 HHS IT 5-year plan states that infrastructure consolidation across the department should be achieved, including standardization. The Agency CIO will be responsible for ensuring that all PDUFA III IT infrastructure and IT investments support the Agency's common IT goals, fit into a common computing environment, and follow good IT management practices.

B. The Agency CIO will chair quarterly briefings on PDUFA IT issues to periodically review and evaluate the progress of IT initiatives against project milestones, discuss alternatives when projects are not progressing, and review proposals for new initiatives. On an annual basis, an assessment will be conducted of progress against PDUFA III IT goals and, established program milestones, including appropriate changes to plans. A documented summary of the assessment will be drafted and forwarded to the Commissioner. A version of the study report redacted to remove confidential commercial or security information, or other information exempt from disclosure, will be made available to the public. The project milestones, assessment and changes will be part of the annual PDUFA III IT report.

C. FDA will implement a common solution in CBER, CDER, ORA and OC for the secure exchange of content including secure e-mail, electronic signatures, and secure submission of, and access to application components.

D. FDA will deliver a single point of entry for the receipt and processing of all electronic submissions in a highly secure environment. This will support CBER, CDER, OC and ORA. The system should automate the current electronic submission processes such as checking the content of electronic submissions for completeness and electronically acknowledging submissions.

E. FDA will provide a specification format for the electronic submission of the Common Technical Document (e-CTD), and provide an electronic review system for this new format that will be used by CBER, CDER and ORA reviewers. Implementation should include training to ensure successful deployment. This project will serve as the foundation for automation of other types of electronic submissions. The review software will be made available to the public.

F. Within the first 12 months, FDA will conduct an objective analysis and develop a plan for consolidation of PDUFA III IT infrastructure and desktop management services activities that will assess and prioritize the consolidation possibilities among CBER, CDER, ORA and OC to achieve technical efficiencies, target potential savings and realize cost efficiencies. Based upon the results of this analysis, to the extent appropriate, establish common IT infrastructure and architecture components according to specific milestones and dates. A documented summary of the analysis will be forwarded to the Commissioner. A version of the study report redacted to remove confidential commercial or security information, or other information exempt from disclosure, will be made available to the public.

G. FDA will implement Capability Maturity Model (CMM) in CBER, CDER, ORA and OC for PDUFA IT infrastructure and investments, and include other industry best practices to ensure that PDUFA III IT products and projects are of high quality and produced with optimal efficiency and cost effectiveness. This includes development of project plans and schedules, goals, estimates of required resources, issues and risks/mitigation plans for each PDUFA III IT initiative.

H. Where common business needs exist, CBER, CDER, ORA and OC will use the same software applications, such as eCTD software, and COTS solutions.

I. Within six months of authorization, a PDUFA III IT 5-year plan will be developed. Progress will be measured against the milestones described in the plan.

XIII. ADDITIONAL PROCEDURES

A. Simplification of Action Letters

To simplify regulatory procedures, CBER and CDER intend to amend their regulations and processes to provide for the issuance of either an "approval" (AP) or a "complete response" (CR) action letter at the completion of a review cycle for a marketing application.

B. Timing of Sponsor Notification of Deficiencies in Applications

To help expedite the development of drug and biologic products, CBER and CDER intend to submit deficiencies to sponsors in the form of an "information request" (IR) letter when each discipline has finished its initial review of its section of the pending application.

XIV. DEFINITIONS AND EXPLANATION OF TERMS

A. The term "review and act on" is understood to mean the issuance of a complete action letter after the complete review of a filed complete application. The action letter, if it is not an approval, will set forth in detail the specific deficiencies and, where appropriate, the actions necessary to place the application in condition for approval.

B. A major amendment to an original application, efficacy supplement, or resubmission of any of these applications, submitted within three months of the goal date, extends the goal date by three months. A major amendment to a manufacturing supplement submitted within two months of the goal date extends the goal date by two months.

C. A resubmitted original application is a complete response to an action letter addressing all identified deficiencies.

D. Class 1 resubmitted applications are applications resubmitted after a complete response letter (or a not approvable or approvable letter) that include the following items only (or combinations of these items):

1. Final printed labeling
2. Draft labeling
3. Safety updates submitted in the same format, including tabulations, as the original safety submission with new data and changes highlighted (except when large amounts of new information including important new adverse experiences not previously reported with the product are presented in the resubmission)
4. Stability updates to support provisional or final dating periods
5. Commitments to perform Phase 4 studies, including proposals for such studies
6. Assay validation data
7. Final release testing on the last 1–2 lots used to support approval
8. A minor reanalysis of data previously submitted to the application (determined
9. Other minor clarifying information (determined by the Agency as fitting the Class 1 category)

10. Other specific items may be added later as the Agency gains experience with the scheme and will be communicated via guidance documents to industry.

E. Class 2 resubmissions are resubmissions that include any other items, including any item that would require presentation to an advisory committee.

F. A Type A Meeting is a meeting which is necessary for an otherwise stalled drug development program to proceed (a "critical path" meeting).

G. A Type B Meeting is a 1) pre-IND, 2) end of Phase 1 (for Subpart E or Subpart H or similar products) or end of Phase 2/pre-Phase 3, or 3) a pre-NDA/BLA meeting. Each requestor should usually only request 1 each of these Type B meetings for each potential application (NDA/BLA) (or combination of closely related products, i.e., same active ingredient but different dosage forms being developed concurrently).

H. A Type C Meeting is any other type of meeting.

I. The performance goals and procedures also apply to original applications and supplements for human drugs initially marketed on an over-the-counter (OTC) basis through an NDA or switched from prescription to OTC status through an NDA or supplement.

SOURCE: FDA. 2005 (July 7). *Enclosure: PDUFA Reauthorization Performance Goals and Procedures.* [Online]. Available: http://www.fda.gov/cder/news/pdufagoals.htm [accessed July 3, 2006].

Appendix D

Committee on the Assessment of the US Drug Safety System Meeting Agendas

MEETING ONE—AGENDA

The National Academies
Institute of Medicine

Committee on the Assessment of the US Drug Safety System
Meeting One

AGENDA

Wednesday, June 8, 2005

OPEN SESSION   **Room 100**

10:00–10:05 a.m.   **Welcome and Introductions**

David Blumenthal
Sheila Burke
Co-Chairs, Committee on the Assessment of the
US Drug Safety System

10:05–10:40 a.m.   **Charge to the Committee**

Steven Galson
Acting Director of the Center for Drug Evaluation
and Research
Food and Drug Administration

Janet Woodcock
Deputy Commissioner of Operations
Food and Drug Administration

10:35–11:00 a.m.   **Questions from the Committee**

11:00–11:45 a.m.   **Perspectives of Pharmaceutical Manufacturers and Payors**

Amit Sachdev
Executive Vice President, Health
Biotechnology Industry Organization (BIO)

Christine Simmon
Vice President of Public Affairs and Development
Generic Pharmaceutical Association (GPhA)

J. Russell Teagarden
Vice President of Clinical Practices &
Therapeutics
Medco Health Solutions, Inc. (on behalf of the
Pharmaceutical Care Management Association)

Alan Goldhammer
Associate Vice President for Regulatory Affairs
Pharmaceutical Research and Manufacturers of
America (PhRMA)

11:45–12:00 p.m.   **Questions from the Committee**

12:00–12:45 p.m.   **Consumer/Patient and Professional Organizations' Perspectives**

David Borenstein
Member, Board of Directors
American College of Rheumatology (ACR)

John A. Gans
Executive Vice-President and Chief Executive
Officer
American Pharmacists Association (APhA)

Bill Vaughan
Senior Policy Analyst
Consumers Union

Jeanne Ireland
Director of Public Policy
Elizabeth Glaser Pediatric AIDS Foundation

| 12:45–1:00 p.m. | Questions from the Committee |
| 1:00 p.m. | Adjourn |

MEETING TWO—AGENDA

The National Academies
Institute of Medicine

Committee on the Assessment of the US Drug Safety System
Meeting Two

AGENDA

Speakers and Times Subject to Change

Tuesday, July 19, 2005

OPEN SESSION   **LECTURE ROOM**

3:00–3:05 p.m.   **Welcome and Introductions**

> *David Blumenthal*
> *Sheila Burke*
> Co-Chairs, Committee on the Assessment of the US Drug Safety System

3:05–6:00 p.m.   **Public Comment**

> *Carla Saxton*
> Professional Affairs Manager
> American Society of Consultant Pharmacists
>
> *Maryann Napoli*
> Center for Medical Consumers
>
> *John J. Pippin*
> Physicians Committee for Responsible Medicine
>
> *Patrick J. Madden*
> *Lesley Maloney*
> American Society of Health-System Pharmacists
>
> *Marc Wheat*
> Chief Counsel and Staff Director
> Subcommittee on Criminal Justice, Drug Policy, and Human Resources
> US House of Representatives

Lindsey Johnson
Consumer Advocate
U.S. Public Interest Research Group (US PIRG)

Alison Rein
Assistant Director
Food & Health Policy National Consumers
League

Beth A. McConnell
Director
PennPIRG and the PennPIRG Education Fund

Marion J. Goff
Donald Klein
American College of Neuropsychopharmacology

Tom Woodward
Director, Alliance for Human Resource Protection
(AHRP)
State Director, International Coalition of Drug
Awareness

6:00 p.m.   **Adjourn**

Wednesday, July 20, 2005

OPEN SESSION   **LECTURE ROOM**

1:00–1:05 p.m. **Welcome and Introductions**

David Blumenthal
Sheila Burke
Co-Chairs, Committee on the Assessment of the
US Drug Safety System

1:05–3:00 p.m. **Food and Drug Administration's (FDA's) Drug Safety
Activities**

Introduction and Overview

Paul J. Seligman
Director, Office of Pharmacoepidemiology and
Statistical Science
Center for Drug Evaluation and Research
Food and Drug Administration

Role of the Office of New Drugs in the Safety Assessment

John K. Jenkins
Director of the Office of New Drugs
Center for Drug Evaluation and Research
Food and Drug Administration

The Postmarketing Safety Assessment and the Office of Drug Safety

Anne E. Trontell
Deputy Director, Office of Drug Safety
FDA Center for Drugs
Food and Drug Administration

Future of Safety Assessment

Paul J. Seligman

3:00–3:30 p.m.	Questions from the Committee
3:30–3:45 p.m.	Break
3:45–4:00 p.m.	The Role of the Agency for Healthcare Research and Quality (AHRQ) in the US Drug Safety System

> *Scott R. Smith*
> Center for Outcomes and Evidence
> Agency for Healthcare Research and Quality

4:00–4:15 p.m.   The Role of the Centers for Medicare and Medicaid Services (CMS) in the US Drug Safety System

> *Speaker TBA*
> Centers for Medicare and Medicaid Services

4:15–4:45 p.m.   Questions from the Committee

4:45–5:15 p.m.   AHRQ-funded Centers for Education and Research on Therapeutics (CERTs)

> and

Contributions of Academia and the Pharmaceutical Industry to Drug Safety Surveillance

> *Hugh Tilson*
> Chair, CERTs Steering Committee

5:15–5:45 p.m.   Questions from the Committee

5:45 p.m.   Adjourn

WORKSHOP—AGENDA

The National Academies
Institute of Medicine

Committee on the Assessment of the US Drug Safety System

**Advancing the Methods and Application of
Risk-Benefit Assessment of Medicines**

January 17, 2006
The Keck Center, Room 100
500 Fifth Street, NW
Washington, DC 20001

Purpose of workshop:

1. Identify methodological approaches for performing integrated and explicit assessments of risk-benefit of pharmaceuticals throughout a product's lifecycle, including identifying the type of information that would be most useful to decision-makers.

2. Obtain expert input on the use of new methodological approaches in pre- and postmarket risk assessment.

3. Identify opportunities and barriers in advancing a public health approach to balancing risks and benefits of pharmaceuticals for drug regulation and risk management.

Tuesday, January 17, 2005

8:15 a.m.   **Opening Remarks**

8:30 a.m.   **Overview of Pharmacoepidemiology: What Is the Evidence Base?**

Session 1: Assessing a product's risk-benefit balance throughout its lifecycle involves the use of a variety of epidemiological resources and methods, including the use of ad hoc data sources, automated data systems, and randomized trials. The choice of specific assessment methods involves a consideration of many factors, including how well it informs decision making intended to optimize a drug's balance between benefits and risks.

Assessing Risks and Benefits of Pharmaceuticals:
Methods and Approaches
Brian Strom, MD, MPH
Chair and Professor
Department of Biostatistics and Epidemiology
University of Pennsylvania

Premarket Assessment of Drug Safety at the FDA
Judith Racoosin, MD, MPH
Safety Team Leader
Division of Neurology Products
Division of Psychiatry Products
Center for Drug Evaluation and Research
U.S. Food and Drug Administration

FDA Postapproval Risk Assessment
Anne Trontell, MD, MPH
Senior Advisor on Pharmaceutical Outcomes
Center for Outcomes and Evidence
Agency for Healthcare Policy and Research

Risk-Benefit Frameworks: Perspectives from the
Field of Environmental Health
Jonathan Samet, MD, MS
Professor and Chair
Department of Epidemiology
Johns Hopkins School of Public Health

9:45 a.m.	Discussion: Q & A with IOM Committee Members & Audience
10:30 a.m.	Break
11:00 a.m.	Case Studies Involving Risk-Benefit Uncertainties

Session 2: This session involves the consideration of two case studies of contemporary drug safety issues, each case involving a different risk-benefit dilemma. The case studies are intended to focus the discussion on the type of information that would be most useful to decision makers, with the case studies selected to address both the preapproval and the postapproval period. The intent is to model not what is or is not actually done at the FDA and by the industry sponsors, but what could or should be done. The proposed format is that speakers for each case study will briefly present the case study, followed by questions of clarification of fact from the IOM Committee and audience. Following lunch, there will be comments from an invited panel and discussion/questions to be posed by the IOM Committee.

Presentation of Case Study 1—Salmeterol
Scott T. Weiss, MD
Professor of Medicine
Harvard Medical School

Presentation of Case Study 2—Muraglitazar
Steve Nissen, MD
Medical Director, Cardiovascular Coordinating
Center
Cleveland Clinic

Questions of Clarification of Fact

12:30 p.m.   Lunch

1:30 p.m.   Reconvene: Panel Discussions

Suggested Discussion Points for the Panelists: Having heard the case studies, what tool or tools (existing or to be developed) would have narrowed the uncertainty about the benefit/risk profile for the drugs? At what point during evidence development should this tool have been brought into play? What would have remained uncertain? How long would it have taken and what effort would it have taken to reduce that uncertainty? How were the risks and benefits identified, evaluated, and weighted? Where were the flaws in this process? What could have/should have been done differently and why? What resources are needed for your approach? How would this approach improve the current risk/benefit evaluation?

Panel:

Judith K. Jones, MD, PhD
President, The Degge Group, Ltd

Wayne Ray, PhD
Professor, Department of Preventive Medicine
Director, Pharmacoepidemiology
Vanderbilt University

Michael P. Stern, MD
Professor, Department of Medicine
Chief, Division of Clinical Epidemiology
University of Texas, San Antonio

Robert B. Wallace, MD, MS
Professor of Epidemiology, College of Public Health
University of Iowa

> Noel Weiss, MD, PhD
> Professor of Epidemiology, School of Public
>   Health and Community Medicine, University of
>   Washington
>
> Discussion: Q & A with IOM Committee Members
>   and Audience

3:00 p.m.   **Break**

3:30 p.m.   **Establishing a framework for risk-benefit methods to reduce uncertainties during pharmacuetical products's lifecycle**

Session 3: This session is designed to session to reflect on what we learned from the case studies and panel discussion and to articulate a framework needed to improve the timing, rigor, and transparency of risk-benefit assessments.

> Janice K. Bush, MD
> VP, Quality, Education & Business Support, Benefit
>   Risk Management
>
> Curt Furberg, MD, PhD
> Professor, Wake Forest University
>
> Louis Garrison, PhD
> Professor of Pharmacy, University of Washington
>
> Joanna Haas, MD, MS
> Vice President, Pharmacovigilance, Genzyme
>   Corporation
>
> Alastair J.J. Wood, MD
> Professor, Vanderbilt University Medical Center
>
> **Discussion—All**

5:00 p.m.   **Adjourn**

MEETING FOUR—AGENDA

The National Academies
Institute of Medicine

Committee on the Assessment of the US Drug Safety System

AGENDA

Thursday, January 19, 2006

OPEN SESSION 8:15–8:25 a.m.	Keck 100 *Welcome and Introductions* *Description of Committee's request to invited speakers*

Many recommendations for strengthening FDA's role in drug safety have been made in the past several years. We have sent today's speakers three sets of recommendations:

- Ganslaw LS. 2005. Drug Safety: New Legal/Regulatory Approaches. FDLI Update: Food and Drug Law, Regulation, and Education.
- FDA Task Force on Risk Management. 1999. Managing the Risks from Medical Product Use: Creating a Risk Management Framework. Report to the FDA Commissioner from the Task Force on Risk Management. http://www.fda.gov/oc/tfrm/riskmanagement.pdf.
- CRS/Thaul. 2005. Drug Safety and Effectiveness: Issues and Action Options After FDA Approval. http://www.law.umaryland.edu/marshall/crsreports/crsdocuments/RL3279703082005.pdf.

Reflecting on these (and other recommendations you find relevant) please comment on the following:

- Which of these or other recommendations are the most important to consider and why?
- Which of these or other recommendations that have been made would you not support and why?

8:25–8:45 a.m.	Geoffrey Levitt *Wyeth Pharmaceuticals*
8:45–9:05 a.m.	Steven Ryder *Pfizer, Inc.*
9:05–9:25 a.m.	James Kotsanos *Eli Lilly and Company*
9:25–9:45 a.m.	James Nickas *Genentech*
9:45–10:15 a.m.	Questions from the Committee
10:15–10:30 a.m.	Break
10:30–10:50 a.m.	Fran Visco *National Breast Cancer Coalition*
10:50–11:10 a.m.	Sid Wolfe *Public Citizen*
11:10–11:30 a.m.	Frank Burroughs Steve Walker *Abigail Alliance for Better Access to Developmental Drugs*
11:30–11:50 a.m.	David H. Campen *Kaiser Permanente (on behalf of America's Health Insurance Plans)*
11:50 a.m.– 12:20 p.m.	Questions from the Committee
12:20–12:30 p.m.	Closing Remarks
12:30 p.m.	Adjourn

Appendix E

Summary

Preventing Medication Errors: Quality Chasm Series
Institute of Medicine

PREVENTING MEDICATION ERRORS

Committee on Identifying and Preventing Medication Errors

Board on Health Care Services

Philip Aspden, Julie A. Wolcott, J. Lyle Bootman, Linda R. Cronenwett,
Editors

INSTITUTE OF MEDICINE
OF THE NATIONAL ACADEMIES

THE NATIONAL ACADEMIES PRESS
Washington, DC
www.nap.edu

THE NATIONAL ACADEMIES PRESS   500 Fifth Street, N.W.   Washington, DC 20001

NOTICE: The project that is the subject of this report was approved by the Governing Board of the National Research Council, whose members are drawn from the councils of the National Academy of Sciences, the National Academy of Engineering, and the Institute of Medicine. The members of the committee responsible for the report were chosen for their special competences and with regard for appropriate balance.

This study was supported by Contract No. HHSM-500-2004-00020C between the National Academy of Sciences and Department of Health and Human Services (Centers for Medicare and Medicaid Services). Any opinions, findings, conclusions, or recommendations expressed in this publication are those of the author(s) and do not necessarily reflect the view of the organizations or agencies that provided support for this project.

Library of Congress Cataloging-in-Publication Data

Preventing medication errors / Committee on Identifying and Preventing Medication Errors, Board on Health Care Services ; Philip Aspden ... [et al.], editors.
    p. ; cm. — (Quality chasm series)
  Includes bibliographical references and index.
  ISBN-13: 978-0-309-10147-9 (hardcover)
  ISBN-10: 0-309-10147-6 (hardcover)
  1. Medication errors—Prevention. I. Aspden, Philip. II. Institute of Medicine (U.S.). Committee on Identifying and Preventing Medication Errors. III. Series.
  [DNLM: 1. Medication Errors—prevention & control—United States. 2. Safety Management—United States. QZ 42 P9435 2006]
  RM146.P744 2006
  615'.6—dc22
                            2006029215

Additional copies of this report are available from the National Academies Press, 500 Fifth Street, N.W., Lockbox 285, Washington, DC 20055; (800) 624-6242 or (202) 334-3313 (in the Washington metropolitan area); Internet, http://www.nap.edu.

For more information about the Institute of Medicine, visit the IOM home page at: **www.iom.edu.**

The serpent has been a symbol of long life, healing, and knowledge among almost all cultures and religions since the beginning of recorded history. The serpent adopted as a logotype by the Institute of Medicine is a relief carving from ancient Greece, now held by the Staatliche Museen in Berlin.

"Knowing is not enough; we must apply.
Willing is not enough; we must do."

—Goethe

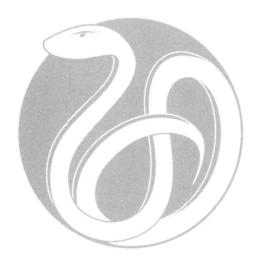

INSTITUTE OF MEDICINE
OF THE NATIONAL ACADEMIES

Advising the Nation. Improving Health.

THE NATIONAL ACADEMIES
Advisers to the Nation on Science, Engineering, and Medicine

The **National Academy of Sciences** is a private, nonprofit, self-perpetuating society of distinguished scholars engaged in scientific and engineering research, dedicated to the furtherance of science and technology and to their use for the general welfare. Upon the authority of the charter granted to it by the Congress in 1863, the Academy has a mandate that requires it to advise the federal government on scientific and technical matters. Dr. Ralph J. Cicerone is president of the National Academy of Sciences.

The **National Academy of Engineering** was established in 1964, under the charter of the National Academy of Sciences, as a parallel organization of outstanding engineers. It is autonomous in its administration and in the selection of its members, sharing with the National Academy of Sciences the responsibility for advising the federal government. The National Academy of Engineering also sponsors engineering programs aimed at meeting national needs, encourages education and research, and recognizes the superior achievements of engineers. Dr. Wm. A. Wulf is president of the National Academy of Engineering.

The **Institute of Medicine** was established in 1970 by the National Academy of Sciences to secure the services of eminent members of appropriate professions in the examination of policy matters pertaining to the health of the public. The Institute acts under the responsibility given to the National Academy of Sciences by its congressional charter to be an adviser to the federal government and, upon its own initiative, to identify issues of medical care, research, and education. Dr. Harvey V. Fineberg is president of the Institute of Medicine.

The **National Research Council** was organized by the National Academy of Sciences in 1916 to associate the broad community of science and technology with the Academy's purposes of furthering knowledge and advising the federal government. Functioning in accordance with general policies determined by the Academy, the Council has become the principal operating agency of both the National Academy of Sciences and the National Academy of Engineering in providing services to the government, the public, and the scientific and engineering communities. The Council is administered jointly by both Academies and the Institute of Medicine. Dr. Ralph J. Cicerone and Dr. Wm. A. Wulf are chair and vice chair, respectively, of the National Research Council.

www.national-academies.org

WILSON D. PACE, Professor of Family Medicine and Green-Edelman Chair for Practice-based Research, University of Colorado; Director, American Academy of Family Physicians National Research Network

KATHLEEN R. STEVENS, Professor and Director, Academic Center for Evidence-Based Practice, University of Texas Health Science Center, San Antonio

EDWARD WESTRICK, Vice President of Medical Management, University of Massachusetts Memorial Health Care

ALBERT W. WU, Professor of Health Policy and Management and Internal Medicine, The Johns Hopkins University

Health Care Services Board

CLYDE J. BEHNEY, Acting Director (June 2005 to December 2005 and from May 2006)

JOHN C. RING, Director (from December 2005 to May 2006)

JANET M. CORRIGAN, Director (September 2004 to May 2005)

ANTHONY BURTON, Administrative Assistant

Study Staff

PHILIP ASPDEN, Study Director

JULIE A. WOLCOTT, Program Officer (to April 2006)

ANDREA M. SCHULTZ, Research Associate (from June 2006)

RYAN L. PALUGOD, Research Assistant (from December 2005)

TASHARA BASTIEN, Senior Program Assistant (to January 2006)

WILLIAM B. MCLEOD, Senior Librarian

GARY J. WALKER, Senior Financial Officer (from December 2005)

TERESA REDD, Financial Advisor (to December 2005)

ELIZABETH E. LAFALCE, Intern (April to May, 2005)

Reviewers

This report has been reviewed in draft form by individuals chosen for their diverse perspectives and technical expertise, in accordance with procedures approved by the NRC's Report Review Committee. The purpose of this independent review is to provide candid and critical comments that will assist the institution in making its published report as sound as possible and to ensure that the report meets institutional standards for objectivity, evidence, and responsiveness to the study charge. The review comments and draft manuscript remain confidential to protect the integrity of the deliberative process. We wish to thank the following individuals for their review of this report:

LOWELL ANDERSON, Watauga Corporation
MARGE BOWMAN, University of Pennsylvania Health System
PATRICIA FLATLEY BRENNAN, School of Nursing and College of Engineering, University of Wisconsin-Madison
DAVID COUSINS, National Patient Safety Organization, London
DON E. DETMER, American Medical Informatics Association and The University of Virginia
WILLIAM EVANS, St. Jude Children's Research Hospital, Memphis
ANN HENDRICH, Ascension Health, St. Louis, MO
CRAIG HOESLEY, University Hospital, University of Alabama at Birmingham
WILLIAM J. KOOPMAN, Department of Medicine, University of Alabama at Birmingham
GERALD D. LAUBACH, Pfizer Inc., Past President

LUCIAN LEAPE, Department of Health Policy and Management, Harvard School of Public Health
ART LEVIN, Center for Medical Consumers, New York, NY
G. STEVE REBAGLIATI, Department of Emergency Medicine, Oregon Health and Sciences University
HUGH TILSON, School of Public Health, University of North Carolina

Although the reviewers listed above have provided many constructive comments and suggestions, they were not asked to endorse the conclusions or recommendations nor did they see the final draft of the report before its release. The review of this report was overseen by **Paul F. Griner**, University of Rochester, Professor Emeritus and **Charles E. Phelps**, University of Rochester. Appointed by the National Research Council and Institute of Medicine, they were responsible for making certain that an independent examination of this report was carried out in accordance with institutional procedures and that all review comments were carefully considered. Responsibility for the final content of this report rests entirely with the authoring committee and the institution.

Preface

In 2000, the Institute of Medicine (IOM) report *To Err Is Human: Building a Safer Health System* raised awareness about medical errors and accelerated existing efforts to prevent such errors. The present report makes clear that with regard to medication errors, we still have a long way to go. The current medication-use process, which encompasses prescribing, dispensing, administering, and monitoring, is characterized by many serious problems and issues that threaten both the safety and positive outcomes of the process. Each of the steps in the process needs improvement and further study.

At the beginning of the medication-use process, prescribers often lack sufficient knowledge about how the drugs they are prescribing will work in specific patient populations. If the balance of medication risks and benefits is not known (as is common, for example, with children and the elderly), it is impossible to say whether medication use is safe. Improving medication use and reducing errors, therefore, requires improving the quality of information generated by the pharmaceutical industry and other researchers regarding drug products and their use in clinical practice. We also need to better understand how to communicate such information to clinicians and patients via packaging, leaflets, and health information technology systems. Lastly, we need to understand how better to prevent medication errors in all care settings and in transitions between care settings. In this report, the IOM Committee on Identifying and Preventing Medication Errors proposes a research agenda for industry and government that can help meet these critical needs.

Despite the lack of data regarding many interventions that might improve the quality and safety of medication use, the committee offers recommendations for change that should be implemented and evaluated. People who use medications to meet their health care needs have a huge stake in that effort. The most powerful strategy for improving safety may be motivating providers and organizations to support the full engagement of patients and surrogates in improving the safety of medication use. In addition, providers and leaders of health care organizations must create the climate and infrastructure necessary to continuously learn about and improve the safety of all steps in the medication-use process. This report provides guidance on the types of error prevention strategies that should be implemented in each care setting. It also presents the committee's recommendations for the pharmaceutical industry, government, and regulatory, certification, and accreditation bodies, each of which has a role to play in improving the quality and safety of medication use.

This report represents the culmination of the dedicated efforts of three groups of people. We would like to thank our fellow committee members who have worked long and diligently on this challenging study, the many experts who provided formal testimony to the committee and informal advice throughout the study, and the staff of the Health Care Services Board who managed the study and coordinated the writing of the final report.

J. Lyle Bootman, Ph.D., Sc.D.
Linda R. Cronenwett, Ph.D., M.A., R.N.
Cochairs
July 2006

Acknowledgments

The Committee on Identifying and Preventing Medication Errors wishes to acknowledge the many people whose contributions and support made this report possible. The committee benefited from presentations made by a number of experts over the past 2 years. The following individuals shared their research, experience, and perspectives with the committee: Tom Abrams, Food and Drug Administration; Bruce Bagley, American Academy of Family Physicians; Robert Ball, Food and Drug Administration; Jim Battles, Agency for Healthcare Research and Quality; Karen Bell, Centers for Medicare and Medicaid Services; Douglas Bierer, Consumer Healthcare Products Association; David Bowen, Office of Senator Edward Kennedy; Bill Braithwaite, eHealth Initiative; Dan Budnitz, Centers for Disease Control and Prevention; Betsy Chrischilles, University of Iowa; John Clarke, ECRI; David Classen, First Consulting Group; Ilene Corina, Patients United Limiting Substandards and Errors in Healthcare; Diane Cousins, U.S. Pharmacopeial Convention; Loriann De Martini, California Department of Health Services; Noel Eldridge, Veterans Health Administration; Frank Federico, Institute for Healthcare Improvement; Susan Frampton, Planetree; David Gustafson, University of Wisconsin; Ed Hammond, Duke University; Mark Hayes, Office of Senator Chuck Grassley; Carol Holquist, Food and Drug Administration; David Hunt, Centers for Medicare and Medicaid Services; Gordon Hunt, Sutter Health; John Jenkins, Food and Drug Administration; Mike Kafrissen, Johnson & Johnson; Ken Kizer, National Quality Forum; Richard Moore, Massachusetts State Senator; Bill Munier, Agency for Healthcare Research and Quality; Dianne Murphy, Food and Drug Administration; Steve Northrop, Office of Senator Chuck Grassley; Jerry

Osheroff, Micromedex; Emily Patterson, Ohio State University; John Reiling, Synergy Health and St. Joseph's Hospital; Lisa Robin, Federation of State Medical Boards; William Rollow, Centers for Medicare and Medicaid Services; Jeffrey Rothschild, Brigham and Women's Hospital Partners Healthcare; Lee Rucker, American Association of Retired Persons; Luke Sato, Harvard Risk Management Foundation; Stephen Schondelmeyer, University of Minnesota; David Schulke, American Health Quality Association; Paul Schyve, Joint Commission on Accreditation of Healthcare Organizations; Paul Seligman, Food and Drug Administration; Vickie Sheets, National Council of State Boards of Nursing; Pat Sodomka, Medical College of Georgia; Scott Stanley, University Health System Consortium; Jonathan Teich, Health Vision; Anne Trontell, Food and Drug Administration; Tim Vanderveen, Alaris & Cardinal Health; and Ed Weisbart, Express Scripts.

The following individuals were important sources of information, generously giving their time and knowledge to further the committee's efforts: Michele Boisse, American Society for Clinical Pharmacology and Therapeutics; Anne Burns, American Pharmacists Association; Francis Dobscha, Advance Med; Melody Eble, Johnson & Johnson; Atheer Kaddis, Blue Cross and Blue Shield of Michigan; Lucinda Maine, American Association of Colleges of Pharmacy; Gary Merica, York Hospital; Joseph Morris, Health Care Improvement Foundation; Richard Park, *IVD Technology* magazine; Ken Reid, Washington Information Source Co.; Ed Staffa, National Association of Chain Drug Stores; Kasey Thompson, American Society of Health-system Pharmacists; Marissa Schlaifer, Academy of Managed Care Pharmacy; Junelle Speller, American Academy of Pediatrics; Sharon Wilson, Center for Nursing Practice; and Charles Young, Massachusetts Board of Registration in Pharmacy.

The committee commissioned eight papers that provided important background information for the report, and would like to thank all the authors for their dedicated work and helpful insights: Harvey J. Murff, Vanderbilt University; Ginette A. Pepper, University of Utah College of Nursing; Grace M. Kuo, Baylor College of Medicine; Marlene R. Miller, Karen A. Robinson, Lisa H. Lubomski, Michael L. Rinke, and Peter J Pronovost, The Johns Hopkins University; Benjamin C. Grasso, The Institute for Self-Directed Care; Albert I. Wertheimer and Thomas M. Santella, Temple University; Eta Berner, University of Alabama at Birmingham with assistance from Lorri Zipperer, Zipperer Project Management; Richard Maisiak, consultant; and Brent Petty, The Johns Hopkins University.

The committee also benefited from the work of other committees and staff of the Institute of Medicine that conducted studies relevant to this report, particularly the Committee on Quality of Health Care in America and the Committee on Identifying Priority Areas for Quality Improvement. The Committee on Quality of Health Care in America produced the 2000 report *To Err Is Human: Building a Safer Health System* and the 2001 report *Crossing the Quality Chasm: A New Health System for the 21st Century*. The committee on Identifying Priority Areas for Quality Improvement produced the 2003 report *Priority Areas for National Action: Transforming Health Care Quality.*

Finally, funding for this project was provided by the Centers for Medicare and Medicaid Services. The committee extends special thanks for that support.

Contents

SUMMARY   1

1   INTRODUCTION   25

PART I: UNDERSTANDING THE CAUSES AND COSTS OF
MEDICATION ERRORS   43

2   OVERVIEW OF THE DRUG DEVELOPMENT, REGULATION,
    DISTRIBUTION, AND USE SYSTEM   50

3   MEDICATION ERRORS: INCIDENCE AND COST   105

PART II: MOVING TOWARD A PATIENT-CENTERED,
INTEGRATED MEDICATION-USE SYSTEM   143

4   ACTION AGENDA TO SUPPORT CONSUMER–PROVIDER
    PARTNERSHIP   151

5   ACTION AGENDA FOR HEALTH CARE ORGANIZATIONS   221

6   ACTION AGENDA FOR THE PHARMACEUTICAL, MEDICAL
    DEVICE, AND HEALTH INFORMATION TECHNOLOGY
    INDUSTRIES   266

7   APPLIED RESEARCH AGENDA FOR SAFE MEDICATION
    USE   310

8   ACTION AGENDAS FOR OVERSIGHT, REGULATION, AND
    PAYMENT   328

APPENDIXES

A BIOGRAPHICAL SKETCHES OF COMMITTEE MEMBERS   349

B GLOSSARY OF TERMS AND ACRONYMS   359

C MEDICATION ERRORS: INCIDENCE RATES   367

D MEDICATION ERRORS: PREVENTION STRATEGIES   409

INDEX   447

Summary

ABSTRACT

The use of medications is ubiquitous. In any given week, more than four of five U.S. adults take at least one medication (prescription or over-the-counter [OTC] drug, vitamin/mineral, or herbal supplement), and almost a third take at least five different medications.[1] Errors can occur with any of these products at any point in the medication-use process and in any care setting. The frequency of medication errors and preventable medication-related injuries represents a very serious cause for concern.

The Centers for Medicare and Medicaid Services sponsored this study by the Institute of Medicine (IOM) with the aim of developing a national agenda for reducing medication errors based on estimates of the incidence of such errors and evidence on the efficacy of various prevention strategies. The study focused on the safe, effective, and appropriate use of medications in the major components of the medication-use system, addressing the use of prescription drugs, OTC drugs, and complementary and alternative medications, in a wide range of care settings—hospital, long-term, and community.

The committee estimates that on average, a hospital patient is subject to at least one medication error per day, with considerable

---

[1]In this report, the terms *medication* and *drug* are used interchangeably.

1

variation in error rates across facilities. The few existing studies of the costs associated with medication errors are limited to the health care costs incurred by preventable injuries, and these are substantial.

At least a quarter of all medication-related injuries are preventable. Many efficacious error prevention strategies are available, especially for hospital care; examples are electronic prescribing and clinical decision-support systems that check dosages and monitor for harmful drug–drug interactions. This report provides guidance on how to implement error prevention strategies in hospitals, long-term care, and ambulatory care.

Establishing and maintaining a strong provider–patient partnership is a key approach for reducing medication errors. The report outlines how such a partnership can be achieved and what roles providers, patients, and third parties must play. For example, consumers should maintain careful records of their medications, providers should review a patient's list of medications at each encounter and at times of transition between care settings (e.g., hospital to outpatient care), and the federal government should seek ways to improve the quality of pharmacy leaflets and medication-related information on the Internet for consumers.

Health care providers in all settings should seek to create high-reliability organizations that constantly improve the safety and quality of medication use. To this end, they should implement active internal monitoring programs so that progress toward improved medication safety can be accurately demonstrated. The report offers guidance on appropriate monitoring systems for each major care setting.

In carrying out this study, the IOM committee identified enormous gaps in the knowledge base with regard to medication errors. Current methods for generating and communicating information about medications are inadequate and contribute to the incidence of errors. Likewise, incidence rates of medication errors in many care settings, the costs of such errors, and the efficacy of prevention strategies are not well understood. The report proposes a research agenda to address these and other knowledge gaps.

STUDY SCOPE

The Institute of Medicine (IOM) report *To Err Is Human: Building a Safer Health System* (IOM, 2000) accelerated existing efforts to prevent medication errors and improve the quality of health care, efforts that are just now gaining acceptance as a discipline requiring investment in individuals who specialize in error prevention and quality improvement. Against this background, at the urging of the Senate Finance Committee, the United States

> ## BOX S-1
> ## Scope of the Study
>
> Congress, through the Medicare Modernization Act of 2003 (Section 107(c)), mandated the Centers for Medicare and Medicaid Services to sponsor the Institute of Medicine to carry out a study:
>
> - To develop a fuller understanding of drug safety and quality issues through the conduct of an evidence-based review of the literature, case studies and analysis. This review will consider the nature and causes of medication errors; their impact on patients; and the differences in causation, impact and prevention across multiple dimensions of health care delivery including patient populations, care settings, clinicians, and institutional cultures.
> - If possible, to develop estimates of the incidence, severity and costs of medication errors that can be useful in prioritizing resources for national quality improvement efforts and influencing national health care policy.
> - To evaluate alternative approaches to reducing medication errors in terms of their efficacy, cost-effectiveness, appropriateness in different settings and circumstances, feasibility, institutional barriers to implementation, associated risk, and quality of evidence supporting the approach.
> - To provide guidance to consumers, providers, payers, and other key stakeholders on high-priority strategies to achieve both short-term and long-term drug safety goals, to elucidate the goals and expected results of such initiatives and support the business case for them, and to identify critical success factors and key levers for achieving success.
> - To assess opportunities and key impediments to broad nationwide implementation of medication error reductions, and to provide guidance to policymakers and government agencies in promoting a national agenda for medication error reduction.
> - To develop an applied research agenda to evaluate the health and cost impacts of alternative interventions, and to assess collaborative public and private strategies for implementing the research agenda through the Agency for Healthcare Research and Quality and other government agencies.

Congress directed the Centers for Medicare and Medicaid Services (CMS) to contract with the IOM for a study to formulate a national agenda for reducing medication errors by developing estimates of the incidence of such errors and determining the efficacy of prevention strategies (see Box S-1).

THE LEVEL AND CONSEQUENCES OF MEDICATION ERRORS ARE UNACCEPTABLE

Rates of Errors and Preventable Harmful Events Are High

The frequency of medication errors and preventable adverse drug events (ADEs) (defined in Box S-2) is a very serious cause for concern. In

---

BOX S-2
Key Definitions

Error: The failure of a planned action to be completed as intended (error of execution) or the use of a wrong plan to achieve an aim (error of planning). An error may be an act of commission or an act of omission (IOM, 2004).

Medication error: Any error occurring in the medication-use process (Bates et al., 1995a). Examples include wrong dosage prescribed, wrong dosage administered for a prescribed medication, or failure to give (by the provider) or take (by the patient) a medication.

Adverse drug event: Any injury due to medication (Bates et al., 1995b). Examples include a wrong dosage leading to injury (e.g., rash, confusion, or loss of function) or an allergic reaction occurring in a patient not known to be allergic to a given medication.

---

hospitals, errors are common during all steps of the medication-use process—procuring the drug, prescribing, dispensing, administering, and monitoring the patient's response. In hospitals, they occur most frequently at the prescribing and administration stages.

Published error rates depend on the intensity and specifics of the error detection methods used. In particular, some methods are better suited to certain stages of the medication-use process. Detection methods addressing all stages but not including direct observation of administration found a rate of 0.1 prescribing errors per patient per day in a study of hospital pediatric units (Kaushal et al., 2001) and a rate of 0.3 prescribing errors per patient per day in a study of hospital medical units (Bates et al., 1995a). A major study using direct observation of administration (Barker et al., 2002) carried out at 36 different health care facilities found an administration error rate of 11 percent, excluding doses administered outside the scheduled time ("wrong-time" errors). Since a hospital patient receives on average at least ten medication doses per day, this figure suggests that on average, a hospital patient is subject to one administration error per day. Further, since prescribing and administration errors account for about three-fourths of medication errors (Leape et al., 1995), the committee conservatively estimates that on average, a hospital patient is subject to at least one medication error per day. Substantial variations in error rates are found, however. For the 36 facilities in the study mentioned above, the administration error rate (excluding wrong-time errors) ranged from 0 to 26 percent, with a median value of 8.3 percent (Barker et al., 2002).

A preventable ADE is a serious type of medication error. ADEs, defined as any injury due to medication (Bates et al., 1995b), are common in hospitals, nursing homes, and the outpatient setting. ADEs associated with a medication error are considered preventable. The committee estimates that at least 1.5 million preventable ADEs occur each year in the United States:

- Hospital care—Classen and colleagues (1997) projected 380,000 preventable ADEs occurring annually, and Bates and colleagues (1995b) 450,000. These are likely underestimates given the higher preventable ADE rate of another study using more comprehensive ADE identification methods (Jha et al., 1998).
- Long-term care—Gurwitz and colleagues (2005) projected 800,000 preventable ADEs, again likely an underestimate given the higher ADE rates of other studies.
- Ambulatory care—Among outpatient Medicare patients alone, Gurwitz and colleagues (2003) projected 530,000 preventable ADEs. Their approach was conservative, however, because it did not involve direct contact with patients, which yields much higher rates (Gandhi et al., 2003).

The above data exclude errors of omission—failure to prescribe medications for which there is an evidence base for the ability to reduce morbidity and mortality. With respect to such errors, the committee found well-documented evidence of inadequate treatments for acute coronary syndromes, heart failure, chronic coronary disease, and atrial fibrillation, as well as inadequate antibiotic and thrombosis prophylaxis in hospitals.

Morbidity Due to Medication Errors Is Costly

Current understanding of the costs of medication errors is highly incomplete. Most of what is known relates to additional health care costs associated with preventable ADEs, which represent the injuries caused by errors.

For hospital care, there is one estimate of the extra costs of inpatient care for a preventable ADE incurred while in the hospital—$5,857 (Bates et al., 1997). This figure excludes health care costs outside the hospital and was derived from 1993 cost data. Assuming conservatively an annual incidence of 400,000 in-hospital preventable ADEs, each incurring extra hospital costs of $5,857, yields an annual cost of $2.3 billion in 1993 dollars or $3.5 billion in 2006 dollars.

For long-term care, as noted earlier, Gurwitz and colleagues (2005) projected an annual incidence of 800,000 preventable ADEs. However, there is no estimate of the associated health care costs for this group of preventable ADEs.

For ambulatory care, the best estimate derives from a study (Field et al., 2005) that calculateed the annual cost of preventable ADEs for all Medicare enrollees aged 65 and older. The cost in 2000 per preventable ADE was estimated at $1,983, while national annual costs were estimated at $887 million.

In addition to the likelihood of underestimation, the above estimates are characterized by some important omissions. First, the costs of some highly common medication errors, such as drug use without a medically valid indication and failure to receive drugs that should have been pre-scribed, were excluded from the Medicare study of ambulatory ADEs (Field et al., 2005). Moreover, the costs of morbidity and mortality arising from the failure of patients to comply with prescribed medication regimens were not assessed. Second, all the studies omitted some important costs: lost earnings, costs of not being able to carry out household duties (lost house-hold production), and compensation for pain and suffering. Third, few data are available for any setting regarding the costs of medication errors that do not result in harm. While no injury is involved, these errors often create extra work, and the costs involved may be substantial.

Effective Error Prevention Strategies Are Available

According to most studies, at least a quarter of all harmful ADEs are preventable. Moreover, many efficacious error prevention strategies are available, especially for hospital care. In the hospital setting, there is good evidence for the effectiveness of computerized order entry with clinical decision-support systems (Bates et al., 1998), for clinical decision-support systems themselves (Evans et al., 1994), and for pharmacist participation on hospital rounds (Leape et al., 1999). Bar coding and smart intravenous (IV) pumps show promise for the hospital setting, but their efficacy has not yet been clearly demonstrated.

Interventions consisting of educational visits appear to hold promise for improving prescribing practices and patient outcomes in nursing homes. Involving pharmacists in the management of medications in nursing homes and ambulatory care also shows promise, but requires additional study. This intervention has been most successful to date in populations with certain conditions, such as diabetes.

IMPROVED PROVIDER–PATIENT COMMUNICATION IS VITAL

Achieving the patient-centered model of care envisioned in the IOM report *Crossing the Quality Chasm: A New Health System for the 21st Century* (IOM, 2001) will require a paradigm shift away from a paternalis-tic, provider-centric model of care. Consumers (and their surrogates) should be empowered as partners in their care, with appropriate communication, information, and resources in place to support them. For medication safety, consumers and providers (including physicians, nurses, and pharmacists) should know and act on patients' rights, providers should engage in meaningful communication about the safe and effective use of medications at multiple points in the medication-use process, and government and other participants should improve consumer-oriented written and electronic information resources.

Patient Rights

Patient rights are the foundation for the safe and ethical use of medications (see Box S-3). Ignoring these rights can have lethal consequences. Millions of Americans take prescription drugs each year without being fully informed by their providers about associated risks, contraindications, and side effects. When clinically significant medication errors do occur, they usually are not disclosed to patients or their surrogates unless injury or death results.

Many but not all patient rights relating to medical care have been established broadly in the U.S. Constitution (Amendments I and XIV) and articulated by the courts through common law. Certain states have instituted a patient bill of rights relating to particular providers or care settings. One important point not specifically addressed by these laws is the right for a patient to be told when an adverse event occurs. Establishing a comprehensive set of patient rights in one document would facilitate patient and

---

BOX S-3
Patient Rights

Patients have the right to:

- Be the source of control for all medication management decisions that affect them (that is, the right to self-determination).
- Accept or reject medication therapy on the basis of their personal values.
- Be adequately informed about their medication therapy and alternative treatments.
- Ask questions to better understand their medication regimen.
- Receive consultation about their medication regimen in all health settings and at all points along the medication-use process.
- Designate a surrogate to assist them with all aspects of their medication management.
- Expect providers to tell them when a clinically significant error has occurred, what the effects of the event on their health (short- and long-term) will be, and what care they will receive to restore their health.
- Ask their provider to report an adverse event and give them information about how they can report the event themselves.

provider understanding and exercise of these rights and improve the safety and quality of medication use.

Actions for Consumers

For sound medication management, providers and consumers[2] should maintain an up-to-date record of medications being administered, including prescription medications, over-the-counter (OTC) drugs, and dietary supplements, as well as all known drug and/or food allergies. Such records are especially important for patients who have chronic conditions, see multiple providers, or take multiple medications.

By becoming more informed and engaged, consumers (and their surrogates) may decrease the probability of experiencing a medication error (Cohen, 2000). Such actions can range from the simple and routine, such as double-checking their prescription when dropping it off and picking it up from the pharmacy, to the more involved, such as forming an active partnership with providers in managing their health care. When using OTC medications, herbal remedies, and dietary supplements, consumers should seek the information they need to make informed decisions. When obtaining medical care, consumers should ask questions and insist on answers from providers to guide their decision making based on their personal values and preferences. They should ensure that their provider explains their medication regimen clearly and speak up if they do not understand. In addition, they should ensure that providers give them written information about their medications, as well as tell them where to obtain information from other sources. Finally, consumers should communicate with their providers if they experience any unexpected changes in the way they feel after initiating a new medication. Some specific actions consumers can take are outlined in Box S-4.

Actions for Providers

Providers can take several specific actions to improve medication safety (see Box S-5). First, they can verify the patient's current medication list for appropriateness at each encounter, and they can ensure that this list is accurate at times of transition between care settings. They can educate their patients about the medication regimen, understanding that patients need different kinds of information at different times and for different purposes. Providers can also respect patients' wishes and inform them of

---

[2]In this report, the term *consumers* is often used in referring to patients to emphasize the active role individuals need to take in ensuring the quality of the health care services they are purchasing.

BOX S-4
Consumer Actions to Enhance Medication Safety

Personal/Home

- Maintain a list of the prescription drugs, nonprescription drugs, and other products, such as vitamins and minerals, you are taking.
- Take the list with you when you visit any medical practitioner, and have him or her review it.
- Be aware of where to find educational material in your local community and at reliable Internet sites.

Ambulatory Care/Outpatient Clinic

- Have the prescriber provide in writing the name of the drug (brand and generic names, if available), what it is for, its dosage, and how often to take it, or provide other written material with this information.
- Have the prescriber explain how to use the drug properly.
- Ask about the side effects of the drug and what to do if you experience a side effect.

Pharmacy

- Make sure the name of the drug (brand or generic) and the directions for use received at the pharmacy are the same as what is written down by the prescriber.
- Know that you can review your list of medications with the pharmacist for additional safety.
- Know that you have the right to counseling by the pharmacist if you have any questions; you can ask the pharmacist to explain how to take the drug properly, what side effects it has, and what to do if you experience them (just as you did with your prescriber).
- Ask for written literature about the drug.

Hospital Inpatient (Patient or Surrogate)

- Ask the doctor or nurse what drugs you are being given at the hospital.
- Do not take a drug without being told the reason for doing so.
- Exercise your right to have a surrogate present whenever you are receiving medication and are unable to monitor the medication-use process yourself.
- Prior to surgery, ask whether there are medications, especially prescription antibiotics, that you should take or any you should stop taking preoperatively.
- Prior to discharge, ask for a list of the medications you should be taking at home, have a provider review them with you, and be sure you understand how the medications should be taken.

BOX S-5
Issues for Discussion with Patients by Providers
(Physicians, Nurses, and Pharmacists)

• Review the patient's medication list routinely and during care transitions.
• Review different treatment options.
• Review the name and purpose of the selected medication.
• Discuss when and how to take the medication.
• Discuss important and likely side effects and what to do about them.
• Discuss drug–drug, drug–food, and drug–disease interactions.
• Review the patient's or surrogate's role in achieving appropriate medication use.
• Review the role of medications in the overall context of the patient's health.

their rights, including the right to have a surrogate present and involved in their medication management whenever they are unable to monitor their own medication use.

When communicating about medication errors that occur with the potential for or actual harm, providers can tell patients how the error may affect their health and what is being done to correct it. The vast majority of patients want and expect to be told about errors, particularly those that cause them harm.

Barriers Experienced by Consumers and Providers

In the current system, a number of barriers affect the ability of consumers to engage in safe and effective use of medications and the ability of providers to change their day-to-day practices to support new consumer-oriented activities (Cohen, 2000). These barriers include (1) knowledge deficits, such as patients lacking sufficient education about their medications and providers lacking the latest pharmacological knowledge about particular drugs; (2) practical barriers, such as patients being unable to pay for their medications and providers having to operate burdensome prescribing arrangements required by payers; and (3) attitudinal factors, such as patients and providers having different cultural norms and beliefs about the use of medications. These barriers often result in errors, such as taking the wrong dose, taking a medication at the wrong time, or taking someone else's medication. Many of these barriers can be overcome by improved consumer-oriented drug information, efforts on the part of providers to respond to the challenges faced by their patients, and actions by health care organizations to adopt a culture of safety and make more extensive use of information technology.

Recommendation 1: To improve the quality and safety of the medication-use process, specific measures should be instituted to strengthen patients' capacities for sound medication self-management. Specifically:

• Patients' rights regarding safety and quality in health care and medication use should be formalized at the state and/or federal levels and ensured at every point of care.

• Patients (or their surrogates) should maintain an active list of all prescription drugs, over-the-counter drugs, and dietary supplements they are taking; the reasons for taking them; and any known drug allergies. Every provider involved in the medication-use process for a patient should have access to this list.

• Providers should take definitive action to educate patients (or their surrogates) about the safe and effective use of medications. They should provide information about side effects, contraindications, and how to handle adverse reactions, as well as where to obtain additional objective, high-quality information.

• Consultation on their medications should be available to patients at key points in the medication-use process (during clinical decision making in ambulatory and inpatient care, at hospital discharge, and at the pharmacy).

Actions for Government and Other Stakeholders

Consumers should be able to obtain high-quality information about medications not only from their providers, but also from the pharmacy and Internet and community-based resources. However, these resources need significant improvement in two overarching areas.

First, current materials (e.g., pharmacy information sheets [leaflets], Internet-based information) are inadequately designed to facilitate consumers' ability to read, comprehend, and act on medication information. Pharmacy leaflets are the source of such information most relied upon by consumers. Yet a number of studies have revealed the inadequate quality of these leaflets, as well as their variable quality from one pharmacy to another and from one drug to another (Svarstad and Mount, 2001). Internet-based health information has proliferated over the last decade, providing consumers with immediate access to valuable resources such as medical journals and libraries, but most consumers are unfamiliar with how to access this information since it usually does not figure prominently during online searches. Rather, consumers are directed to a multitude of other sources of information with differing standards for the content provided.

The federal government should develop mechanisms for improving pharmacy leaflets and the quality of Internet information for consumers.

Second, there is a need for additional resources beyond pharmacy leaflets and Internet information that can be provided on a national scale. In particular, a national drug information telephone helpline and community-based health resource centers should be developed to promote consumer education. Further, communication networks already in place, such as those associated with the public health infrastructure (e.g., the Centers for Disease Control and Prevention's National Center for Health Marketing) and consumer networks should be used for broad dissemination of national medication safety initiatives.

> **Recommendation 2: Government agencies (i.e., the Agency for Healthcare Research and Quality [AHRQ], the Centers for Medicare and Medicaid Services [CMS], the Food and Drug Administration [FDA], and the National Library of Medicine [NLM]) should enhance the resource base for consumer-oriented drug information and medication self-management support.** Such efforts require standardization of pharmacy medication information leaflets, improvement of online medication resources, establishment of a national drug information telephone helpline, the development of personal health records, and the formulation of a national plan for the dissemination of medication safety information.
>
> • Pharmacy medication information leaflets should be standardized to a format designed for readability, comprehensibility, and usefulness to consumers. The leaflets should be made available to consumers in a manner that accommodates their individual needs, such as those associated with variations in literacy, language, age, and visual acuity.
> • The NLM should be designated as the chief agency responsible for Internet health information resources for consumers. Drug information should be provided through a consumers' version of the DailyMed program, with links to the NLM's Medline Plus program for general health and additional drug information.
> • CMS, the FDA, and the NLM, working together, should undertake a full evaluation of various methods for building and funding a national network of drug information helplines.
> • CMS, the FDA, and the NLM should collaborate to confirm a minimum dataset for personal health records and develop requirements for vendor self-certification of compliance. Vendors should take the initiative to improve the use and functionality of personal health records by incorporating basic tools to support consumers' medication self-management.

• A national plan should be developed for widespread distribution and promotion of medication safety information. Health care provider, community-based, consumer, and government organizations should serve as the foundation for such efforts.

ELECTRONIC PRESCRIBING AND MONITORING FOR ERRORS IN ALL CARE SETTINGS ARE ESSENTIAL

Safe medication use requires that clinicians synthesize several types of information, including knowledge of the medication itself, as well as understanding of how it may interact with coexisting illnesses and medications and how its use might be monitored. Several electronic supports can help providers absorb and apply the necessary information.

Access to Automated Point-of-Care Reference Information

The underlying knowledge base is constantly changing, creating a situation in which it is almost impossible for health care providers to have current knowledge of every medication they prescribe. Clinicians therefore need access to critical syntheses of the evidence base. The Cochrane Collaboration (CC, 2005) is one such resource. In addition, many software applications now being developed provide decision support for prescribing clinicians (Epocrates, 2005). Applications of this type are typically available via the Internet or on personal digital assistants (PDAs). All prescribers should use point-of-care reference information.

Electronic Prescribing

Paper-based prescribing is associated with high error rates (Kaushal et al., 2003). Having all pharmacies receive prescriptions electronically would result in fewer errors than occur with current paper or oral approaches (Bates, 2001). Electronic prescribing is safer (Bates et al., 1998) because it eliminates handwriting and ensures that the key fields (for example, drug name, dose, route, and frequency) include meaningful data. More important, as noted above, computerization enables the delivery of clinical decision support (Evans et al., 1998), including checks for allergies, drug–drug interactions, overly high doses, and clinical conditions, as well as suggestions for appropriate dosages given the patient's level of renal function and age. It should be noted that recent studies have identified implementation problems and the unintended occurrence of new types of errors with these computerized approaches (for example, pharmacy inventory displays of available drug doses being mistaken for the usual or minimally effective doses). Avoiding these problems requires addressing business and cultural issues before such strategies are implemented and aggressively solving technological problems during the implementation process. Regulatory issues must also be addressed for electronic transmission of prescriptions to be practical.

Effective Use of Well-Designed Technologies

To deliver safe drug care, health care organizations should make effective use of well-designed technologies, which will vary by setting. Although the evidence for this assertion is strongest in the inpatient setting (AHRQ, 2005), the use of technology will undoubtedly lead to major improvements in all settings. In acute care, technologies should target prescribing by including computerized provider order entry with clinical decision support. Administration is also a particularly vulnerable stage in the medication-use process, and several technologies are likely to be especially important in this stage. These include electronic medication administration records, which can improve documentation of what medications have been given and when, as well as machine-readable identification, such as bar coding, and smart IV infusion pumps. All these technologies should be linked electronically.

In nursing homes, computerized prescribing with decision support will likely be important, although there has been little research on its efficacy (Gurwitz et al., 2005). Moreover, implementation of computerized prescribing in this setting will be challenging since most nursing homes have very limited resources.

Some evidence suggests that computerized prescribing will be important in the outpatient setting as well (Gandhi et al., 2003), although it may not yield significant safety benefits without added decision support. Equally important are likely to be approaches that improve communication between patients and providers.

Communication of Patient-Specific Medication-Related Information

The delivery of care often involves moving the locus of care among sites and providers. These "handoffs" are fraught with errors. One strategy for reducing errors during these care transitions is to reconcile medication orders between transition points, especially between care settings such as hospital and outpatient, but also between points within organizations, such as the intensive care unit and a general care unit. This reconciliation involves comparing what a patient is taking in one setting with what is being provided in another to avoid errors of transcription and omission, duplication of therapy, and drug–drug and drug–disease interactions. This process typically reveals many discrepancies (Pronovost et al., 2003).

Reconciliation is facilitated when medication data are transmitted electronically among providers, with confirmation by the patient. Three important steps are required. First, a complete and accurate medication list must be compiled. Second, the data must be structured into components such as the medication name, dose, route, frequency, duration, start date, and so on. Third, these data must be formatted in a way that allows disparate computer systems to understand both their structure and content.

The power of interoperable health care data was demonstrated after the devastation of Hurricane Katrina. Pharmacy chains were able to make patients' medication lists available quickly to care providers, and states with immunizations registries were able to retrieve immunization records, enabling the enrollment of children in new schools.

Monitoring for Errors

All health care provider groups should seek to be high-reliability organizations preoccupied with the possibility of failure (Reason, 2000). They should implement active internal monitoring programs so that progress toward improved medication safety can be accurately demonstrated. Voluntary internal reporting systems have recognized limitations for evaluating the true frequency of medication errors and ADEs (Flynn et al., 2002). Error detection methods that complement such systems should be used in all care settings. These include computerized detection of ADEs, observation of medication passes in hospitals to assess administration errors, and audits of filled prescriptions in community pharmacies to monitor dispensing errors.

Many external programs exist to which patients and providers can report a medication error or hazardous situation (IOM, 2004). Voluntary practitioner reporting to an external program will continue to be important, as it is often the only way practitioners can effect change outside their organizations. Errors need to be reported and analyzed if improvements in care are to be achieved.

Adopting a Safety Culture

Patient safety can best be achieved through the adoption of a culture of safety—an organizational commitment to continually seeking to improve safety. To achieve a safety culture, senior management of health care organizations must devote sufficient attention to safety, as well as make sufficient resources available for quality improvement and safety teams (IOM, 2004). Senior management must also authorize the investment of resources in technologies that have been demonstrated to be effective but are not yet widely implemented in most organizations, such as computerized provider order entry systems and electronic health records. It has become increasingly clear that the introduction of any of these technologies requires close attention to business processes and ongoing maintenance. As noted above, studies have shown that these tools can have unintended and adverse consequences, and that avoiding these consequences requires addressing both business and cultural issues.

Recommendation 3: All health care organizations should immediately make complete patient-information and decision-support tools available to clinicians and patients. Health care systems should capture information on medication safety and use this information to improve the safety of their care delivery systems. Health care organizations should implement the appropriate systems to enable providers to:

- Have access to comprehensive reference information concerning medications and related health data.
- Communicate patient-specific medication-related information in an interoperable format.
- Assess the safety of medication use through active monitoring and use these monitoring data to inform the implementation of prevention strategies.
- Write prescriptions electronically by 2010. Also by 2010, all pharmacies should be able to receive prescriptions electronically. By 2008, all prescribers should have plans in place to implement electronic prescribing.
- Subject prescriptions to evidence-based, current clinical decision support.
- Have the appropriate competencies for each step of the medication-use process.
- Make effective use of well-designed technologies, which will vary by setting.

ENORMOUS KNOWLEDGE DEFICITS MUST BE ADDRESSED

Current methods for generating and communicating information about medications are inadequate and contribute to a growing rate of medication errors. Likewise, error incidence rates, costs to the health system, and prevention strategies are not well understood. As a result, there are enormous gaps in the knowledge required to implement a safe medication-use system.

Risk/Benefit Information for Prescription Drugs

Being able to determine whether a medication error has been made depends on knowing the correct dose of the drug for that patient at that time and whether the indication for that drug is correct in comparison with alternative approaches to treatment. Over the past several decades, however, drug evaluations have not been sufficiently comprehensive. As a result, the balance of risk and benefit for a drug frequently is not known for a given population. Such gaps in therapeutic knowledge often result in devastating effects on clinical practice and patient health, as exemplified by adverse events involving hormone replacement therapy, cyclooxygenase-2 (COX-2) inhibitors, and nonsteroidal anti-inflammatory drugs that resulted in increased morbidity and mortality.

These issues are magnified in specific patient populations. For example, the majority of prescriptions written for children are off label—not based on empirical demonstration of safety and efficacy. Among those over age 80, the fastest-growing segment of the population, almost nothing is known about the balance of risks and benefits. Patients with renal dysfunction are another large and growing group for whom more comprehensive studies are needed. And patients with multiple comorbidities are typically excluded from premarketing clinical trials, yet many of the major problems with drug toxicity have occurred in those taking multiple medications because of multiple diseases. Thus the numbers and types of patients for whom clinical outcomes are measured must be greatly increased to elucidate the proper dosing of drugs in individuals and within subgroups.

Of critical concern is the need for transparency through the publication of clinical studies in a national repository to advance medication safety, error prevention, and public knowledge. Such a repository should include postmarket studies. The goal of such studies is to generate new data about a drug's effects in the population; often, however, these studies place insufficient emphasis on safety information. There is a need for comprehensive redesign and expansion of the mechanisms for undertaking clinical studies to improve understanding of the risks and benefits of drug therapies, prevent errors and ADEs, and meet the health needs of the population.

Communication of Drug Information

How information about a drug is communicated to providers and consumers can directly affect the frequency of medication errors and ADEs (see Box S-6). Drug information is communicated through labeling and packaging, marketing practices, and advertisements. Poorly designed materials and inadequate representation of the risks and benefits to providers and consumers have led to many errors, including inappropriate prescribing;

BOX S-6
Drug Naming, Labeling, and Packaging Problems

- Brand names and generic names that look or sound alike
- Different formulations of the same brand or generic drug
- Multiple abbreviations to represent the same concept
- Confusing word derivatives, abbreviations, and symbols
- Unclear dose concentration/strength designations
- Cluttered labeling—small fonts, poor typefaces, no background contrast, overemphasis on company logos
- Inadequate prominence of warnings and reminders
- Lack of standardized terminology

confusion among products, affecting dispensing and administration; and compromised ability to monitor the effects of drugs adequately.

In particular, drug names that look or sound alike increase the risk of medication errors. Abbreviations, acronyms, certain dose designations, and other symbols used for labeling also have caused errors. Even the layout and presentation of drug information on the drug container or package label can be visually confusing, particularly if it is designed for marketing rather than clinical purposes.

Unit-of-use packaging—containers that provide enough medication for a particular period, such as blister packs containing 30 individually wrapped doses—is not widely employed in the United States but is used extensively elsewhere. This form of packaging brings important safety and usage benefits. The committee believes the expanded implementation of unit-of-use packaging in this country warrants further investigation.

Another issue related to medication safety is the common practice of providers offering free samples of prescription drugs to patients to start them on their medications quickly, to adjust prescribed doses before the full prescription is filled, and to offset medication costs for indigent and underinsured patients. However, there has been growing unease about the way free samples are distributed. In particular, concern exists about the resulting lack of documentation of medication use and the bypassing of standard prescribing and dispensing services, which incorporate drug-interaction checking and pharmacy counseling services. There is a need for resarch on the impact of differing sample distribution methods on medication safety.

Recommendation 4: Enhancing the safety and quality of the medication-use process and reducing errors requires improved methods for labeling drug products and communicating medication information to providers and consumers. For such improve-

ments to occur, materials should be designed according to designated standards to meet the needs of the end user. Industry, AHRQ, the FDA, and others as appropriate (e.g., U.S. Pharmacopeia, Institute for Safe Medication Practices) should work together to undertake the following actions to address labeling, packaging, and the distribution of free samples:

• The FDA should develop two guidance documents for industry: one for drug naming and another for labeling and packaging. The FDA and industry should collaborate to develop (1) a common drug nomenclature that standardizes abbreviations, acronyms, and terms to the extent possible, and (2) methods of applying failure modes and effects analysis to labeling and packaging.

• Additional study of optimum designs for all drug labeling and information sheets to reflect human and cognitive factors should be undertaken. Methods for testing and measuring the effects of these materials on providers and consumers should also be established, including methods for field testing of the materials. The FDA, the NLM, and industry should work with consumer and patient safety organizations to improve the nomenclature used in consumer materials.

• The FDA, the pharmaceutical industry, and other stakeholders should collaborate to develop a strategy for expanding unit-of-use packaging for consumers to new therapeutic areas. Studies should be undertaken to evaluate different unit-of-use packaging and design approaches that will best support various consumer groups in their medication self-management.

• AHRQ should fund studies to evaluate the impact of free samples on overall patient safety, provider prescribing practices, and consumer behavior (e.g., adherence to the medication regimen), as well as alternative methods of distribution that can improve safety, quality, and effectiveness.

Health Information Technology

Realization of the full benefits of many health information technologies (such as decision-support systems, smart IV pumps, bar code administration systems, and pharmacy database systems) is hampered by the lack of common data standards for system integration and well-designed interfaces for end users.

Problems with data standards for drug information are threefold. First, there is no complete, standardized set of terms, concepts, and codes to represent drug information. Second, there is no standardized method for presenting safety alerts according to severity and/or clinical importance. Instead, providers are sometimes inundated with too many alerts, which can result in "alert fatigue." Third, many systems lack intelligent mechanisms for relating patient-specific data to allowable overrides, such as those associated with a particular patient and drug allergy alert or duplicate therapy request.

The ability of clinicians to use health information technologies successfully depends on how well the technologies have been designed at the level of human-machine interaction (i.e., the user interface). Displaying information in a cluttered, illogical, or confusing manner leads to decreased user performance and satisfaction. Moreover, a poorly designed user interface can contribute to medication errors. Addressing user interface issues requires greater attention to the cognitive and social factors influencing clinicians in their daily workflow and interaction with technologies (van Bemmel and Musen, 1997).

> **Recommendation 5: Industry and government should collaborate to establish standards affecting drug-related health information technologies. Specifically:**
>
> • **The NLM should take the lead in developing a common drug nomenclature for use in all clinical information technology systems, based on standards for the national health information infrastructure.**
>
> • **AHRQ should take the lead in organizing mechanisms for safety alerts according to severity, frequency, and clinical importance to improve clinical value and acceptance.**
>
> • **AHRQ should take the lead in developing intelligent prompting mechanisms specific to a patient's unique characteristics and needs; provider prescribing, ordering, and error patterns; and evidence-based best-practice guidelines.**
>
> • **AHRQ should take the lead in developing user interface designs based on the principles of cognitive and human factors and the context of the clinical environment.**
>
> • **AHRQ should support additional research to determine specifications for alert mechanisms and intelligent prompting, as well as optimum designs for user interfaces.**

Research on Medication Errors: Incidence Rates, Costs, and Prevention Strategies

In reviewing the research literature, the committee concluded that large gaps exist in our understanding of medication error incidence rates, costs, and prevention strategies. The committee believes the nation should invest about $100 million annually in the research proposed below.

The primary focus of research on medication errors in the next decade should be prevention strategies, recognizing that to plan an error prevention study, it is essential to be able to measure the baseline rate of errors. Evidence on the efficacy of prevention strategies for improving medication safety is badly needed in a number of settings, including care transitions, ambulatory care (particularly home care, self-care, and medication use in schools), pediatric care, psychiatric care, and the use of OTC and complementary and alternative medications. For hospitals, key areas are further investigation of some prevention strategies (particularly bar coding and smart IV pumps) and how to integrate electronic health records with computerized provider order entry, clinical decision support, bar coding, and smart IV pumps.

Overall, most data on medication error incidence rates come from the inpatient setting, but the magnitude of the problem is likely to be greater outside the hospital. Areas of priority for research on medication error and ADE incidence rates are care transitions, specialty ambulatory clinics, psychiatric care, the administering of medications in schools, and the use of OTC and complementary and alternative medications. Much more research is needed as well on the patient's role in the prevention of errors, specifically, what systems provide the most cost-effective support for safe and effective medication self-management or for surrogate participation in medication use when a patient is unable to self-manage.

Most studies of the costs of medication errors relate to hospitals, and some report data more than 10 years old (Bates et al., 1997). A better understanding of the costs and consequences of medication errors in all care settings is needed to help inform decisions about investing in medication error prevention strategies.

Recommendation 6: AHRQ should take the lead, working with other government agencies such as CMS, the FDA, and the NLM, in coordinating a broad research agenda on the safe and appropriate use of medications across all care settings, and Congress should allocate the funds necessary to carry out this agenda. This agenda should encompass research methodologies, incidence rates by type and severity, costs of medication errors, reporting systems, and in particular, further testing of error prevention strategies.

OVERSIGHT, REGULATION, AND PAYMENT

Improving medication safety will require key changes in oversight, regulation, and payment. Accordingly, the following recommendation is addressed to the stakeholders that shape the environment in which care is delivered, including legislators, regulators, accreditors, payers, and patient safety organizations.[3]

Recommendation 7: Oversight and regulatory organizations and payers should use legislation, regulation, accreditation, and payment mechanisms and the media to motivate the adoption of practices and technologies that can reduce medication errors, as well as to ensure that professionals have the competencies required to deliver medications safely.

- Payers and purchasers should continue to motivate improvement in the medication-use process through explicit financial incentives.
- CMS should evaluate a variety of strategies for delivering medication therapy management.
- Regulators, accreditors, and legislators should set minimum functionality standards for error prevention technologies.
- States should enact legislation consistent with and complementary to the Medicare Modernization Act's electronic prescribing provisions and remove existing barriers to such prescribing.
- All state boards of pharmacy should undertake quality improvement initiatives related to community pharmacy practice.
- Medication error reporting should be promoted more aggressively by all stakeholders (with a single national taxonomy used for data storage and analysis).
- Accreditation bodies responsible for the oversight of professional education should require more training in improving medication management practices and clinical pharmacology.

MOVING FORWARD

The American people expect safe medication care. In this report, the committee proposes an ambitious agenda for making the use of medications safer. This agenda requires that all stakeholders—patients, care providers, payers, industry, and government, working together—commit to preventing medication errors. Given that a large proportion of injurious drug events are preventable, this proposed agenda should deliver early and measurable benefits.

---

[3]Patient safety organizations are regulated through the Patient Safety and Quality Improvement Act of 2005 (P.L. 109-41). Broadly, they are organizations separate from health care providers that collect, manage, and analyze patient safety data, and advocate safety improvements on the basis of analysis of the patient safety data they receive.

REFERENCES

AHRQ (Agency for Healthcare Research and Quality). 2005. *Advances in Patient Safety: From Research to Implementation.* Vols. 1–4. Rockville, MD: AHRQ.

Barker KN, Flynn EA, Pepper GA, Bates DW, Mikeal RL. 2002. Medication errors observed in 36 health care facilities. *Archives of Internal Medicine* 162(16):1897–1903.

Bates DW. 2001. A 40-year-old woman who noticed a medication error. *Journal of the American Medical Association* 285(24):3134–3140.

Bates DW, Boyle DL, Vander Vliet MB, Schneider J, Leape L. 1995a. Relationship between medication errors and adverse drug events. *Journal of General Internal Medicine* 10(4): 100–205.

Bates DW, Cullen DJ, Laird N, Petersen LA, Small SD, Servi D, Laffel G, Sweitzer BJ, Shea BF, Hallisey R, Vander Vliet M, Nemeskal R, Leape LL. 1995b. Incidence of adverse drug events and potential adverse drug events. Implications for prevention. ADE Prevention Study Group. *Journal of the American Medical Association* 274:29–34.

Bates DW, Spell N, Cullen DJ, Burdick E, Laird N, Petersen LA, Small SD, Sweitzer BJ, Leape L. 1997. The costs of adverse drug events in hospitalized patients. Adverse Drug Events Prevention Study Group. *Journal of the American Medical Association* 277(4):307–311.

Bates DW, Leape LL, Cullen DJ, Laird N, Petersen LA, Teich JM, Burdick E, Hickey M, Kleefield S, Shea B, Vander Vliet M. 1998. Effect of computerized physician order entry and a team intervention on prevention of serious medication errors. *Journal of the American Medical Association* 280(15):1311–1316.

CC (Cochrane Collaboration). 2005. *What Is the Cochrane Collaboration?* [Online]. Available: http://www.cochrane.org/docs/descrip.htm [accessed October 6, 2005].

Classen DC, Pestotnik SL, Evans RS, Lloyd JF, Burke JP. 1997. Adverse drug events in hospitalized patients. Excess length of stay, extra costs, and attributable mortality. *Journal of the American Medical Association* 277(4):301–306.

Cohen MR. 2000. *Medication Errors: Causes, Prevention, and Risk Management.* Sudbury, MA: Jones and Bartlett Publishers.

Epocrates. 2005. *All-One-Guide to Drugs, Diseases and Diagnostics.* [Online]. Available: http://www2.epocrates.com [accessed October 6, 2005].

Evans RS, Classen DC, Pestotnik SL, Lundsgaarde HP, Burke JP. 1994. Improving empiric antibiotic selection using computer decision support. *Archives of Internal Medicine* 154(8):878–884.

Evans RS, Pestotnik SL, Classen DC, Clemmer TP, Weaver LK, Orme JF, Lloyd JF, Burke JP. 1998. A computer-assisted management program for antibiotics and other antiinfective agents. *New England Journal of Medicine* 338(4):232–238.

Field TS, Gilman BH, Subramanian S, Fuller JC, Bates DW, Gurwitz JH. 2005. The costs associated with adverse drug events among older adults in the ambulatory setting. *Medical Care* 43(12):1171–1176.

Flynn EA, Barker KN, Pepper GA, Bates DW, Mikeal RL. 2002. Comparison of methods for detecting medication errors in 36 hospitals and skilled-nursing facilities. *American Journal of Health-System Pharmacy* 59(5):436–446.

Gandhi TK, Weingart SN, Borus J, Seger AC, Peterson J, Burdick E, Seger DL, Shu K, Federico F, Leape LL, Bates DW. 2003. Adverse drug events in ambulatory care. *New England Journal of Medicine* 348(16):1556–1564.

Gurwitz JH, Field TS, Harrold LR, Rothschild J, Debellis K, Seger AC, Cadoret C, Garber L, Fish LS, Kelleher M, Bates DW. 2003. Incidence and preventability of adverse drug events among older person in the ambulatory setting. *Journal of the American Medical Association* 289(94):1107–1116.

Gurwitz JH, Field TS, Judge J, Rochon P, Harrold LR, Cadoret C, Lee M, White K, LaPrino J, Mainard JF, DeFlorio M, Gavendo L, Auger J, Bates DW. 2005. The incidence of adverse drug events in two large academic long-term care facilities. *American Journal of Medicine* 118(3):251–258.

IOM (Institute of Medicine). 2000. *To Err Is Human: Building a Safer Health System.* Washington, DC: National Academy Press.

IOM. 2001. *Crossing the Quality Chasm: A New Health System for the 21st Century.* Washington, DC: National Academy Press.

IOM. 2004. *Patient Safety: Achieving a New Standard for Care.* Washington, DC: The National Academies Press.

Jha AK, Kuperman GJ, Teich JM, Leape L, Shea B, Rittenberg E, Burdick E, Seger DL, Vander Vliet M, Bates DW. 1998. Identifying adverse drug events: Development of a computer-based monitor and comparison with chart review and stimulated voluntary report. *Journal of the American Medical Informatics Association* 5(3):305–314.

Kaushal R, Bates DW, Landrigan C, McKenna KJ, Clapp MD, Federico F, Goldmann DA. 2001. Medication errors and adverse drug events in pediatric inpatients. *Journal of the American Medical Association* 285(16):2114–2120.

Kaushal R, Shojania KG, Bates DW. 2003. Effects of computerized physician order entry and clinical decision support systems on medication safety: A systematic review. *Archives of Internal Medicine* 163(12):1409–1416.

Leape LL, Bates DW, Cullen DJ, Cooper J, Demonaco HJ, Gallivan T, Hallisey R, Ives J, Laird N, Laffel G, Nemeskal R, Petersen L, Porter K, Servi D, Shea B, Small S, Weitzer B, Thompson B, Vander Vleit M. 1995. Systems analysis of adverse drug events. *Journal of the American Medical Association* 274(1):35–43.

Leape LL, Cullen DJ, Clapp MD, Burdick E, Demonaco HJ, Erickson JI, Bates DW. 1999. Pharmacists participation on physician rounds and adverse drug events in the intensive care unit. *Journal of the American Medical Association* 282(3):267–270.

Pronovost P, Weast B, Schwarz M, Wyskiel RM, Prow D, Milanovich SN, Berenholtz S, Dorman T, Lipsett P. 2003. Medication reconciliation: A practical tool to reduce the risk of medication errors. *American Journal of Critical Care* 18(4):201–205.

Reason J. 2000. Human error: Models of management. *British Medical Journal* 320(7237): 768–770.

Svarstad BL, Mount JK. 2001. *Evaluation of Written Prescription Information Provided in Community Pharmacies, 2001.* Rockville, MD: U.S. FDA.

van Bemmel JH, Musen MA. 1997. *Handbook of Medical Informatics.* Heidelberg, Germany: Springer-Verlag.

Appendix F

Committee Biographies

COMMITTEE ON THE ASSESSMENT OF
THE US DRUG SAFETY SYSTEM

Sheila Burke (Chair), MPA, RN, is deputy secretary and chief operating officer of the Smithsonian Institution. Ms. Burke is also the vice chair of the Robert Wood Johnson Health Policy Fellowships Board. She is a member of the Medicare Payment Advisory Commission and serves as chair of the Kaiser Family Foundation, the Kaiser Commission on the Future of Medicaid and the Uninsured, WellPoint Health Networks, Chubb Corporation, and the University of San Francisco. She is an adjunct lecturer in public policy at the Kennedy School of Government, Harvard University. She previously was executive dean and a lecturer in public policy at Harvard University's John F. Kennedy School of Government. From 1986 to 1996, Ms. Burke was chief of staff to Senate Majority Leader Robert Dole. In 1995, she was also elected to serve as secretary of the Senate. Before joining Senator Dole's personal office, she served the Senate Committee on Finance as a professional staff member and as deputy staff director. Early in her career, she worked as a staff nurse in Berkeley, California, and was director of program and field services for the National Student Nurses Association in New York. She received her MPA from Harvard University and her BS in nursing from the University of San Francisco. Ms. Burke is a member of the Institute of Medicine.

David Blumenthal, MD, MPP, is the Samuel O. Thier Professor of Medicine and Professor of Health Care Policy at Harvard Medical School and director of the Institute for Health Policy at Massachusetts General Hospital and Partners HealthCare System. Dr. Blumenthal is also the director of the Harvard University Interfaculty Program for Health Systems Improvement. Harvard University receives about $1 million per year from the Merck Foundation to support the research and convening activities of the Program for Health System Improvement. Dr. Blumenthal serves on several editorial boards, including those of the *American Journal of Medicine* and the *Journal of Health Politics, Policy and Law*. He is a national correspondent for the *New England Journal of Medicine*. Dr. Blumenthal was the founding chairman of AcademyHealth (formerly the Academy for Health Services Research and Health Policy), the national organization of health services researchers, and is a member of its board of directors. During the late 1970s, he was a professional staff member on Senator Edward Kennedy's Subcommittee on Health and Scientific Research. Dr. Blumenthal previously was the chair of the Institute of Medicine (IOM) Committee on Department of Veterans Affairs Pharmacy Formulary Analysis. His research interests include academic-industrial relationships in the life sciences, quality management in health care, the role and influence of health information technology, determinants of physician behavior, and access to health services. He received his MD and his MPP from Harvard University. Dr. Blumenthal is a member of the IOM.

Sir Alasdair Breckenridge, CBE, is chairman of the UK Medicines and Healthcare Products Regulatory Agency (MHRA). MHRA is the executive agency of the UK Department of Health that is responsible for protecting and promoting public health and patient safety by ensuring that medicines, healthcare products, and medical equipment meet appropriate standards of safety, quality, performance, and effectiveness and are used safely. In 2004, he was awarded a knighthood for his service to medicine in recognition of his role in ensuring that British patients receive safe medical treatment. Prof. Breckenridge has played a leading role in monitoring the safety of medicines for many years. He previously was the chairman of the UK Committee on the Safety of Medicines (CSM) and was a member of the CSM Adverse Reactions Group and the Subcommittee on Adverse Reactions to Vaccines and Immunisation. He is a former professor of clinical pharmacology at the University of Liverpool and headed its Department of Pharmacology and Therapeutics for 26 years. Prof. Breckenridge has been both a member and chairman of a regional health authority and a member of a local health authority. His research interests include the pharmacology of HIV drugs.

R. Alta Charo, JD, is the Warren P. Knowles Professor of Law and Bioethics at the University of Wisconsin Law School and its Medical School's Department of Medical History & Bioethics. She teaches in the areas of Food and

Drug Administration law, biotechnology law, bioethics, and reproductive rights. In addition, she has served on the UW Hospital clinical-ethics committee, the UW institutional review board for the protection of human subjects in medical research, and the UW Bioethics Advisory Committee. Prof. Charo is the author of nearly 100 articles, book chapters, and government reports on such topics as voting rights, environmental law, medical-genetics law, reproductive rights law, science policy and bioethics. She is a member of the board of directors of the Alan Guttmacher Institute and the program board of the American Foundation for AIDS Research (amfAR). She serves on several expert advisory boards of organizations with an interest in stem-cell research, including WiCell and the California Institute for Regenerative Medicine. She has served as a consultant to the Institute of Medicine (IOM) and the National Institutes of Health (NIH) former Office of Protection from Research Risks. In 1994, Prof. Charo served on the NIH Human Embryo Research Panel, and from 1996–2001, on the presidential National Bioethics Advisory Commission where she participated in drafting its reports on such topics as cloning, stem cell research, and research ethics. She is a member of the National Research Council (NRC) Board on Life Sciences and the IOM Board on Population Health and Public Health Practices. She currently co-chairs the NRC-IOM Human Embryonic Stem Cell Research Advisory Committee.

Susan Edgman-Levitan, PA, is executive director of the John D. Stoeckle Center for Primary Care Innovation at Massachusetts General Hospital (MGH). She is a lecturer in the Department of Medicine of Massachusetts General Hospital and an associate in health policy at Harvard Medical School. Before going to MGH, Ms. Edgman-Levitan was the founding president of the Picker Institute. She has been the coprincipal investigator on the Harvard Consumer Assessment of Health Plans Study (CAHPS) from 1995 to the present, which is funded by the Agency for Healthcare Research and Quality. She has served as chair of the Institute for Healthcare Improvement (IHI) Breakthrough Series Collaborative on Improving Service Quality and is the IHI fellow for patient and family-centered care. She is an editor of *Through the Patient's Eyes* (a book on creating and sustaining patient centered care), *The CAHPS Improvement Guide,* and has written many papers and other publications on patient-centered care. She serves on several boards, including those of the National Patient Safety Foundation (NPSF), the Center for Information Therapy, the Foundation for Informed Medical Decision Making, Planetree, and the American Academy on Physician and Patient. She has co-chaired the annual NPSF congress on patient safety since 2002. She received the Distinguished Alumni Award from the Duke Physician Assistant Program and was inducted into the Duke University Medical Center Hall of Fame in 2004. She received her PA degree from Duke University.

Susan Ellenberg, PhD, is professor of biostatistics and associate dean for clinical research at the University of Pennsylvania School of Medicine. Previously, Dr. Ellenberg was director of the Office of Biostatistics and Epidemiology at the Center for Biologics Evaluation and Research of the Food and Drug Administration (FDA), chief of the Biostatistics Research Branch in the Division of AIDS of the National Institute of Allergy and Infectious Diseases, and mathematical statistician in the Biometrics Research Branch of the Cancer Therapy Evaluation Program at the National Cancer Institute. Before her federal government service, she had positions at the EMMES Corporation and the George Washington University. She serves as associate editor of *Clinical Trials* and of the *Journal of the National Cancer Institute*. Dr. Ellenberg is a fellow of the American Statistical Association and the American Association for the Advancement of Science and an elected member of the International Statistical Institute. Her recent book on clinical trials data monitoring committees, of which Thomas Fleming (University of Washington) and David DeMets (University of Wisconsin) were coauthors, was named WileyEurope Statistics Book of the Year for 2002. Dr. Ellenberg's research interests include issues in the design and analysis of clinical trials and assessment of medical product safety, particularly focusing on efficient trial designs, interim monitoring and the operation of data monitoring committees, evaluation of surrogate endpoints, ethical issues in clinical research, and special issues in trials of cancer and AIDS therapies and of vaccines. She serves on two National Institutes of Health-sponsored data monitoring committees, and one for Curagen. She received her PhD in mathematical statistics from George Washington University.

Robert D. Gibbons, PhD, is a professor of biostatistics and psychiatry and director of the Center for Health Statistics at the University of Illinois at Chicago. He received his doctorate in statistics and psychometrics from the University of Chicago in 1981. He received a Young Scientist Award from the Office of Naval Research (1981), a Career Scientist Award from the National Institutes of Health (NIH) (1995), and numerous other NIH grants. His research spans medical, biologic, and environmental statistics, with emphasis on statistical problems in mental health, health services research, longitudinal data analysis, and environmental regulatory statistics. Dr. Gibbons is a fellow of the American Statistical Association and received two the Youden Prizes for statistical contributions to chemistry and the Harvard Award for contributions to psychiatric epidemiology and biostatistics. Dr. Gibbons has served on several Institute of Medicine (IOM) committees, including the Committee on Halcion and the Committee on Organ Procurement and Transplantation, and served on the IOM Board on Health Sciences Policy. He has written over 150 peer-reviewed papers and four books. Dr. Gibbons recently has conducted statistical work focusing on the reanalysis of data on selective serotonin reuptake inhibitors and suicide. Dr. Gibbons is a member of the IOM.

George Hripcsak, MD, MS, is professor and vice chair of Columbia University's Department of Biomedical Informatics, associate director of medical informatics services for New York-Presbyterian Hospital, and senior informatics advisor at the New York City Department of Health and Mental Hygiene. He led the effort to create the Arden Syntax, a language for representing health knowledge that has become a national standard. His Applied Informatics project—funded by the US Department of Commerce to link the medical center, a home care agency, and the New York City Department of Health to improve inner-city tuberculosis care—won the National Information Infrastructure award. Dr. Hripcsak's current research focus is on the clinical information stored in electronic medical records. Using data mining techniques, such as machine learning and natural language processing, he is developing the methods necessary to support clinical research and patient safety initiatives. Dr. Hripcsak was a elected fellow of the American College of Medical Informatics in 1995 and served on the Board of Directors of the American Medical Informatics Association (AMIA). As chair of the AMIA Standards Committee, he coordinated the medical-informatics community response to the Department of Health and Human Services for the health-informatics standards rules under the Health Insurance Portability and Accountability Act of 1996. He chaired the Biomedical Library and Informatics Review Committee of the National Library of Medicine through 2005. He is associate editor of the *Journal of the American Medical Informatics Association* and of *Computers in Biology and Medicine*, and he is an editorial board member of the *Journal of Biomedical Informatics*. He received his MD and his MS in biostatistics from Columbia University.

David Korn, MD, is senior vice president for biomedical and health sciences research at the Association of American Medical Colleges. He served as Carl and Elizabeth Naumann Professor and dean of the Stanford University School of Medicine from 1984 to 1995, and as vice president of Stanford University from 1986 to 1995. Earlier, he had served as professor and chairman of the Department of Pathology at Stanford from 1968. Dr. Korn was appointed by President Ronald Reagan as chairman of the National Cancer Advisory Board from 1984 to 1991. He has been chairman of the Stanford University Committee on Research, president of the American Association of Pathologists (now the American Society for Investigative Pathology), president of the Association of Pathology Chairmen; member of the Board of Directors and the Executive Committee of the Federation of American Societies for Experimental Biology, and member of the Board of Directors of the Association of Academic Health Centers. He was also a founder of the

California Transplant Donor Network, the Clinical Research Roundtable of the Institute of Medicine (IOM), and the Association for the Accreditation of Human Research Protection Programs. Dr. Korn has been a member of the editorial boards of the *American Journal of Pathology*, *The Journal of Biological Chemistry*, and *Human Pathology*, and for many years he was an associate editor of the latter. He received his MD from Harvard University. Dr. Korn is a member of the IOM.

David O. Meltzer, MD, PhD, is associate professor of medicine and affiliated faculty of the Department of Economics and Graduate School of Public Policy at the University of Chicago. He is director of the Center for Health and Social Sciences and the Centers for Disease Control and Prevention's Chicago Center of Excellence in Health Promotion Economics at the University of Chicago. He is codirector of the Section of General Internal Medicine research program, the Robert Wood Johnson Clinical Scholars Program, and the MD/PhD Program in the Social Sciences at the University of Chicago. Dr. Meltzer is a faculty research fellow for the National Bureau of Economic Research. His awards include the Lee Lusted Prize of the Society for Medical Decision Making, the Health Care Research Award of the National Institute for Health Care Management, the Young Investigator Award of the Society for Hospital Medicine, the Robert Wood Johnson Generalist Physician Award, the Eugene Garfield Economic Impact Award from Research America, and the Leaders in General Medicine Award from the Midwest Society for General Internal Medicine. Dr. Meltzer's research interests include the theoretical foundations of medical cost-effectiveness analysis, the effects of medical specialization and prospective payment systems on the cost and quality of care, and the effects of Food and Drug Administration regulation on innovation in the pharmaceutical industry. He is completing work on a small grant from TAP Pharmaceuticals on risk factors for gastrointestinal bleeding and on a small grant from a consortium of pharmaceutical companies on methods to assess the cost effectiveness of treatment for diabetes. The Center for Health and the Social Sciences at the University of Chicago received about $25,000 from the Merck Foundation last year for general support. Dr. Meltzer received his MD and PhD in economics from the University of Chicago.

Woodrow A. Myers, Jr., MD, MBA, is the former executive vice president and chief medical officer of WellPoint Health Networks. Dr. Myers managed WellPoint's Healthcare Quality Assurance Division, including medical policy, clinical affairs, and health services operations. He was also responsible for strategic initiatives designed to enhance the healthcare experience for the company's members and to simplify administration and improve communications with physicians and other healthcare professionals. Before joining WellPoint, he was director of healthcare management at Ford Motor Company. Dr. Myers also served as the corporate medical director for Anthem Blue Cross Blue Shield, commissioner of health for the state of Indiana, and commissioner of health for New York City. During the time Dr. Myers served as the commissioner of health in the State of Indiana, he advocated on behalf of Ryan White, a young boy afflicted with HIV who wanted to attend school. After a laborious process, Dr. Myers helped to change the law so that Indiana became the sole determiner of who attended school, thereby setting an important legal precedent. Earlier in his career, he was an assistant professor of medicine at the University of California San Francisco and a fellow in critical care medicine at the Stanford University Medical Center. Dr. Myers has received numerous medical and community-service awards and has published extensively on medical issues important to public health. He has served on the Board of Directors of the Stanford Hospital and is a former university trustee. He served as a member of the Harvard University Board of Overseers. He received his MD from Harvard University and his MBA from Stanford University. Dr. Myers is a member of the Institute of Medicine.

Mary K. Olson, PhD, is an associate professor of economics and political economy at Tulane University. Before working at Tulane University, she was associate professor of health policy and administration in the Yale University School of Medicine Department of Epidemiology and Public Health. Dr. Olson has expertise on Food and Drug Administration (FDA) regulation. She has published articles that examine new-drug approval policies, FDA enforcement strategies, FDA advisory committees, the effects of prescription drug user fees on FDA, the effects of faster drug reviews on the safety of new medicines, and the risks associated with novel and less novel drugs. Her research interests include pharmaceutical regulation and new drug safety, and gender-related risks among newly approved drugs. Dr. Olson is completing work on a small grant from the Agency for Healthcare Research and Quality for a project to examine the association between the length of FDA review times and adverse drug reaction counts among the 1990–1998 new-drug approvals. Dr. Olson received her PhD in political economics from Stanford University.

Bruce M. Psaty, MD, PhD, is a professor of medicine, epidemiology, and health services, and co-director of the Cardiovascular Health Research Unit, University of Washington, Seattle, and an affiliate investigator in the Center for Health Studies at Group Health, Seattle, WA. He is the principal investigator on four large epidemiologic studies and has had a major roles in National Institutes of Health (NIH)-funded multi-center studies, including the Cardiovascular Health Study, the Multi-Ethnic Study of Atherosclerosis, and the Women's Health Initiative. He is the chair of the NIH Cardiovascular Disease and Sleep Epidemiology Study Section and chair of the Group Health Research Committee. Earlier in his career, he was a Robert Wood Johnson Clinical Scholar at the University of Washington. Dr. Psaty is a member of the American Epidemiological Society as well as the American Heart Association Council on Epidemiology and Prevention. In 2005, he received the University of Washington Outstanding Public Service award. He publishes regularly in peer-reviewed journals, including many articles and editorials on the risks and benefits of a variety of drug therapies. Dr. Psaty's research interests include cardiovascular epidemiology, drug safety, hypertension, epidemiologic methods, pharmacogenetics, and pharmacoepidemiology. He has served on three NIH-funded data monitoring committees. He received his MD and PhD from Indiana University and his MPH from the University of Washington.

Christopher H. Schroeder, MDiv, JD, is Charles S. Murphy Professor of Law and Public Policy Studies and Director of the Program in Public Law at Duke University Law School. He has served as acting assistant attorney general in the Office of Legal Counsel in the US Department of Justice, and as Chief Counsel to the Senate Judiciary Committee. He teaches environmental law; government, business, and public policy; environmental litigation; toxic-substances regulation; and philosophy of environmental protection. He has written on the philosophic foundations of risk regulation and liability, the regulation of toxic substances, American environmental policy, and a variety of topics in public law and theory. He is coauthor of a leading environmental-law casebook (5th edition, 2006), *Environmental Regulation: Law, Science, and Public Policy.* His most recent book is *A New Progressive Agenda for the Public Health and the Environment* (2005), coedited with Rena Steinzor. His research interests include risk regulation, democratic theory, legislative institutions and separation of powers. Mr. Schroeder received his BA from Princeton University, his MDiv from Yale University, and his JD from the University of California, Berkeley.

Andy Stergachis, PhD, MS, RPh, is professor of epidemiology, adjunct professor of pharmacy and the former interim chairman of the Department of Pathobiology in the School of Public Health and Community Medicine, University of Washington. He was chairman of the University's Department of Pharmacy and director of the Program in Pharmaceutical Outcomes Research and Policy. He is affiliated with the University's Northwest Center for Public Health Practice. Dr. Stergachis has served on the National Institutes of Health Epidemiology and Disease Control Study Section, the Agency for Healthcare Research and Quality Health Systems Research Study Section, committees of the National Committee on Quality Assurance, and the

Institute of Medicine's Committee on Poison Prevention and Control and Committee to Study the Interactions of Drugs, Biologics, and Chemicals in the US Military. He held several positions with Group Health Cooperative of Puget Sound and served on its Pharmacy and Therapeutics Committee and the board of the Group Health Community Foundation. In 1998, he joined *drugstore.com* and served as vice president and chief pharmacist; now serves as pharmacy adviser. He cofounded and served as principal of Formulary Resources and serves as a consultant on managed care pharmacy for that company. Dr. Stergachis was consultant to United HealthCare for its pharmacoepidemiology cooperative agreement with the Food and Drug Administration. He was the 1990 American College of Preventive Medicine/Burroughs Wellcome Scholar in Pharmacoepidemiology. The American Association of Pharmaceutical Research Scientists awarded Dr. Stergachis the 1994 Research Achievement Award in Economic, Marketing and Management Sciences. In 1999, he was selected as one of the 50 Most Influential Pharmacists in the United States by *American Druggist*. He was awarded the 2002 Pinnacle Award by the American Pharmaceutical Association Foundation. He serves as board member of the American Pharmacists Association Foundation and he is a fellow in the International Society for Pharmacoepidemiology. He received his PhD and MS from the University of Minnesota and his BPharm from Washington State University.

Index

A

AAMC. *See* Association of American Medical Colleges
Abbreviated NDAs, 32
"Academic detailing," 183
Academic research enterprise, 2, 5, 28, 146. *See also* Professional societies
Accelerated approval, 165
Accountability, by the FDA, need for greater, 4
Accutane, 120
ACE inhibitors, 38
Adverse drug reactions monitoring, 98
Adverse event (AE) reporting, 54, 167
    background incidence of, 114
    electronic submission of, 109
    prevalence of, 113
    recommendations concerning, 7, 114–115
    substantial under-reporting, 55, 109
Adverse Event Reporting System (AERS), 53–56, 98, 157, 184
Advertising. *See* Direct-to-consumer advertising; Pharmaceutical advertising
Advisory committees, 44–46, 179, 211
    on communication with the public, 188
    and the credibility of safety science, 131–142

recommendations concerning, 9–10, 12, 133–134, 188–189
    timeline for planning meetings of, 45
Advocacy movements, 177
    for AIDS treatment, 22, 75
AE. *See* Adverse event reporting
AERS. *See* Adverse Event Reporting System
The agency. *See* Food and Drug Administration
Agency for Healthcare Research and Quality (AHRQ), 21, 25, 113, 180, 183, 212
AIDS treatment advocacy movement, 22, 75
ALLHAT. *See* Antihypertensive and Lipid-Lowering Treatment to Prevent Heart Attack Trial
Alosetron (Lotronex), 59
Amlodipine, 115
Antidepressants, warnings added to labels on, 17, 50
Antihypertensive and Lipid-Lowering Treatment to Prevent Heart Attack Trial (ALLHAT), 115
Appropriations
    as source of FDA funding, 13, 19, 23, 118, 193, 196, 198
Approval process, 27
    accelerated, 165
    confirmatory studies, 115–119
    safety signal generation, 108–110

safety signal strengthening and testing, 110–115
shortening, 107–119
speed of, 16
APPROVe trials, 55
Association of American Medical Colleges (AAMC), 142, 211
Automated healthcare databases, 7, 114–115
Azidothymidine (AZT), 37

B

Bain report, 32
Bayesian analysis, 109–110
Best Pharmaceuticals for Children Act, 57, 152, 165
"Best practices," disseminating, 87–88
Bias, intellectual, 141
Biologics license application (BLA) submissions, 42
numbers of new approvals, 42
Biotechnology Industry Organization (BIO), 88
Bioterrorism and Preparedness and Response Act, 23
BLA. See Biologics license application submissions
Black box warnings, 50, 58–59
Black triangle, 170–171
Booz Allen Hamilton, 211
Boston Consulting Group, 123
British National Formulary, 170
Bromfenac, 38
Bureau of Labor Statistics, 92
Bush, President George W., 88, 207

C

C-Path Institute, 213
Calcium-channel blockers, 115
Cardiovascular risks, 112, 116
CBER. See Center for Biologics Evaluation and Research
CDC. See Centers for Disease Control and Prevention
CDER. See Center for Drug Evaluation and Research
CDRH. See Center for Devices and Radiological Health

Celecoxib, 17
Center for Biologics Evaluation and Research (CBER), 49, 129, 188
Center for Devices and Radiological Health (CDRH), 188
Center for Drug Evaluation and Research (CDER), ix–x, 15, 21, 31, 46–47, 49, 65, 105, 179, 193–202, 205. See also Organizational dysfunction in the CDER culture; Solutions proposed for CDER's organizational dysfunction
credibility of, 85
history of funding, 194
IT needs within, 202
organizational culture in, 4, 66
press coverage of internal problems in, 2
recommendations concerning review teams, 10, 146–147
relevant changes at, 210
shepherding products through trials, 154
staffing, 195, 199–200
Center for Outcomes and Evidence, 212
Centers for Disease Control and Prevention (CDC), 81, 112, 128
Centers for Education and Research on Therapeutics (CERTs), 109
Centers for Medicare and Medicaid Services (CMS), 21, 25, 115, 180–181, 201
Central Hudson Gas & Electric Corp. v. Public Service Commission, 159–160
Cerivastatin, 17, 109
CERTs. See Centers for Education and Research on Therapeutics
CFR. See Code of Federal Regulations
Changes at the FDA
during course of study, 205–215
Critical Path Initiative and partnerships, 212–213
Drug Safety Initiatives, 205
Drug Safety Oversight Board, 205–206
Drug Watch Web page, 206
labeling, 210
leadership changes in the FDA, 207–208
other relevant changes at the FDA and CDER, 210
program reviews or evaluations, 211–212

recent materials from the FDA, 208–209
structural changes and leadership changes in the CDER, 206–207
Changes in the broad context of drug regulation, 19–21
The charge (to the committee), 21–24
defining and meeting, 21–28
disclaimers, 24–25
the shifting landscape of drug safety, 26
study process, 25–26
toward a new vision of drug safety, 26–28
Chlorthalidone, 115
Cisapride, 50, 109, 168
Citizens' Advisory Committee, 130
Clinical development, PDUFA goal for, 42
Clinical holds, 154
Clinical investigation (phase 2) studies, 35
Clinical pharmacology (phase 1) studies, 35
Clinical review templates, in postmarketing, 79–80
Clinical trials, 76, 153
early, and related studies, 34–35
formal (phase 3), 35
in IND submission and review, and their limitations, 37–39
premarket, 38
recommendations regarding, 10, 144–145
clinicaltrials.gov, 143, 145
Clozapine, 168
CMS. *See* Centers for Medicare and Medicaid Services
Code of Federal Regulations (CFR), 153, 159
COI. *See* Conflict of interest considerations
Commissioner of the FDA, 5–6, 9, 92–93, 131. *See also* individual commissioners
instability in the office of, 5, 88–89
Committee on Identifying and Preventing Medication Errors, 24
Committee on Patient Education, 187
Committee on the Assessment of the US Drug Safety System, 2, 17, 65, 105, 178
charge to, 21–24
Communication about safety, 27, 177–192
FDA's challenges in, 4, 184–190
how industry communicates to the public and patients, 184, 188

improving, 187–190
between providers and the drug safety system, 181–184
between the public and the drug safety system, 178–179
recommendations concerning, 12–13, 188–189
roles and needs of providers and patients, 178–184
structure needed to support an effective drug safety system, 4
Confirmatory studies, 143n
reducing uncertainty about risk and benefit after approval, 115–119, 122
Conflict of interest (COI) considerations, 45, 86, 93, 134–142
appearance of, 73
"cover memos" regarding, 135–139
recommendations concerning, 141–142
zero-tolerance policy regarding, 140–141
Congress, 2, 4, 8, 48, 66, 69, 95, 97, 117–119, 153
ensuring that CDER receives needed authority and assets, x, 18
periodic reports to, 23, 71, 197, 202
recommendations to, 6–8, 11–13, 98–100, 117–119, 169–172, 197–203
"Consults," 78–79, 82
Consumer Bill of Rights, 177
Consumer medication information, 185–187
criteria for useful, 187
Consumer Price Index, 23
Consumer Product Safety Commission, 114
Consumers. *See also* AIDS treatment advocacy movement; The public
empowering, 20
organizations of, 4, 66
representatives of, 179
Council of Public Representatives (COPR), 190
"Cover memos" regarding COI considerations, 135–139
CPI. *See* Critical Path Initiative
Crawford, Acting FDA Commissioner Lester M., 207
Credibility of safety science, 126–147
advisory committees, 131–142
expertise in the CDER, 127–131
transparency, 142–147

Critical Path Initiative (CPI), 33, 70n, 105,
    201, 207, 211–213
    report on, 20
Critical Path Opportunities Report, 212–213
Culture of safety in CDER, 27, 65–104
    difficulties changing, 90
    the external environment, 68–75
    organizational challenges, 65–100
    solutions proposed for CDER's
        organizational dysfunction, 90–100
    structural factors, policies, and
        procedures, 75–90

                    D

"DailyMed" health information
    clearinghouse, 210
Data management, 39–40
Databases
    automated, 56
    mining, 57, 157
DCLG. See Director's Consumer Liaison
    Group
DDMAC. See Division of Drug Marketing
    and Communication
DDRE. See Division of Drug Risk Evaluation
"Dear Health Practitioner" letters, 58, 158
DEcIDE. See Developing Evidence
    to Inform Decisions about
    Effectiveness Network
Decision-making
    concerning postmarket safety of a
        drug, ix, 47
    political considerations in, 90
    regulatory, by the FDA, ix
    science-based, 66, 129
Department of Defense (DoD), 118
Department of Health and Human Services
    (DHHS), 2, 18, 41, 71, 74n, 93n,
    113, 153, 180, 205. See also
    Secretary of Health and Human
    Services
Department of Health, Education, and
    Welfare (DHEW), 74n
Department of Veterans Affairs (VA), 21,
    92, 112–113, 201
"Detailing," 18, 158, 183–184
    academic, 183
Developing Evidence to Inform Decisions
    about Effectiveness (DEcIDE)
    Network, 113, 180

Development cost, of drugs, 32
DHEW. See Department of Health,
    Education, and Welfare
DHHS. See Department of Health and
    Human Services
Dietary supplements, 153
Differing professional opinion (DPO)
    procedure, 47n
Direct-to-consumer (DTC) advertising, 21,
    52–53, 158–164, 167, 171–172
    court challenges to restricting, 159
    deterrence of excessive, 198
    need for more robust standards of
        assessment, 189
    recommendations concerning, 11–12,
        169–172
Director's Consumer Liaison Group
    (DCLG), 190
Disagreement in the face of uncertainty, 127
    nurturing a culture that values, 94
    scientific, 85–87
Discipline reviews, 79
    different perspectives of, 86
Disclaimers, 24–25
Disclosure requirements, 141
Dispute resolution, 84
    in NDAs, 47–48
Division of Drug Marketing and
    Communication (DDMAC), 52,
    78, 159, 163, 179
    "DDMAC Watch," 162
Division of Drug Risk Evaluation (DDRE),
    32, 36, 51, 56
Division of Neurology Products (DNP), 36
DoD. See Department of Defense
DPO. See Differing professional opinion
    procedure
Drug approval process
    limitations on, 59
    pressure to speed up, 22, 40
Drug Development Science Obstacles and
    Opportunities for Collaborations,
    211
Drug industry. See Pharmaceutical industry
Drug Price Competition and Patent Term
    Extension Act, 152
Drug Regulation Reform Act, 156
Drug safety
    communication about, 27, 177–192
    culture of safety in CDER, 27
    experts in, 66

regulatory process and agency able to protect the public health, 27
rigorous science of, 27
the shifting landscape of, 26
toward a new vision of, 26–28
warning the public about risks, 1
Drug safety activities, actionable performance goals for, 97
Drug Safety and Risk Management (DSaRM) Advisory Committee, 46, 87, 112, 133–134, 187
Drug Safety Initiative, 205
Drug Safety Management Board, 144
Drug Safety Oversight Board (DSB), 47, 82, 86–87, 99, 185, 187–188, 205–206
Drug safety system, 3–4, 17
    committee convened to assess, 2
    communicating with providers, 181–184
    communicating with the public, 178–179
    communication structure needed to support effectively, 4
    financial resources required to enable CDER to support the FDA mission, 4
    impairment in, 4
    organizational culture of CDER, 4
    regulatory authority necessary to provide for drug safety, 4
    regulatory science and processes necessary to enhance drug safety, 4
    resources for, 4–5, 13–14, 166, 193–204
Drug Watch Web site, 57, 99, 179, 185, 187, 205–206
Drugs. *See also* New drugs; Prescription drugs; Sponsors of drugs; individual drugs cited
    conditions linked to, 54
    cost of, 178
    development costs, 32
    effectiveness of, 107
    generics, 159
    life-saving for specific patients, 1
    "lifestyle," 21
    mechanisms of action, 2
    milestones in lifecycle of, 167
    over-the-counter, 90
    pediatric, 165
    potential benefit of, 34

promotion and information, postmarket, 52–53
promotion to patients greatly increased, 21
DSaRM. *See* Drug Safety and Risk Management Advisory Committee
DSB. *See* Drug Safety Oversight Board
DTC advertising. *See* Direct-to-consumer advertising

E

Economic impact of drugs, 32
Electronic medical records, 117
Electronic submission, of adverse event reports, 109
"End of phase 2 meeting," in IND submission and review, 35–36
Enforcement tools, 163, 166–167
    decisions about, 58
Enhancing Drug Safety and Innovation Act, 201n
Environmental Protection Agency, 197n
Epidemic Intelligence Service program, 128
Epidemiologic studies, 76, 86, 115, 201
Epidemiologists, safety teams of, 88
European Medicines Agency, 54, 158, 173, 211
Evaluation of FDA's First Cycle Review Performance—Retrospective Analysis, 209
Exceptions, in FDA's regulatory authority, 165
Expectations of multiple constituencies, conflicting, 69
Expertise
    in the CDER, and the credibility of safety science, 127–131
    in preapproval evaluation for the PDUFA IV, 98
External environment in CDER's organizational dysfunction, 68–75, 97–100
    the FDA-industry interface, 70–75

F

Fast track studies, 39
FDA. *See* Food and Drug Administration
FDA Science Board, 129

FDAMA. *See* Food and Drug
Administration Modernization Act
FD&C. *See* Food, Drug, and Cosmetic Act
Federal Advisory Committee Act, 116, 146,
190
Federal advisory committees, on consumer
issues, examples of, 190
Federal Aviation Administration,
organizational problems at, 67, 91
Federal Communications Commission, 92,
197n
Federal Register, 45, 156, 161, 186
Federal Trade Commission (FTC), 160
Financial resources. *See* Resources for the
drug safety system
First Amendment protections, of truthful
commercial speech, 159, 161–162,
171, 183
Food and Drug Administration (FDA),
ix–x, 1–12, 15, 23–25, 65, 105,
177, 180–181, 205. *See also*
Commissioner of the FDA; Recent
FDA materials
approval but not a lifetime guarantee, 2
challenges in communicating to the
public and patients, 184–190
consumer medication information
from, 185–187
credibility of, 4–5, 70, 85, 88, 132
filing and review of submitted
marketing applications, PDUFA
goal for, 43
history of drug regulation by, 152–153
history of DTC advertising regulation
by, 160–161
improving communication with the
public, 187–190
increasingly dependent on industry
funding, 71
interface with industry, 70–75
need for greater accountability and
transparency by, 4
need for increased resources, 151, 193
oversight and review of clinical trial
protocols during development,
PDUFA goal for, ix, 42
public confidence in eroded, 15
"regulatory capture" of, 73–74, 155,
196–197
regulatory decision-making by, ix
relevant changes at, 210
reports from, 20, 209

response to public meeting input, 185
Science Board, 129
Food and Drug Administration (FDA)
authority, 51, 151. *See also* Direct-
to-consumer (DTC) advertising;
Strengthening FDA's regulatory
authority
after approval, 155–164
to compel completion of
postmarketing commitments,
155–157
exceptions in, 165
guidance documents, 41, 208–209
oversight of sponsor promotional
activities, 158–164
preapproval, 37, 154–155
recommendations concerning, 11, 170
to unilaterally impose risk-reducing
remedies, such as label changes and
distribution restrictions, 157–158
Food and Drug Administration
Modernization Act (FDAMA), 143,
152, 156
Food, Drug, and Cosmetic (FD&C) Act, 16,
22–23, 48, 51, 69, 90, 152, 156,
159, 184
Drug Amendments to, 16, 152
Food Research Laboratory, 129
FTC. *See* Federal Trade Commission
Funding. *See* Resources for the drug safety
system; User-fee funding system

G

Galson, CDER Director Steven, 207
GAO. *See* Government Accountability
Office
Gates Foundation, 212
"General applicability" matters, 134n
General Practice Research Database
(GPRD), 112, 200
Generic drugs, 159
Goals. *See* Performance goals
Government Accountability Office (GAO),
36, 57, 66, 71–72, 92, 158, 163
Government agencies
compared with private-sector
counterparts, 68–69
roles of, 180–181
GPRD. *See* General Practice Research
Database

GRMP. *See Guidance for Review Staff and Industry: Good Review Management Principles and Practices for PDUFA Products*
Guidance documents, 208–209
compared to MAPPs, 77n
writing, 41
Guidance for Industry: Consumer-Directed Broadcast Advertisements, 161
Guidance for Industry: Development and Use of Risk Minimization Action Plans, 119, 208
Guidance for Industry: Good Pharmacovigilance Practices and Pharmacoepidemiologic Assessment, 208
Guidance for Industry: Investigators, and Reviewers Exploratory IND Studies, 208
Guidance for Industry: Premarketing Risk Assessment, 208
Guidance for Review Staff and Industry: Good Review Management Principles and Practices for PDUFA Products (GRMP), 78
Guidance on Conflict of Interest for Advisory Committee Members, Consultants and Experts, 134

H

Health, commodification of, 184n
Health care delivery system, 2, 5, 28, 69, 177
Health care entities, 4–5
Healthcare databases, automated, 7, 114–115
Henney, FDA Commissioner Jane, 16, 89
Hinchey Amendment, 45
History of the Food and Drug Administration (FDA)
CDER funding, 194
CDER staffing, 195
drug regulation by, 152–153
DTC advertising regulation, 160–161
milestones in, 22–23
HIV/AIDS crisis, 22. *See also* AIDS treatment advocacy movement
HMO Research Network, 111–112
Human subjects, protecting, 33–34
Hypothesis-testing studies, 143

I

ICH. *See* International Conference on Harmonisation
IND. *See* Investigational New Drug submission and review process
Indications, re-examination for new, 167
The industry. *See* Pharmaceutical industry
Infliximab, 109
Information technology (IT). *See also* Databases; Medication information; Reference information
needs within the CDER, 202
Ingenix Inc., 111–112
Initial filing review, 40–41
in NDAs, 40–41
Innovation or Stagnation?—Challenge and Opportunity on the Critical Path to New Medical Products, 212
Instability at the top, and CDER's organizational dysfunction, 88–90
Institute of Medicine (IOM), ix–x, 2–3, 21, 24, 50, 66–67, 178, 182
Committee on Identifying and Preventing Medication Errors, 24
workshops, 143
Institutional review boards (IRBs), 33
Integrated Promotional Services, 56
Intellectual bias, 141
Interdisciplinary tension, 76
International Conference on Harmonisation (ICH), 54, 145, 208
International Society of Pharmacoepidemiology (ISPE), 112, 128
Interoffice polarization, and CDER's organizational dysfunction, 83–85
Investigational New Drug (IND) submission and review process, 25–26, 33–39
completion of clinical trials and their limitations, 37–39
early clinical trials and related studies, 34–35
"end of phase 2 meeting" and phase 3 trials, 35–36
pre-new drug application submission meeting, 33, 39
roles of the OND and the ODS/OSE premarket, 36–37
IOM. *See* Institute of Medicine
iPLEDGE, 121, 167–168
IRBs. *See* Institutional review boards

Isotretinon, 50, 120, 167–168
ISPE. *See* International Society of
    Pharmacoepidemiology
IT. *See* Information technology

K

Kaiser Foundation Research Institute,
    111–112

L

Labeling, 49–51, 167–168. *See also* Off-
    label use; Symbol needed to denote
    limited knowledge about new drugs
    changes, 167
    FDA authority to unilaterally impose
        changes, 157–158
    negotiations, 50
    recommendations concerning, 11–12,
        169–172
    relevant changes at the FDA and
        CDER, 210
Leadership
    changes at the CDER, 206–207
    changes at the FDA, 207–208
    in solving CDER's organizational
        dysfunction, 91–94
Letters
    "Dear Health Practitioner," 58, 158
    sent to drug sponsors in NDAs, 51
Lifecycle approach
    to drug safety, conditions and
        restrictions on distribution
        throughout, 96, 167–170
    to drugs, 26, 126
    to risk and benefit, 28, 96
"Lifestyle" drugs, 21
Lotronex, 59

M

Management Advisory Board, appointing
    an external, 6, 93–94
Management issues in CDER's
    organizational dysfunction, 79–90
    performance goals for the PDUFA IV,
        100
    solving, 90–91
Management studies, 68, 89–90, 95

*Manual of Administrative Policies and
    Procedures* (MAPPs), 47n, 77, 95
Mechanisms of action. *See also* New
    molecular entities
    of drugs, 2
MedDRA. *See* Medical Dictionary for
    Regulatory Activities
MedGuides, 50, 157, 186
Medical Dictionary for Regulatory
    Activities (MedDRA), 54, 57
Medical Officer Retention Subcommittee,
    82
Medical records, move toward electronic,
    117
Medicare Modernization Act, 113
Medicare Part D, 19, 113
Medication guide, 157. *See also* MedGuides
Medication information, private-sector
    developers of, 186
Medicine Plus program, 181
Medicines and Health products Regulatory
    Agency (MHRA), 170
MedWatch reporting system, 53–54,
    109–110, 184
MHRA. *See* Medicines and Health products
    Regulatory Agency
Murglitazar, 107

N

NAS. *See* National Academy of Sciences
Natalizumab, 168
National Academies Public Access Records
    Office, 26n
National Academy of Sciences (NAS), 92
National Aeronautics and Space
    Administration, organizational
    problems at, 67, 82
National Cancer Institute (NCI), 190
National Disease and Therapeutic Index, 56
National Electronic Injury Surveillance
    System–Cooperative Drug Adverse
    Event Surveillance System (NEISS–
    CADES), 114
National Health Service, 171
National Institute for Health and Clinical
    Excellence (UK), 125
National Institute of General Medical
    Sciences, 128
National Institutes of Health (NIH), 20–21,
    55, 81, 92, 116, 118, 180, 190

National Library of Medicine (NLM), 143, 145, 180–181, 183
National Prescription Audit, 56
National Science Foundation (NSF), 92
Natural history of a drug, 31–64
  economic impact of drugs, 32
  IND submission and review, 33–39
  new drug applications, 39–51
  postmarket period, 51–59
NCI. *See* National Cancer Institute
NDAs. *See* New Drug Applications
Needs, of providers and patients, 178–184
Negotiations, about label wording, 50
NEISS–CADES. *See* National Electronic Injury Surveillance System–Cooperative Drug Adverse Event Surveillance System
New Drug Applications (NDAs), 22–23, 32, 39–51, 106. *See also* Abbreviated NDAs; Supplemental NDAs
  advisory committees, 44–46
  assembly of review team and beginning of review, 41, 43–44, 77, 96
  composition of review teams, 78, 83
  dispute resolution, 47–48
  initial filing review, 40–41
  key review meetings, 48
  letters sent to sponsors, 51, 79
  PDUFA timetables and performance goals triggered, 40
  postapproval requirements and labeling, 49–51
  review teams, 6, 41, 43–44, 77, 96
  RiskMAPs, 48–49
  safety tracking, 46–47
  site inspections, 51
New drugs, 2, 38, 107–119, 165
New molecular entities (NMEs), 41–44, 98, 106, 166
  numbers of priority and standard approvals, 42
  priority reviews of, 41, 133
  recommendations concerning, 9, 12, 133–134, 173
New vision of drug safety, 26–28
NIH. *See* National Institutes of Health
NLM. *See* National Library of Medicine
NMEs. *See* New molecular entities
NSF. *See* National Science Foundation

O

ODS/OSE. *See* Office of Drug Safety/Office of Surveillance and Epidemiology
Off-label use, 122
Office of Drug Safety/Office of Surveillance and Epidemiology (ODS/OSE), 32, 48–57, 67, 75–78, 83–86, 129, 146, 207
  role in IND submission and review, 36–39
  staffing, 107
Office of Drug Safety Policy and Communication. *See* Office of Safety Policy and Communication
Office of Generic Drugs, 32
Office of the Inspector General (OIG), 71, 156
Office of Management and Budget, 18, 95
Office of New Drug Chemistry, 78
Office of New Drugs (OND), 32–36, 51, 56–57, 67, 75–79, 82–86, 105, 146, 194–195, 206–207
  role in IND submission and review, 36–37
Office of Safety Policy and Communication, 13, 185, 187, 189, 207
OIG. *See* Office of the Inspector General
OND. *See* Office of New Drugs
Opinion differences and CDER's organizational dysfunction, 85–87
Organizational dysfunction in the CDER culture, 4, 65–100. *See also* Solutions proposed for CDER's organizational dysfunction
  inconsistency, 87–88
  instability and politicization, 88–90
  internal disagreements about handling of safety issues, 47
  interoffice polarization, 83–85
  management issues, 79–81
  mass media coverage of, 66, 84
  policies, and procedures in solving, 77–90
  recommendations concerning, 5–7
  scientific disagreement and differences of opinion, 85–87
  structural factors, 75–77
  suboptimal work environment, 81–83
Orphan Drug Act, 152
Over-the-counter (OTC) drugs, 90, 153

P

Package inserts, for patients, 185
Patient Health Advisories, 206
Patient package inserts, 185
Patients, 2, 5
    access to drugs, 16
    advocacy movements for, 177
    more engaged and knowledgeable, 21
    need to reassure, 147
    roles and needs of, 178–184
PDUFA. See Prescription Drug User Fee Act
Pediatric drugs, 165
Peer-review, 118
    recommendations concerning, 12, 173
Performance goals (suggested for) PDUFA
        IV, 98–100
    in performance report to Congress,
        98–100
    safety-related, 98–100
Pharmaceutical advertising. See also Direct-
        to-consumer advertising
    tax deductibility of, 199
Pharmaceutical drugs. See Drugs
Pharmaceutical industry, 2, 146, 177. See
        also Sponsors of drugs; User-fee
        funding system
    communications with the public and
        patients, 158, 184, 186
    credibility of, 4–5, 70
    social responsibility of, 119
Pharmaceutical Research and
        Manufacturers of America
        (PhRMA), 89, 123, 143, 162–163,
        196
    guiding principles on DTC advertising,
        164
Pharmacoepidemiology
    need for career-development awards
        in, 128
    recommendations concerning, 9,
        134–141
Pharmacogenomics, 34
Pharmacovigilance, 208
Phases of clinical trials and medicine
        development, 35
    phase 1–clinical pharmacology studies,
        34–35, 37
    phase 2–clinical investigation studies,
        34–35, 37
    phase 3–formal clinical trials, 35–36,
        124

phase 4–postmarketing surveillance,
        including further formal
        therapeutic trials, 35, 55, 106, 111,
        117, 133, 157, 211
Plan B (emergency contraceptive), 89–91
Planning advisory committee meetings,
        timeline for, 45
Polarization, interoffice, 66, 68, 80–85
Policies and procedures, and CDER's
        organizational dysfunction, 77–79
Political considerations, in decision-making,
        90–91
Politicization, and CDER's organizational
        dysfunction, 88–90
Postmarketing safety of a drug, 51–59, 95–97
    decision-making concerning, ix, 47
    drug promotion and information,
        52–53
    identifying and evaluating spontaneous
        safety signals, 56–58
    need to monitor, 59, 74, 156
    postmarket data, 55–56
    recommendations concerning, 8,
        127–131
    regulatory actions, 58–59
    requirements and labeling, in NDAs,
        25, 49–51
    risk communication activities and risk
        management for the PDUFA IV, 99
    spontaneous adverse event reporting
        system, 53–55
Postmarketing study commitments, 155,
        172–173, 211
    for the PDUFA IV, 99
Postmarketing surveillance, including
        further formal therapeutic trials
        (phase 4), 35
PPP. See Pregnancy Prevention Program;
        Public-private partnership
Pre-new drug application submission
        meeting, 39
Preapproval period, 37, 123, 154–155
    safety conferences during, 48
Predictive Safety Testing Consortium, 213
Pregnancy Prevention Program (PPP), 120
Premarket clinical trials, 38
Prescribers' understanding, 5
Prescription Drug User Fee Act (PDUFA),
        15, 66, 70–74, 116, 154–155, 193.
        See also User-fee funding system
    clinical development of, 42
    deadlines in, 49

FDA filing and review of submitted marketing applications, 43
FDA oversight and review of clinical trial protocols during development, 42
goals of, 42–43
in NDAs, 40
PDUFA I, 16, 23, 72
PDUFA II, 16, 23, 35–36, 40, 72–73
PDUFA III, 35–36, 40, 48–49, 73, 121
PDUFA IV, 98–100
Reauthorization Performance Goals and Procedures, 23
short history of, 72–73
sponsor-requested meetings with FDA during clinical development, 42–43
sunset of approaching, 19
timetables and performance goals triggered, 40
Prescription Drug User Fee Act (PDUFA): Adding Resources and Improving Performance in FDA Review of New Drug Applications, 209
Prescription drugs
off-label use, 122
providers' knowledge about, 179
safety of, 1–2
taking multiple, 153
Prescriptions, taxing, 198
Preventing Medication Errors, 50, 178, 182
recommendations from, 180–183
Princeton Survey Research Associates, 162
Priority reviews, 133
of new molecular entities, 41
Product seizures, 58
Product submissions, reductions in, 133
Professional opinions. *See* Differing professional opinion procedure
Professional societies, 4–5
Program reviews or evaluations, 211–212
advisory committees, 211
partnerships, 211–212
postmarketing study commitments, 211
Project managers, 34
Promotion of drugs to patients. *See also* Direct-to-consumer advertising; Pharmaceutical advertising
increases in, 21
Propulsid, 17
Protection of human subjects, 33
Providers, roles and needs of, 178–184

The public, 2, 5, 28
improving communication with, 187–190
perspectives on DTC advertising, 162
Public Employees for Environmental Responsibility, 86n
Public Health Advisories, 206
Public-private partnership (PPP), 8, 117–119, 201
Pure Food and Drug Act, ix, 19n, 22, 152, 184

Q

Quality-adjusted life years (QALYs), 125

R

Randomized controlled trials, 86
Rationale for strengthening drug regulation, 164–166
realistic regulatory action on safety needed, without the "last call" of approvals, 166
Reauthorization Performance Goals and Procedures (PDUFA), 23, 196–199
Recent FDA materials, 208–209
guidance documents, 41, 208–209
reports, 209
Recommendations, 5–14
adverse event reporting, 7, 114–115
advisory committees, 9–10, 12, 133–142, 188–189
AERS, 7, 110
amending the FD&C Act, 5–6, 92–93
automated healthcare databases, 7, 114–115
better science and expertise, 7–10
CDER review teams, 10, 146–147
clinical trials, 10, 144–145
for the Commissioner of the FDA, 5–6, 9, 92–93, 131
communication about safety, 12–13, 188–189
conflicts of interest, 10, 141–142
for Congress, 6–8, 11–13, 98–100, 117–119, 169–172, 197–203
for consumers, 180–181
direct-to-consumer advertising, 11–12, 169–172

external Management Advisory Board, 6, 93–94
FDA authority, 11, 170
labeling, 11, 169–170
NDA, 10, 144–146
NDA review teams, 6, 96
new molecular entities, 9, 12, 133–134, 173
Office of Drug Safety Policy and Communication, 13, 189
organizational culture, 5–7
peer-review, 12, 173
pharmacoepidemiology, 9, 134–141
postmarketing safety of a drug, 8, 127–131
from *Preventing Medication Errors,* 180–183
for providers and patients, 182–183
public-private partnership, 8, 117–119
regulation, 10–12
resources, 13–14, 197–203
risk-benefit analyses, 8, 125–126
risk management, 11, 169–170
RiskMAPs, 8, 121
safety-related performance goals for the PDUFA IV, 6–7, 98–100
for the Secretary of DHHS, 6, 8, 93–94, 117–119
Reference information, access to comprehensive, 182
Regulatory activities for safety, 4, 31. *See also* Enforcement tools
in the postmarket period, 58–59
realistic needed, without the "last call" of approvals, 166
recommendations concerning, 10–12
Regulatory authority necessary to provide for drug safety, 4, 27, 151–176. *See also* Food and Drug Administration authority
an aging and inadequate statutory framework, 153–166
history of FDA drug regulation, 152–153
strengthening FDA's regulatory authority, 167–173
"Regulatory briefings," 46
"Regulatory capture" of the FDA, 73–74, 155, 196–197
Regulatory "tool kit," 168, 213
Research. *See* Academic research enterprise

Resources for the drug safety system, 5, 166, 193–204
levels required to enable CDER to support the FDA mission, 4
recommendations concerning, 13–14, 197–203
Review elements for new drug approval beginning in NDAs, 41, 43–44
current, 52
data on NMEs, 172–173
meetings key in NDAs, 48
Review Panel on New Drug Regulation, 74, 155–156, 172
Review teams, 34
composition of, 78, 83
in NDAs, assembling, 41, 43–44
Risk-benefit analyses
for approval decisions, 106–107, 166
evolving throughout the drug's lifecycle, 2, 4, 96, 121–126
recommendations concerning, 8, 125–126
Risk communication activities, 27
postmarket, 97
Risk management
postmarket, 97
recommendations concerning, 11, 169–170
Risk Minimization Action Plans (RiskMAPs), 119–121, 146, 167
developing and assessing, 57, 158
in NDAs, 48–49
Rofecoxib, 17, 55, 168
Roles, of providers and patients (in drug safety system), 5, 178–184
Rolling reviews, 39–40

S

Safety data, gaps in, 37
Safety officers, 37
Safety-related performance goals for the PDUFA IV, 98–100
expertise in preapproval evaluation, 98
monitoring of adverse drug reactions and the AERS, 98
performance management, 100
postmarketing risk communication activities and risk management, 99
postmarketing study commitments, 99

Safety signals, 27, 84. *See also* Spontaneous safety signals in the postmarket period
  in generation, 108–110
  reducing uncertainty about and benefit after approval, 108–115
  in strengthening and testing, 110–115
Safety teams, of epidemiologists, 88
Safety "tool kits," 213
Safety tracking, 46–47
  in NDAs, 46–47
Science-based decision-making, 66, 129
Science of safety, 27, 105–150
  benefits after approval, 107–119, 122
  credibility of, 126–147
  generating, 106–126
  and recommendations concerning expertise, 7–10
  reducing uncertainty about, 107–119, 122
  rigor in, 27
  risk-benefit analyses throughout the drug's lifecycle, 121–126
  risk minimization action plans, 119–121
  understanding risk and benefit for approval decisions, 66, 106–107
Scientific advances, 28. *See also* Academic research enterprise
  increasing the numbers of targeted drugs, 20
Scientific disagreement, and CDER's organizational dysfunction, 85–87
Scientific reviewers, 34
Secretary of Health and Human Services, 6, 45, 93–94, 97
Sector maps, 110
Signals. *See* Safety signals
Site inspections, 51
  in NDAs, 51
SMART (System to Manage Accutane Related Teratogenicity), 120–121
Social Security Administration, 92
Solutions proposed for CDER's organizational dysfunction, 90–100
  agency leadership, 91–94
  external environment, 97–100
  management, 90–91
  structural factors, 94–97
"Special Government Employees," 131, 211

Special symbol needed to denote limited knowledge about new drugs, 170–172. *See also* Black triangle
Sponsors of drugs
  letters sent to, 51
  materials generated by, 52
  meeting with FDA during clinical development, PDUFA goal for, 42–43
  non-compliance by, 18
  obligations of, 34
Spontaneous safety signals in the postmarket period
  AERS, 53–55
  identifying and evaluating, 56–58
Stakeholders, 2, 4, 177. *See also* individual stakeholders
Statement of task. *See* The charge (to the committee)
Statutory framework (for drug regulation)
  aging of, 153–166
  FDA authority after approval, 155–164
  FDA authority preapproval, 154–155
  inadequacy of, 153–166
  rationale for strengthening, 164–166
Steering Committee for the Collaborative Development of a Long-Range Action Plan for the Provision of Useful Prescription Medicine Information, 186
Strengthening FDA's regulatory authority, 167–173
  conditions and restrictions on distribution throughout the drug lifecycle, 167–170
  greater regulatory flexibility post approval, 166
  periodic review of data on NMEs, 172–173
  special symbol needed to denote limited knowledge about new drugs, 170–172
Structural changes in the CDER, 206–207
Structural factors in CDER's organizational dysfunction, 75–77
  solving, 94–97
Study process, 25–26
Supplemental NDAs, 31
Supplements, dietary, 153
Surrogate endpoints, 107
Suspension of approval, 173

T

Taxing prescriptions, 198
"Team approach," 76. *See also* Review
    teams; Safety teams
Terfenadine, 109
Terminology coding, 54
Thompson v. Western States Medical
    Center, 160
Throckmorton, CDER Deputy Director
    Douglas, 207
Timeline, for planning advisory committee
    meetings, 45
Toxicologic studies, 44
Transparency
    and the credibility of safety science,
        142–147
    need for greater, 4–5, 124, 127
Troglitazone, 17, 50, 109
Tufts Center for the Study of Drug
    Development, 71

U

Uncertainty, disagreement in the face of,
    127
Under-reporting of adverse events,
    substantial, 55, 109
Union of Concerned Scientists, 86n
University of Arizona, 213
US drug safety system. *See also* Committee
    on the Assessment of the US Drug
    Safety System
    impaired by, 4
    an improved, 13–14
    a transformed, 4
Useful consumer medication information,
    criteria for, 187
User-fee funding system, 16, 23, 40, 70, 83,
    196–197

V

VA. *See* Department of Veterans Affairs
Vaccine Safety Datalink (VSD), 112
Valdecoxib, 17
Vanderbilt University, 111
Veterans Health Administration, 92
Vioxx, 65
Virginia State Board of Pharmacy v.
    Virginia Citizens Consumer
    Council, Inc., 159
Vision. *See* New vision of drug safety
von Eschenbach, FDA Acting Commissioner
    Andrew, 86n
VSD. *See* Vaccine Safety Datalink

W

Wall Street Journal, 162
Warning the public about drug safety risks,
    1. *See also* Black box warnings;
    Labeling
Washington Legal Foundation, 162
Web sites, 25, 140, 142–143, 159, 172,
    179, 181, 187, 190, 210
WHI. *See* Women's Health Initiative
WHO. *See* World Health Organization
Withdrawals, 1–2, 16, 165, 173
Women's Health Initiative (WHI), 55, 115,
    123–124, 181
World Health Organization (WHO), 143,
    145, 212

Z

Zero-tolerance policy, regarding COI
    considerations, 140–141